Dosage Form Formulation Technologies for Improving Bioavailability

Dosage Form Formulation Technologies for Improving Bioavailability

Editors

Gábor Vasvári
Ádám Haimhoffer

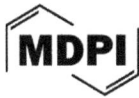

Basel • Beijing • Wuhan • Barcelona • Belgrade • Novi Sad • Cluj • Manchester

Editors

Gábor Vasvári
Department of
Pharmaceutical Technology,
Faculty of Pharmacy
University of Debrecen
Debrecen
Hungary

Ádám Haimhoffer
Department of
Pharmaceutical Technology,
Faculty of Pharmacy
University of Debrecen
Debrecen
Hungary

Editorial Office
MDPI AG
Grosspeteranlage 5
4052 Basel, Switzerland

This is a reprint of articles from the Special Issue published online in the open access journal *Pharmaceutics* (ISSN 1999-4923) (available at: www.mdpi.com/journal/pharmaceutics/special_issues/4IEDR453W2).

For citation purposes, cite each article independently as indicated on the article page online and as indicated below:

Lastname, A.A.; Lastname, B.B. Article Title. *Journal Name* **Year**, *Volume Number*, Page Range.

ISBN 978-3-7258-1570-8 (Hbk)
ISBN 978-3-7258-1569-2 (PDF)
doi.org/10.3390/books978-3-7258-1569-2

© 2024 by the authors. Articles in this book are Open Access and distributed under the Creative Commons Attribution (CC BY) license. The book as a whole is distributed by MDPI under the terms and conditions of the Creative Commons Attribution-NonCommercial-NoDerivs (CC BY-NC-ND) license.

Contents

About the Editors vii

Ildikó Bácskay, Boglárka Papp, Péter Pártos, István Budai, Ágota Pető, Pálma Fehér, et al.
Formulation and Evaluation of Insulin-Loaded Sodium-Alginate Microparticles for Oral Administration
Reprinted from: *Pharmaceutics* 2024, 16, 46, doi:10.3390/pharmaceutics16010046 1

Ildikó Bácskay, Zsolt Hosszú, István Budai, Zoltán Ujhelyi, Pálma Fehér, Dóra Kósa, et al.
Formulation and Evaluation of Transdermal Patches Containing BGP-15
Reprinted from: *Pharmaceutics* 2024, 16, 36, doi:10.3390/pharmaceutics16010036 17

Boglárka Papp, Marc Le Borgne, Florent Perret, Christelle Marminon, Liza Józsa, Ágota Pető, et al.
Formulation and Investigation of CK2 Inhibitor-Loaded Alginate Microbeads with Different Excipients
Reprinted from: *Pharmaceutics* 2023, 15, 2701, doi:10.3390/pharmaceutics15122701 35

Jaylen C. Mans and Xiaowei Dong
The Development of Lipid-Based Sorafenib Granules to Enhance the Oral Absorption of Sorafenib
Reprinted from: *Pharmaceutics* 2023, 15, 2691, doi:10.3390/pharmaceutics15122691 53

Ibrahim Ashraf, Pierre A. Hanna, Shadeed Gad, Fathy I. Abd-Allah and Khalid M. El-Say
Enhancing Pharmacokinetics and Pharmacodynamics of Rosuvastatin Calcium through the Development and Optimization of Fast-Dissolving Films
Reprinted from: *Pharmaceutics* 2023, 15, 2640, doi:10.3390/pharmaceutics15112640 64

Yulia Svenskaya and Tatiana Pallaeva
Exploiting Benefits of Vaterite Metastability to Design Degradable Systems for Biomedical Applications
Reprinted from: *Pharmaceutics* 2023, 15, 2574, doi:10.3390/pharmaceutics15112574 79

Nada M. El Hoffy, Ahmed S. Yacoub, Amira M. Ghoneim, Magdy Ibrahim, Hussein O. Ammar and Nermin Eissa
Computational Amendment of Parenteral In Situ Forming Particulates' Characteristics: Design of Experiment and PBPK Physiological Modeling
Reprinted from: *Pharmaceutics* 2023, 15, 2513, doi:10.3390/pharmaceutics15102513 112

Anna Stasiłowicz-Krzemień, Piotr Szulc and Judyta Cielecka-Piontek
Co-Dispersion Delivery Systems with Solubilizing Carriers Improving the Solubility and Permeability of Cannabinoids (Cannabidiol, Cannabidiolic Acid, and Cannabichromene) from *Cannabis sativa* (Henola Variety) Inflorescences
Reprinted from: *Pharmaceutics* 2023, 15, 2280, doi:10.3390/pharmaceutics15092280 128

Liza Józsa, Dániel Nemes, Ágota Pető, Dóra Kósa, Réka Révész, Ildikó Bácskay, et al.
Recent Options and Techniques to Assess Improved Bioavailability: In Vitro and Ex Vivo Methods
Reprinted from: *Pharmaceutics* 2023, 15, 1146, doi:10.3390/pharmaceutics15041146 152

Stefania Marano, Manish Ghimire, Shahrzad Missaghi, Ali Rajabi-Siahboomi, Duncan Q. M. Craig and Susan A. Barker
Development of Robust Tablet Formulations with Enhanced Drug Dissolution Profiles from Centrifugally-Spun Micro-Fibrous Solid Dispersions of Itraconazole, a BCS Class II Drug
Reprinted from: *Pharmaceutics* **2023**, *15*, 802, doi:10.3390/pharmaceutics15030802 . . . . **177**

Laura Di Renzo, Antonella Smeriglio, Mariarosaria Ingegneri, Paola Gualtieri and Domenico Trombetta
The Pharmaceutical Formulation Plays a Pivotal Role in Hydroxytyrosol Pharmacokinetics
Reprinted from: *Pharmaceutics* **2023**, *15*, 743, doi:10.3390/pharmaceutics15030743 . . . . **205**

Kunchorn Kerdmanee, Thawatchai Phaechamud and Sucharat Limsitthichaikoon
Thermoresponsive Azithromycin-Loaded Niosome Gel Based on Poloxamer 407 and Hyaluronic Interactions for Periodontitis Treatment
Reprinted from: *Pharmaceutics* **2022**, *14*, 2032, doi:10.3390/pharmaceutics14102032 . . . . **219**

About the Editors

Gábor Vasvári

Gabor Vasvari is the assistant professor of pharmaceutical technology at the University of Debrecen. His research areas include the development of novel lipid-based drug delivery systems such as solid dispersions, gastroretentive and lipid-based microparticle systems, dissolution and solubility enhancement of APIs, and the complexation of APIs with cyclodextrin polymers and their in vitro investigation. After obtaining his degree in pharmacy from the University of Debrecen in 2013, he took a postgraduate specialist training course. After that, he continued his research on melt dosage forms, obtaining his Ph.D. in 2020. Over the years, he has participated in many scientific conferences and successfully presented the development steps and related results at national and international conferences and forums.

Ádám Haimhoffer

Adam Haimhoffer is the assistant professor of pharmaceutical technology at the University of Debrecen. Adam has published several papers about improving the bioavailability of drugs. He is an expert in the science of cyclodextrin, cyclodextrin polymer, and gastro-retentive dosage forms. After obtaining his degree in pharmacy from the University of Debrecen in 2018, he spent half a year as a research assistant in the Department of Drug Science and Technology at the University of Turin. After that, he continued his research on gastro-retentive dosage forms and cyclodextrin, obtaining his Ph.D. in 2022. Over the years, he has participated in many scientific conferences and in several domestic and international research projects.

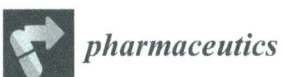

Article

Formulation and Evaluation of Insulin-Loaded Sodium-Alginate Microparticles for Oral Administration

Ildikó Bácskay [1,2], Boglárka Papp [1], Péter Pártos [1], István Budai [3], Ágota Pető [1,2], Pálma Fehér [1], Zoltán Ujhelyi [1] and Dóra Kósa [1,2,*]

[1] Department of Pharmaceutical Technology, Faculty of Pharmacy, University of Debrecen, Nagyerdei Körút 98, 4032 Debrecen, Hungary; feher.palma@pharm.unideb.hu (P.F.); ujhelyi.zoltan@pharm.unideb.hu (Z.U.)
[2] Institute of Healthcare Industry, University of Debrecen, Nagyerdei Körút 98, 4032 Debrecen, Hungary
[3] Faculty of Engineering, University of Debrecen, Ótemető Utca 2-4, 4028 Debrecen, Hungary; budai.istvan@eng.unideb.hu
* Correspondence: kosa.dora@pharm.unideb.hu; Tel.: +36-52-512-900

Abstract: The development of oral insulin drug delivery systems is still an ongoing challenge for pharmaceutical technology researchers, as the formulation process has to overcome a number of obstacles due to the adverse characteristics of peptides. The aim of this study was to formulate different sodium-alginate microparticles as a possible method for oral insulin administration. In our previous studies, the method has been successfully optimized using a small model peptide. The incorporation of insulin into alginate carriers containing nonionic surfactants has not been described yet. In order to enhance the absorption of insulin through biological barriers, Labrasol ALF and Labrafil M 2125 CS were selected as permeation-enhancing excipients. They were applied at a concentration of 0.10% (v/v%), along with various combinations of the two, to increase oral bioavailability. Encapsulation efficiency showed sufficient drug incorporation, as it resulted in over 80% in each composition. In vitro dissolution and enzymatic stability test results proved that, as a pH-responsive polymer, alginate bead swelling and drug release occur at higher pH, thus protecting insulin against the harsh environment of the gastrointestinal tract. The remaining insulin content was 66% due to SIF degradation after 120 min. Permeability experiments revealed the impact of permeation enhancers and natural polymers on drug absorption, as they enhanced drug transport significantly through Caco-2 cells in the case of alginate microparticle formulations, as opposed to the control insulin solution. These results suggest that these formulations are able to improve the oral bioavailability of insulin.

Keywords: microbead; oral bioavailability; absorption enhancement; Labrasol ALF; Labrafil M 2125 CS; Caco-2 cells

1. Introduction

According to the World Health Organization, 422 million people worldwide have diabetes, and 1.5 million deaths are directly attributed to diabetes each year. Both the number of cases and the prevalence of diabetes have been constantly increasing over the past decades. The most effective therapy for patients living with diabetes mellitus to control high blood sugar level is insulin administration [1]. However, insulin administration is available almost exclusively in injectable form, despite the fact that it has several drawbacks [2]. Continuous injections are painful, inconvenient, and lead to low patient compliance [3,4]. In the long-term, access to an affordable and more comfortable treatment would be crucial. However, the development of oral insulin drug delivery systems is still an ongoing challenge for pharmaceutical technology researchers, as the formulation process has to overcome a number of obstacles due to the adverse characteristics of peptide-type drugs [5]. The frequent enzymatic degradation in the gastrointestinal tract, the low permeability and the physical barriers, all make the formulation of oral dosage forms difficult [6]. To overcome the abovementioned limiting factors associated with oral insulin delivery, several strategies have been investigated in the last decades [7,8]. Orally administered formulations must meet the following requirements: they must protect the drug from the harsh acidic conditions and degrading action of pepsin in the stomach, and several other proteolytic enzymes in the intestinal lumen [9]. Chemical modification of the peptide and enzyme inhibitors helps address this challenge [10]. In order to reach the site of action and achieve the required pharmacological effect when administered orally, we have to face the biological membranes as well. Absorption enhancers temporarily interrupt membrane integrity in order to improve drug permeation through the intestinal and basal membranes [11]. For this purpose, non-ionic surfactants are commonly used, as they are relatively less toxic than other excipients [12]. For many years, extensive research has been conducted to investigate innovative methods for administering insulin, including approaches like micro- and nanoparticles. Among the many options, polymer-based delivery systems gained more focus due to their easy formulation process. Both natural and synthetic polymers have been used to formulate polymer-based delivery systems for oral insulin administration [13,14]. However, natural polymers have been of greater interest due to their high biocompatibility and low toxicity [15]. The two most investigated natural polymers are alginate and chitosan. In recent years, several studies have investigated different alginate-based insulin formulations that seem promising for increasing the oral bioavailability of insulin [16–19]. The great benefit of sodium-alginate lies in its status a non-toxic, biocompatible and biodegradable polysaccharide. The mucoadhesive property of sodium alginate increases the absorption of oral insulin, making it a potential excipient for designing drug delivery dosage forms [20]. In the presence of divalent cations, such as calcium, sodium alginate crosslinks and forms a polymer matrix that controls drug release at specific pH [21]. Lower pH inhibits the release of drugs, as sodium alginate microparticles are stable in acidic conditions, while higher pH promotes the disintegration of the microsphere structure, thus increasing release rate [22]. The formulation of insulin-loaded calcium cross-linked sodium-alginate microparticles containing different non-ionic surfactants has not been particularly investigated.

Incorporation of insulin into alginate carriers containing nonionic surfactants has not been described yet. For this purpose, we intended to formulate and investigate different sodium-alginate formulations containing two polyoxylglyceride-type permeation-enhancing agents. Labrasol ALF and Labrafil M 2125 CS were selected in order to improve the absorption of the active ingredient through the intestinal mucosa [23]. Microbeads contained these excipients at a concentration of 0.10% (v/v%), as well as combinations of them. The efficacy and safety of these excipients have been investigated in several studies [24–27]. Cross-linking of alginate with calcium occurred with the help of a semi-automated instrument, making the formulation process much easier and faster, based on our previous experiments [28]. A number of in vitro investigations were carried out to characterize the microbeads and investigate the protective effect of the polymer in simulated gastrointestinal conditions. Since safety is an essential aspect of pharmaceutical developments, the biological properties of the excipients and compositions were evaluated as well [29]. Overall, the aim of our research was to formulate suitable delivery systems for oral insulin delivery with improved bioavailability.

2. Materials and Methods

2.1. Materials

Human recombinant insulin, pepsin ($\geq$400 unit/mg protein), and pancreatin ($\geq 3\times$ USP specifications) were obtained from Sigma-Aldrich (St. Louis, MO, USA). Sodium alginate was purchased from BÜCHI Labortechnik AG (Flawil, Switzerland). Calcium chloride dihydrate was ordered from VWR International (Debrecen, Hungary). Labrasol ALF (Caprylocaproyl Prolyoxyl-8-glycerides) and Labrafil M2125 CS (Linoleoyl Polyoxyl-6 glycerides) were purchased from Gattefossé (Saint-Priest, France). The Caco-2 cell line was obtained from the European Collection of Cell Cultures (ECACC, Public Health England,

Salisbury, UK). MTT dye (3-(4,5-Dimethylthiazol-2-yl)-2,5-diphenyltetrazolium bromide), phosphate buffered saline (PBS) buffer solution, Dulbecco's Modified Eagle's Medium (DMEM), heat-inactivated fetal bovine serum (FBS), L-glutamine, non-essential amino acids solution, and penicillin-streptomycin solution were obtained from Sigma-Aldrich (St. Louis, MO, USA). TrypLE™ Express Enzyme (no phenol red) and Pierce™ Detergent Compatible Bradford Assay Kit were ordered from Thermo Fisher Scientific (Waltham, MA, USA).

2.2. Methods

2.2.1. Formulation of Insulin-Loaded Sodium-Alginate Microparticles

Insulin-loaded alginate microparticles were formulated using the controlled polymerization method with the Büchi Encapsulator B-395 Pro apparatus. This process is based on the fact that the controlled, laminar liquid flow is cracked into equally sized beads due to the vibration at the optimal frequency [30]. For the preparation, the peptide was distributed in 20 mL of the polymer 1.50 $w/v\%$ sodium-alginate solution combined with 0.10 $v/v\%$ of penetration enhancers when needed. The polymer–peptide mixture then was loaded into a syringe and forced into the pulsation chamber of the apparatus at the rate of 5.00 mL/min and passed through an electrical field between the nozzle, with an average diameter of 200 µm, and the electrode set at 1000 V, resulting in a surface charge. Due to electrostatic repulsion, the beads dropped into the hardening 100 mM calcium-chloride dihydrate solution separately. Microparticles were then washed with distilled water, filtered with a vacuum pump and dried by lyophilization for 24 h.

2.2.2. Bradford Assay

The insulin content of the formulations was determined with the help of the Pierce™ Detergent Compatible Bradford Assay Kit, which is a rapid and ready-to-use colorimetric method for quantitative analysis of peptides and proteins [31]. Compared to the traditional Bradford reagent, which is incompatible with most detergents, the modified assay reagent is compatible with most of the commonly used detergents and lysis reagents. Similar to the Bradford method, an immediate shift in absorption maximum occurs, from 465 nm to 595 nm, when the dye binds to a protein, resulting in a color change from green to blue [32]. A total of 150 µL of each sample and 150 µL of assay reagent were pipetted into a 96-well plate. For the standard calibration curve, BSA standard solutions were used in predetermined concentrations. In addition, the assay is complete in just 10 min. The assay can be used with samples that contain or do not contain detergent as well.

2.2.3. Encapsulation Efficiency and Drug-Loading Capacity

Insulin encapsulation efficiency was determined indirectly. To define the amount of insulin encapsulated in the beads, 150 µL of undiluted sample was measured from the hardening solution after formulation. Insulin content was calculated via the Bradford Assay. The encapsulation efficiency of insulin was determined by the equation underneath [33]:

$$EE = \frac{Qt - Qh}{Qt} \times 100 \qquad (1)$$

where Qt is the theoretic drug content encapsulated in the beads, and Qh is the insulin content that remained in the hardening solution.

Loading capacity was defined as the difference between the amount of initial insulin and drug left uncapsulated in the hardening solution, expressed as a percentage of the weight of dry microbeads (Wd) [17]:

$$LC = \frac{Qt - Qh}{Wd} \times 100 \qquad (2)$$

2.2.4. Swelling Behavior

The water absorption capacity of insulin-loaded sodium alginate microbeads was determined gravimetrically. A total of 50 mg of dry beads were placed in 50 mL distilled water at room temperature for 2 h. The swollen beads were then filtered with vacuum filtration. The swelling behavior was calculated from the change in dry and swollen mass of the beads using the following equation [34]:

$$S = \frac{Ws - Wd}{Ws} \times 100 \qquad (3)$$

where Ws is the weight of swollen particles and Wd is the weight of dry beads.

2.2.5. Morphology

The morphology, shape, size and surface area of the particles were characterized using a scanning electron microscope (SEM) with the Hitachi Tabletop microscope (TM3030 Plus). For the analysis, samples were attached to a plate covered with double-sided adhesive tape. The accelerating voltage was 5–15 kV during micrography [35].

2.2.6. In Vitro Dissolution

In order to determine drug release from the formulated microbeads, an in vitro dissolution assay was carried out using the USP dissolution apparatus (Erweka DT 800). Dry beads were placed in freshly prepared HCl (pH 1.2) and phosphate (pH 6.8) buffer solution at 37 °C temperature, with the paddle speed set at 100 rpm. A total of 1 mL aliquots from both dissolution media were collected at predetermined time intervals. Fresh-release media were replaced after each sampling. Drug concentration was analyzed using the Bradford assay.

2.2.7. Enzymatic Stability

Enzymatic degradation was performed in the presence of pepsin and pancreatin proteolytic enzymes. Microparticles were placed into 100 mL of simulated gastric fluid (SGF) containing pepsin for 1 h and into simulated intestinal fluid (SIF) containing pancreatin for 2 h, according to the European Pharmacopoeia specifications. The beads were incubated at 37 °C under moderate stirring in both media. The enzymatic reaction was stopped with an equivalent volume of ice-cold reagent (0.1 M NaOH for SGF and 0.1 M HCl for SIF) [36]. The samples were analyzed using the Bradford assay.

2.2.8. Caco-2 Cell Culture

The immortalized human adenocarcinoma Caco-2 cell line was selected for MTT and permeability assays [37]. Cells were maintained through weekly passaging in plastic cell culture flasks in Dulbecco's Modified Eagel's medium (DMEM), supplemented with 2 mM of L-glutamine, 100 mg/L gentamycin and 10% heat-inactivated fetal bovine serum. The cells were stored in a 5% CO_2 cell incubator at 37 °C.

2.2.9. Caco-2 Cell Viability Assay

The cell viability of immortalized human colon adenocarcinoma Caco-2 cells was evaluated through the MTT assay. The cells were seeded at a density of 10^4 cells/well on flat bottom 96-well tissue culture plates and allowed to grow for 7 days. For the MTT assay, the DMEM medium was removed, and the cells were treated with the excipients used for the formulation (sodium-alginate, calcium-chloride dihydrate, Labrasol ALF, Labrafil M2125 CS) and with the bead compositions as well. The mitochondrial activity of viable cells was determined after a 3 h incubation with MTT dye. The formed formazan crystal precipitate was dissolved in acidic isopropanol, and absorbance was measured with the FLUOstar OPTIMA Microplate Reader (BMG LABTECH, Offenburg, Germany) at 570 nm against a 690 nm reference. Cell viability was demonstrated as the percentage of the untreated control [38].

2.2.10. Permeability Experiments

For the permeability experiments, the Caco-2 cell line was selected, as it perfectly models the human intestinal absorption of drugs administered orally [39]. Cells were seeded on 24-well ThinCert™ polyester inserts with a 0.40 µm pore size at a density of 4×10^4 cells. Measurements started when the transepithelial electrical resistance (TEER) values reached 800–1000 $\Omega \times cm^2$ in each insert [40]. The DMEM culture medium was replaced with test solutions in the apical chamber, and phosphate buffer solution was added to the basal chamber. In permeability tests, all the four compositions have been studied. For this experiment the same amount of dry microbead samples were dissolved in PBS buffer for 120 min. As control, insulin solution was used. After 120 min, samples were collected from the basolateral compartment to determine the permeated amount of insulin. The samples were analyzed using the Bradford assay.

2.2.11. Transepithelial Electrical Resistance Measurements

To follow membrane function and integrity during the permeability experiments, transepithelial electrical resistance (TEER) was measured with Millipore Millicell-ERS 00001 equipment [41]. As a follow-up, measurements were carried out 12 h after incubation to study cell membrane recovery.

2.2.12. Statistical Analysis

Data were analyzed using the GraphPad Prism 8 and herein presented as means ± SD. The results were compared using one-way ANOVA and repeated-measures ANOVA followed by Tukey's or Dunnett's post hoc testing. Difference of means was regarded as significant in case of $p < 0.05$ and signed with asterisks. All experiments were carried out in quintuplicates and repeated at least five times.

3. Results

3.1. Formulation of Insulin-Loaded Sodium-Alginate Microparticles

Insulin was encapsulated in different alginate formulations containing penetration enhancer excipients in a concentration of 0.1% (v/v%). The selected compositions are described in Table 1.

Table 1. Composition of the selected alginate formulations.

Composition	Sodium-Alginate Solution	Labrasol ALF	Labrafil M2125 CS
Insulin beads	20 mL	-	-
Insulin beads + Labrasol ALF	20 mL	0.1% (v/v%)	-
Insulin beads + Labrafil M2125 CS	20 mL	-	0.1% (v/v%)
Combination	20 mL	0.1% v/v%	0.1% (v/v%)

3.2. Encapsulation Efficiency and Drug-Loading Capacity

The encapsulation efficiency of insulin in the beads was over 80% in each case. A significant difference was evaluated between the EE of the compositions with both excipients. The lowest value was observed in the case of insulin beads containing both penetration enhancers, as the surfactant content was twice as high in those particles. The insulin beads supplemented with only one of the excipients (Labrasol ALF or Labrafil M2125 CS) showed almost the same EE. The drug-loading capacity results were between 1.28 and 1.49%. The results are presented in Figure 1 and Table 2.

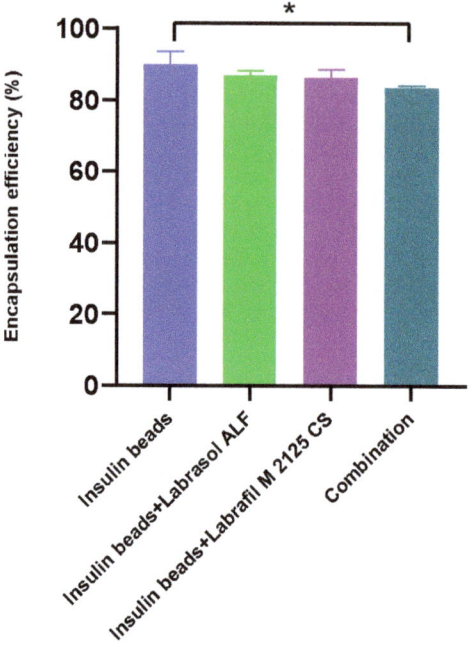

Figure 1. Encapsulation efficiency of insulin. EE measurements showed at least 80% in each case. A significant difference was observed between the formulations without surfactants and those that contained the combination of them. Each data point represents the mean ± SD, $n = 5$. One-way ANOVA with Tukey's post hoc test was performed to compare the different groups. Significant differences are marked with asterisks. * Indicates statistically significant differences at $p < 0.05$.

Table 2. Loading capacity of the formulated insulin-alginate compositions.

Composition	LC (±SD; %)
Insulin beads	1.45 ± 0.15
Insulin beads + Labrasol ALF	1.49 ± 0.14
Insulin beads + Labrafil M2125 CS	1.34 ± 0.03
Combination	1.28 ± 0.09

3.3. Swelling Behavior

The swelling behavior of the beads formulated with a 200 µm nozzle was approximately 70%. Bead swelling was 3.5–4 times their dry mass, regardless of the formulation and excipient content. It has been shown that bead swelling is not affected by the excipients. The results of swelling capacity are presented in Figure 2.

3.4. Morphology

The morphology of the lyophilized insulin-loaded alginate microparticles is depicted in Figure 3. The SEM images of dry microspheres present flattened sphere-shaped beads with squashes due to the drying process. Small calcium-chloride crystals can be observed on the bead surface as well. SEM analysis also confirmed that the diameter of the microbeads is close to 200 µm. The average diameter of the formulated microparticles is presented in Table 3.

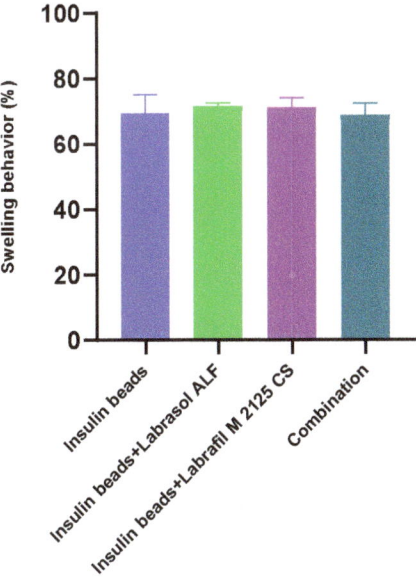

Figure 2. Swelling behavior of the formulated beads after 2 h. Excipient content did not affect equilibrium water uptake significantly. Each data point represents the mean ± SD, $n = 5$. One-way ANOVA was carried out to compare the groups. No significant difference was observed in swelling behavior of the beads.

Table 3. Average diameter and polydispersity index (PDI) of the formulated microparticles.

Composition	Diameter of Lyophilized Microspheres (±SD; μm)
Insulin beads	277.8 ± 11.95
Insulin beads + Labrasol ALF	292.9 ± 9.56
Insulin beads + Labrafil M2125 CS	296.3 ± 10.19
Combination	298.4 ± 8.21

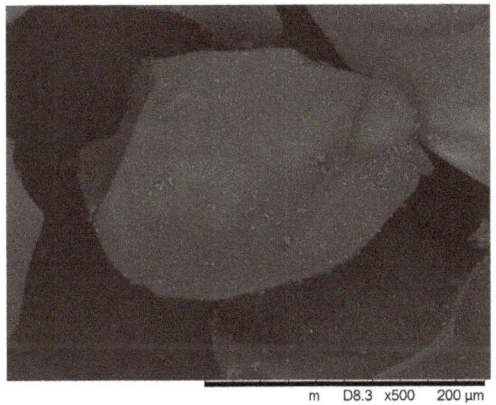

(a)

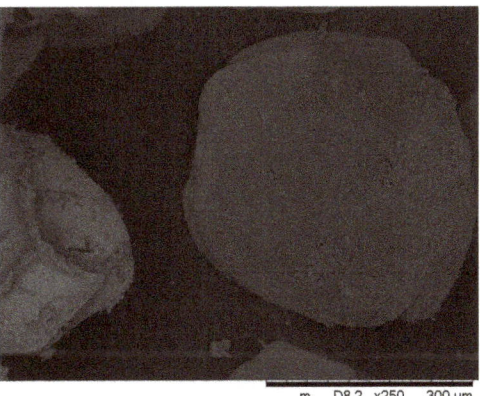

(b)

Figure 3. *Cont.*

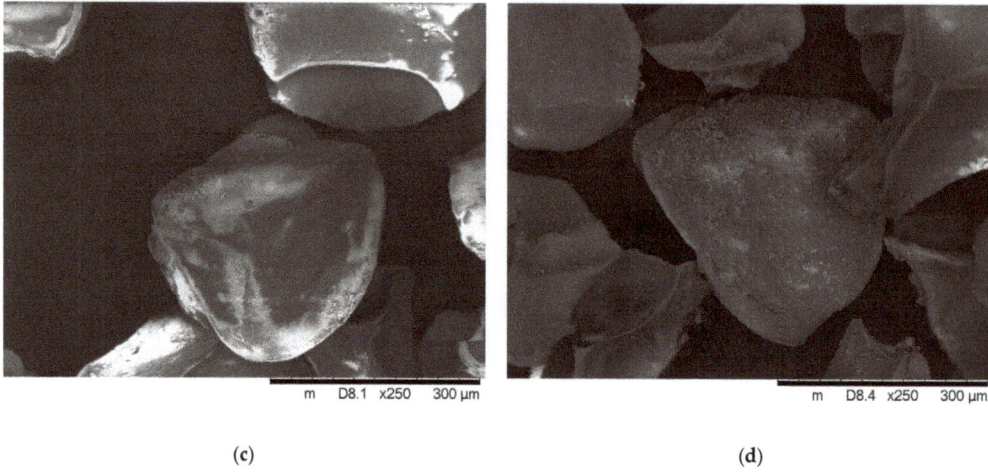

(c)   (d)

Figure 3. SEM micrographs of insulin-loaded alginate beads: (**a**) insulin beads; (**b**) insulin beads containing Labrasol ALF; (**c**) insulin beads containing Labrafil M2125 CS; (**d**) insulin beads containing both excipients.

3.5. In Vitro Dissolution

In vitro dissolution experiments were carried out in HCl (pH 1.2) and phosphate buffer solution (pH = 6.80). Insulin release at pH 1.2 was very slow, with less than 13% of drug content released within 120 min. At higher pH, in the first 2 h, a burst release of insulin was observed, where insulin release from the microparticles was over 66%. After 2 h, the insulin release rate was much lower. The excipient content did not affect insulin dissolution significantly. Figure 4 shows the percentage of released drug from sodium-alginate beads by time.

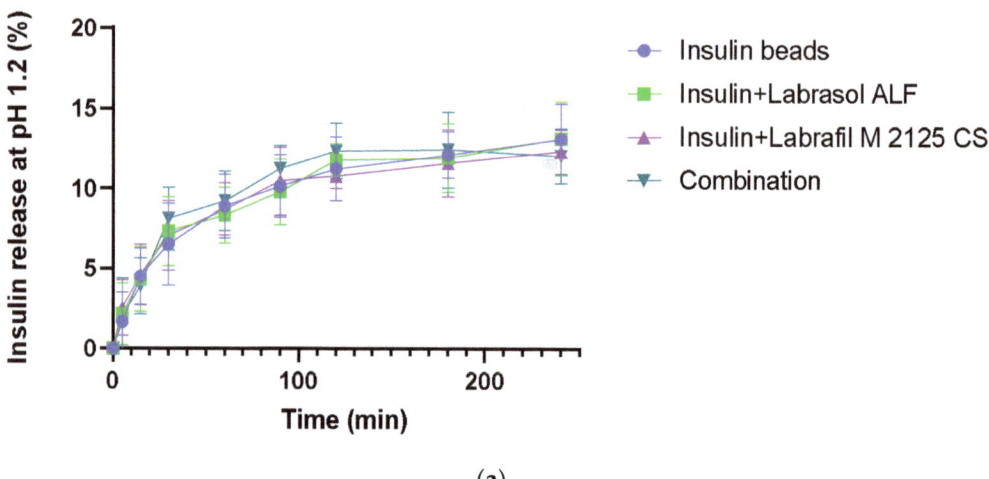

(a)

Figure 4. *Cont.*

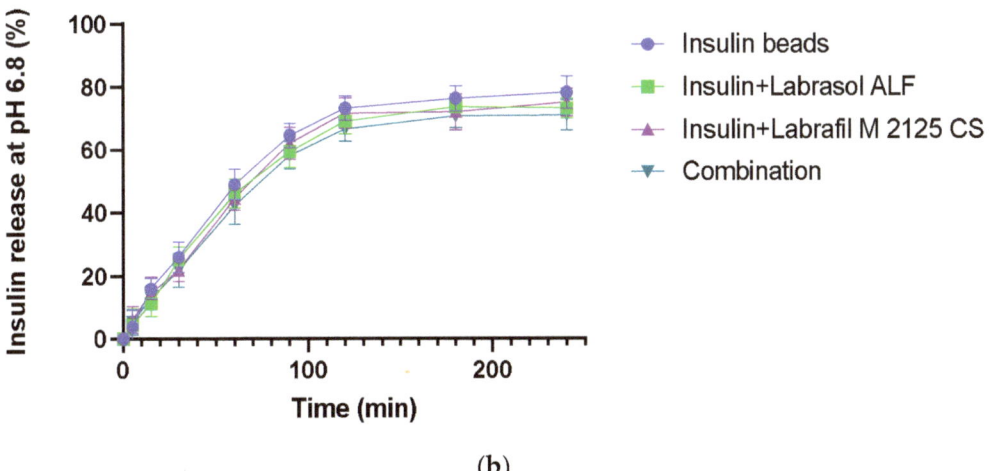

(b)

Figure 4. In vitro dissolution of insulin: (**a**) in HCl (pH = 1.2); (**b**) in phosphate buffer solution (pH = 6.8). Each data point represents the mean ± SD, n = 5.

3.6. Enzymatic Stability

In simulated gastric fluid, less than 2.50% of insulin remained after a 30 min incubation in the case of the non-formulated insulin samples, and free insulin was completely degraded within 1 h of incubation. In simulated intestinal conditions, less than 2% of active insulin was measured after 2 h incubation. According to the results, our formulations were able to protect insulin against the enzymatic conditions of GIT, as at least 80% of insulin remained protected from SGF degradation after 60 min and 66% from SIF degradation after 120 min. Figure 5 represents the results of the study.

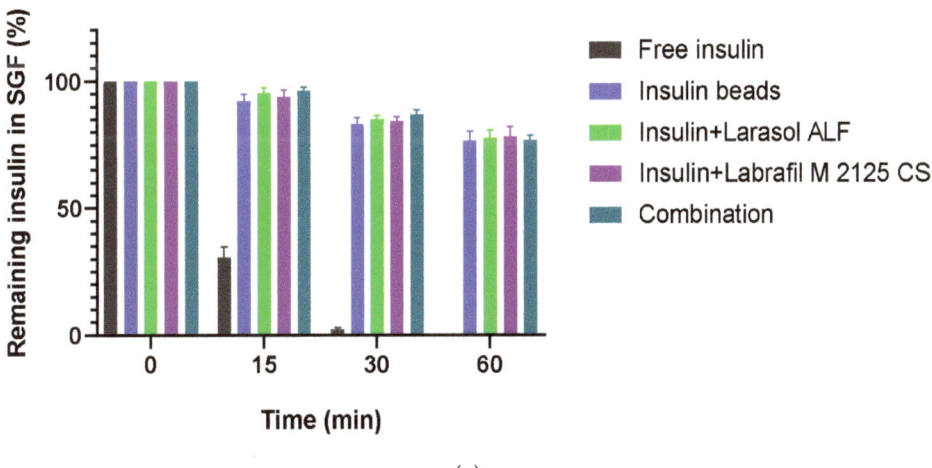

(a)

Figure 5. *Cont.*

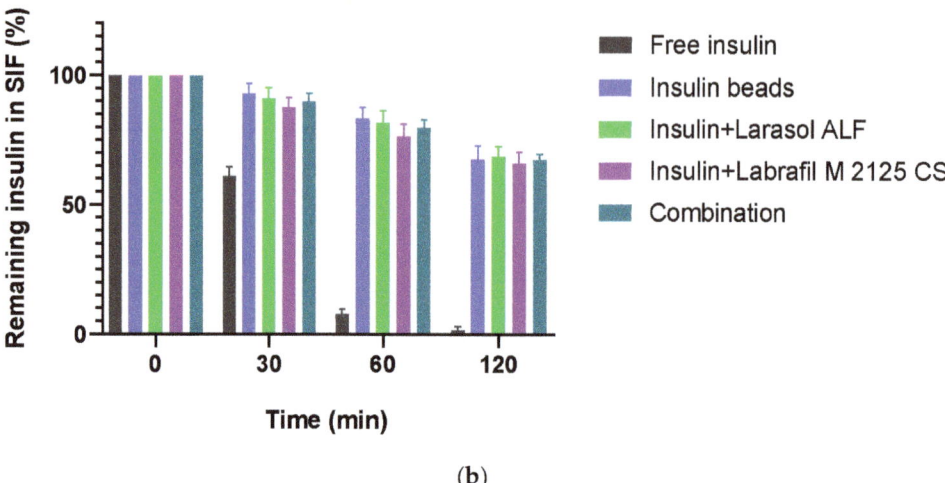

(**b**)

Figure 5. Enzymatic stability of insulin encapsulated in sodium-alginate microparticles: (**a**) in simulated gastric fluid containing pepsin; (**b**) in simulated intestinal fluid containing pancreatin. The control was free insulin. Each data point represents the mean ± SD, $n = 5$. Compared to free insulin, all four alginate formulations significantly protected insulin from enzymatic degradation.

3.7. Caco-2 Cell Viability Assay

The Caco-2 cell viability assay results demonstrate that the selected excipients are all safe at the applied 0.10% (v/v%) concentration. The bead-forming polymer and the hardening solution did not seem to be toxic, even at higher concentrations, in contrast with the permeation enhancers. As for the formulations, the 0.10% (v/v%) penetration enhancer content did not result in cell damage; all four formulations proved to be safe under in vitro conditions. Overall, cell viability was over 70% in each case, in line with the ISO 10993-5 [42] recommendation. Figure 6a demonstrates the results of the MTT assay regarding excipients, while Figure 6b represents the results of the formulated compositions.

3.8. Permeability Experiments

Figure 7 demonstrates the results of insulin permeability experiments. The permeability of encapsulated insulin was significantly higher than that of the control insulin solution. In the case of the formulations containing penetration enhancers, increased drug permeability was measured, suggesting the opening of tight junctions. The best API permeability was reached with beads containing both penetration enhancer excipients.

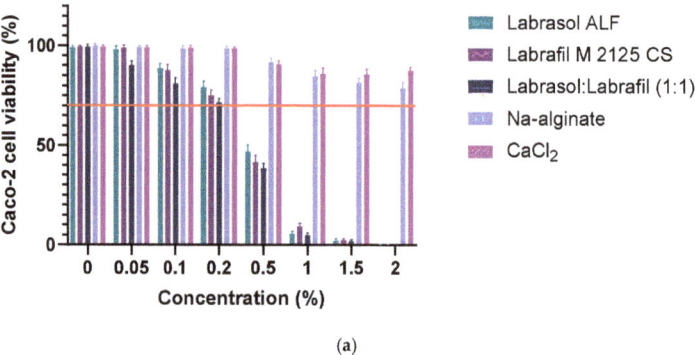

(**a**)

Figure 6. *Cont.*

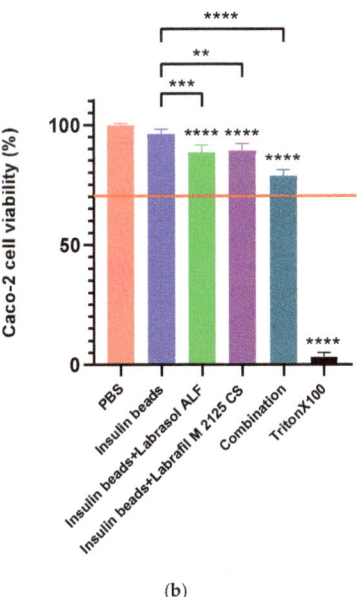

(b)

Figure 6. Results of MTT cell viability measurements of: (**a**) the applied excipients; (**b**) the formulated sodium-alginate microbeads containing insulin. Neither the selected excipients nor the bead formulations showed toxicity at the applied concentration according to ISO 10993-5 recommendation, while Labrasol ALF and Labrafil M 2125 CS seemed to be toxic at higher concentrations. The positive control was Triton X-100, the negative control was a phosphate-buffered solution (PBS). Each data point represents the mean ± SD, n = 5. One-way ANOVA with Tukey's post hoc test was carried out to compare the groups. Significant differences are marked with asterisks. The asterisks **, *** and **** indicate statistically significant differences at $p < 0.01$, $p < 0.001$ and $p < 0.0001$.

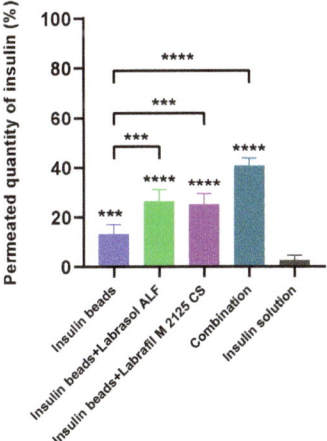

Figure 7. Permeated quantity of insulin via Caco-2 cell monolayer. Insulin solution was applied as control. The results demonstrate an increased peptide permeability in case of formulations containing penetration enhancer excipients. Each data point represents the mean ± SD, n = 5. To compare the groups, one-way ANOVA with Dunnett's multiple comparisons test was performed. Significant differences are marked with asterisks. The asterisks *** and **** indicate statistically significant differences at $p < 0.001$ and $p < 0.0001$.

3.9. Transepithelial Electrical Resistance Measurements

The permeability test started when the Caco-2 monolayer reached high (800 Ω × cm^2) TEER values. During the drug permeability investigation, the membrane integrity of Caco-2 cells was monitored through TEER measurements. After 30 min, the formulations started to cause a decrease in TEER values, suggesting the opening of tight junctions. Follow-up measurements confirmed that the TEER values started to increase after the treatment. At the end of the experiment, TEER was above 90% of the baseline. Figure 8 presents the results of TEER measurements.

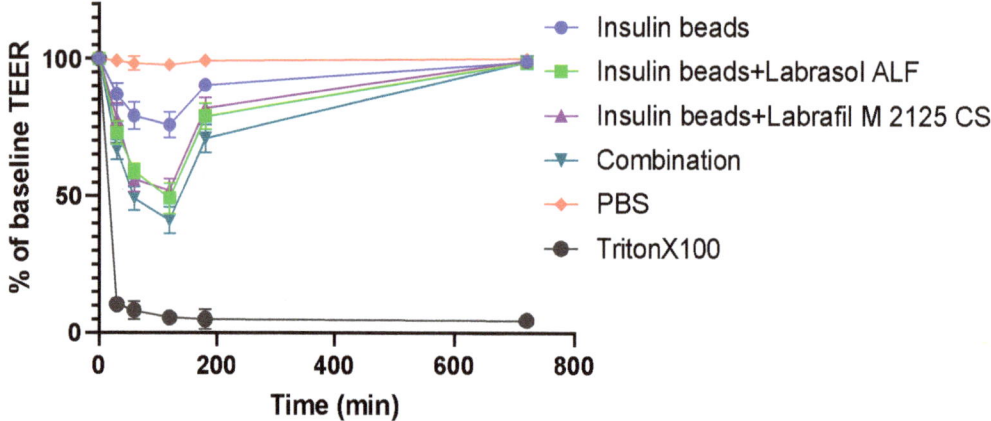

Figure 8. Transepithelial electrical resistance of Caco-2 cells during permeability assessment and 12 h after treatment. The follow-up measurements confirmed that TEER values started to increase after the treatment. At the end of the experiment TEER was above 90% of the baseline. Each data point represents the mean ± SD, n = 5.

4. Discussion

The oral bioavailability of hydrophilic macromolecular drugs, such as peptides and proteins, is extremely low due to their low stability and poor membrane permeability in the gastrointestinal tract. Natural polysaccharides have been widely investigated as potential delivery systems to improve the oral bioavailability of peptides and proteins in the last decades, still remaining a subject of great interest [43]. The objective of this investigation was to formulate optimal delivery systems for oral insulin administration. For this purpose, sodium-alginate was selected as a drug carrier polymer due to its beneficial properties in combination with two non-ionic surfactants as permeation enhancers. Insulin-loaded alginate microbeads were prepared using a controlled-gelification method with the help of the Büchi Encapsulator B-395 Pro apparatus.

The encapsulation efficiency of insulin exceeded 80% in each composition. The EE was significantly lower in the case of beads containing the combination of surfactants. Higher surfactant content changes the wetting angle of sodium-alginate solution when it falls into the calcium-chloride solution, resulting in an increase of surface area [44–46]. Water uptake was also investigated by swelling the beads in distilled water, as it influences drug release and further application as well. Swelling behavior resulted in at least 70% and was not affected by the excipients.

The performed scanning electron microscopy images confirmed that the morphology and shape of the beads are rather a flattened sphere, which is in contrast with the expected spherical morphology. This phenomenon is caused by the abovementioned increase in the wetting angle caused by the permeation enhancers. Squashes and tiny calcium crystals were also observed on the surface due to lyophilization, as the surface of the beads remains wet after vacuum filtration [34]. The average particle size seemed to be close to the theoretical

200 µm; according to the operation manual of the Büchi apparatus, the diameter of calcium-alginate beads is usually bigger than the nozzle diameter.

Insulin release from microbeads was investigated at pH 1.2 and 6.8 as well, and showed pH dependence, as expected [47]. Being a pH-responsive polymer, the relatively intact microstructure of alginate in acidic conditions, due to alginic acid, resulted in a slow-release rate at pH 1.2. In contrast, at higher pH, alginate forms a soluble salt, causing matrix swelling and disintegration, leading to higher drug release [48]. The stability of insulin in SGF containing pepsin and in SIF containing pancreatin was also studied. Compared to free insulin, a significant amount of API remained intact in both media after incubation time, suggesting the protective effect of the alginate matrix. A relatively higher degradation was observed in SIF than in SGF, which might be explained by bead swelling and drug release at higher pH.

In order to improve the intestinal absorption of insulin, different non-ionic surfactants and their combination were incorporated as absorption enhancers [49,50]. These excipients have the ability to modulate tight-junctions reversibly, thus increasing paracellular transport and intestinal permeability [51]. Our results have demonstrated the beneficial effects of surfactants in increasing permeability, as significantly more insulin permeated through Caco-2 cells seeded on the artificial membrane in the case of sodium-alginate microparticle formulations ($p < 0.0001$). Among the four compositions, those containing permeation enhancers supported significantly better API transport than insulin beads ($p < 0.001$). Applying the combination of Labrasol ALF and Labrafil M 2125 CS reached the highest permeated insulin quantity indicating improved bioavailability ($p < 0.0001$). Furthermore, alginate and other natural polymers have the ability to open epithelial cell tight junctions temporary as well, thus modulating the paracellular permeability of cell monolayers [52]. The significant difference between the control insulin solution and the insulin beads indicates that microparticulate systems are able to exert this effect. The TEER measurements performed confirmed our results, as the decreased TEER values during incubation suggest the modulation of cell integrity, while follow-up measurements confirmed that neither alginate nor the applied surfactants altered tight junctions irreversibly.

The cytotoxicity of the applied polymer solution, hardening solution and surfactants has been evaluated on Caco-2 cells using the well-known MTT assay. It is still one of the most popular in vitro methods to investigate cell viability [53]. Our results confirmed that neither the selected excipients nor the bead formulations showed toxicity at the applied concentration. Since safety is important in pharmaceutical dosage forms, the MTT assay was performed for the microbead formulations as well. This analysis proved their safety for cells under in vitro conditions.

Our results suggest that the incorporation of non-ionic surfactants with calcium cross-linked alginate microparticles is a promising option to improve the oral bioavailability of insulin. The carefully selected excipients and alginate are both able to enhance the intestinal absorption of the active substance as well as protecting it from the enzymatic degradation of the gastrointestinal tract.

5. Conclusions

The aim of the study was to formulate stable oral delivery systems that allow for enhanced in vitro drug release and intestinal absorption of insulin and to create a well-tolerated drug formulation that provides a high degree of protection against drug degradation. In our previous research, we successfully formulated alginate microparticles containing surfactants with a small model peptide as promising delivery systems for peptide-type active substances. In order to achieve better oral bioavailability, we selected other excipients, as well as their combination, and increased the concentrations tenfold. According to the results, our formulations were still safe under in vitro conditions. Further in vivo studies could demonstrate the importance of these formulations in insulin therapy. Formulations developed with such an approach would increase patient compliance with insulin therapy, thus playing an important role in the treatment of a leading disease.

Author Contributions: Conceptualization, I.B. (Ildikó Bácskay) and D.K.; methodology, Z.U. and D.K.; software, Á.P.; validation, I.B. (Ildikó Bácskay); formal analysis, Á.P.; investigation, B.P., P.P., I.B. (István Budai) and D.K.; resources, I.B. (Ildikó Bácskay); data curation, D.K.; writing—original draft preparation, I.B. (Ildikó Bácskay) and D.K.; writing—review and editing, D.K.; visualization, P.F.; supervision, D.K.; project administration, I.B. (Ildikó Bácskay); funding acquisition, I.B. (Ildikó Bácskay). All authors have read and agreed to the published version of the manuscript.

Funding: This research was supported by the ÚNKP-22-4-I National Excellence Program of the Ministry for Innovation and Technology through the National Research, Development and Innovation Fund. Project No. TKP2021-EGA-19 has been implemented with the support provided by the Ministry of Culture and Innovation of Hungary, from the National Research, Development and Innovation Fund, financed under the TKP2021-EGA funding scheme. The publication was supported by the GINOP-2.3.1-20-2020-00004 and GINOP-2.3.4-15-2016-00002 projects. The project was co-financed by the European Union and the European Regional Development Fund.

Institutional Review Board Statement: Not applicable.

Informed Consent Statement: Not applicable.

Data Availability Statement: The data that support the findings of this study are available from the corresponding author (kosa.dora@pharm.unideb.hu) with the permission of the head of the department, upon reasonable request.

Conflicts of Interest: The authors declare no conflicts of interest.

References

1. Petersmann, A.; Müller-Wieland, D.; Müller, U.A.; Landgraf, R.; Nauck, M.; Freckmann, G.; Heinemann, L.; Schleicher, E. Definition, Classification and Diagnosis of Diabetes Mellitus. *Exp. Clin. Endocrinol. Diabetes* **2019**, *127*, S1–S7. [CrossRef] [PubMed]
2. Khafagy, E.-S.; Morishita, M.; Onuki, Y.; Takayama, K. Current Challenges in Non-Invasive Insulin Delivery Systems: A Comparative Review. *Adv. Drug Deliv. Rev.* **2007**, *59*, 1521–1546. [CrossRef] [PubMed]
3. Wong, C.Y.; Martinez, J.; Dass, C.R. Oral Delivery of Insulin for Treatment of Diabetes: Status Quo, Challenges and Opportunities. *J. Pharm. Pharmacol.* **2016**, *68*, 1093–1108. [CrossRef] [PubMed]
4. Peyrot, M.; Rubin, R.R.; Kruger, D.F.; Travis, L.B. Correlates of Insulin Injection Omission. *Diabetes Care* **2010**, *33*, 240–245. [CrossRef] [PubMed]
5. Iyer, H.; Khedkar, A.; Verma, M. Oral Insulin—A Review of Current Status. *Diabetes Obes. Metab.* **2010**, *12*, 179–185. [CrossRef] [PubMed]
6. Spoorthi Shetty, S.; Halagali, P.; Johnson, A.P.; Spandana, K.M.A.; Gangadharappa, H.V. Oral Insulin Delivery: Barriers, Strategies, and Formulation Approaches: A Comprehensive Review. *Int. J. Biol. Macromol.* **2023**, *242*, 125114. [CrossRef] [PubMed]
7. Gedawy, A.; Martinez, J.; Al-Salami, H.; Dass, C.R. Oral Insulin Delivery: Existing Barriers and Current Counter-Strategies. *J. Pharm. Pharmacol.* **2018**, *70*, 197–213. [CrossRef] [PubMed]
8. Kumar, V.; Choudhry, I.; Namdev, A.; Mishra, S.; Soni, S.; Hurkat, P.; Jain, A.; Jain, D. Oral Insulin: Myth or Reality. *Curr. Diabetes Rev.* **2018**, *14*, 497–508. [CrossRef]
9. Karsdal, M.A.; Riis, B.J.; Mehta, N.; Stern, W.; Arbit, E.; Christiansen, C.; Henriksen, K. Lessons Learned from the Clinical Development of Oral Peptides. *Br. J. Clin. Pharmacol.* **2015**, *79*, 720–732. [CrossRef]
10. Choonara, B.F.; Choonara, Y.E.; Kumar, P.; Bijukumar, D.; du Toit, L.C.; Pillay, V. A Review of Advanced Oral Drug Delivery Technologies Facilitating the Protection and Absorption of Protein and Peptide Molecules. *Biotechnol. Adv.* **2014**, *32*, 1269–1282. [CrossRef]
11. Maher, S.; Brayden, D.; Casettari, L.; Illum, L. Application of Permeation Enhancers in Oral Delivery of Macromolecules: An Update. *Pharmaceutics* **2019**, *11*, 41. [CrossRef] [PubMed]
12. Jones, L.S.; Bam, N.B.; Randolph, T.W. Surfactant-Stabilized Protein Formulations: A Review of Protein-Surfactant Interactions and Novel Analytical Methodologies. In *Therapeutic Protein and Peptide Formulation and Delivery*; American Chemical Society: Washington, DC, USA, 1997; pp. 206–222.
13. Mansoor, S.; Kondiah, P.P.D.; Choonara, Y.E.; Pillay, V. Polymer-Based Nanoparticle Strategies for Insulin Delivery. *Polymers* **2019**, *11*, 1380. [CrossRef] [PubMed]
14. Wang, M.; Wang, C.; Ren, S.; Pan, J.; Wang, Y.; Shen, Y.; Zeng, Z.; Cui, H.; Zhao, X. Versatile Oral Insulin Delivery Nanosystems: From Materials to Nanostructures. *Int. J. Mol. Sci.* **2022**, *23*, 3362. [CrossRef] [PubMed]
15. Gao, S.; Tang, G.; Hua, D.; Xiong, R.; Han, J.; Jiang, S.; Zhang, Q.; Huang, C. Stimuli-Responsive Bio-Based Polymeric Systems and Their Applications. *J. Mater. Chem. B* **2019**, *7*, 709–729. [CrossRef] [PubMed]
16. Xu, Z.; Chen, L.; Duan, X.; Li, X.; Ren, H. Microparticles Based on Alginate/Chitosan/Casein Three-dimensional System for Oral Insulin Delivery. *Polym. Adv. Technol.* **2021**, *32*, 4352–4361. [CrossRef]

17. Li, J.; Wu, H.; Jiang, K.; Liu, Y.; Yang, L.; Park, H.J. Alginate Calcium Microbeads Containing Chitosan Nanoparticles for Controlled Insulin Release. *Appl. Biochem. Biotechnol.* **2021**, *193*, 463–478. [CrossRef] [PubMed]
18. Sarmento, B.; Ribeiro, A.; Veiga, F.; Sampaio, P.; Neufeld, R.; Ferreira, D. Alginate/Chitosan Nanoparticles Are Effective for Oral Insulin Delivery. *Pharm. Res.* **2007**, *24*, 2198–2206. [CrossRef]
19. Chen, Y.; Song, H.; Huang, K.; Guan, X. Novel Porous Starch/Alginate Hydrogels for Controlled Insulin Release with Dual Response to PH and Amylase. *Food Funct.* **2021**, *12*, 9165–9177. [CrossRef]
20. George, A.; Shah, P.A.; Shrivastav, P.S. Natural Biodegradable Polymers Based Nano-Formulations for Drug Delivery: A Review. *Int. J. Pharm.* **2019**, *561*, 244–264. [CrossRef]
21. Xie, J.; Li, A.; Li, J. Advances in PH-Sensitive Polymers for Smart Insulin Delivery. *Macromol. Rapid Commun.* **2017**, *38*, 1700413. [CrossRef]
22. Wang, X.; Sun, H.; Mu, T. Materials and Structure of Polysaccharide-Based Delivery Carriers for Oral Insulin: A Review. *Carbohydr. Polym.* **2024**, *323*, 121364. [CrossRef] [PubMed]
23. Mccartney, F.; Jannin, V.; Brayden, D.J. Investigation of Labrasol ®ALF as an Intestinal Permeation Enhancer: Ussing Chambers and Intestinal Instillations Labrasol ®Increases P App of FITC Dextrans in MW-Dependent Fashion. 2019. Available online: https://www.researchgate.net/publication/332978723_Investigation_of_LabrasolR_ALF_as_an_intestinal_permeation_enhancer_Ussing_chambers_and_intestinal_instillations?channel=doi&linkId=5cd517ff299bf14d9586dd16&showFulltext=true (accessed on 6 November 2023).
24. Tarsitano, M.; Cristiano, M.C.; Mancuso, A.; Barone, A.; Torella, D.; Paolino, D. Lipid-Based Formulations Containing Labrafil M2125-CS: A Deep Investigation on Nanosystem Stability. *Nanomanufacturing* **2022**, *2*, 41–52. [CrossRef]
25. McCartney, F.; Jannin, V.; Chevrier, S.; Boulghobra, H.; Hristov, D.R.; Ritter, N.; Miolane, C.; Chavant, Y.; Demarne, F.; Brayden, D.J. Labrasol®Is an Efficacious Intestinal Permeation Enhancer across Rat Intestine: Ex Vivo and In Vivo Rat Studies. *J. Control. Release* **2019**, *310*, 115–126. [CrossRef] [PubMed]
26. Eaimtrakarn, S.; Rama Prasad, Y.V.; Ohno, T.; Konishi, T.; Yoshikawa, Y.; Shibata, N.; Takada, K. Absorption Enhancing Effect of Labrasol on the Intestinal Absorption of Insulin in Rats. *J. Drug Target.* **2002**, *10*, 255–260. [CrossRef]
27. Dubray, O.; Jannin, V.; Demarne, F.; Pellequer, Y.; Lamprecht, A.; Béduneau, A. In-Vitro Investigation Regarding the Effects of Gelucire ®44/14 and Labrasol®ALF on the Secretory Intestinal Transport of P-Gp Substrates. *Int. J. Pharm.* **2016**, *515*, 293–299. [CrossRef]
28. Kósa, D.; Pető, Á.; Fenyvesi, F.; Váradi, J.; Vecsernyés, M.; Budai, I.; Németh, J.; Fehér, P.; Bácskay, I.; Ujhelyi, Z. Oral Bioavailability Enhancement of Melanin Concentrating Hormone, Development and In Vitro Pharmaceutical Assessment of Novel Delivery Systems. *Pharmaceutics* **2021**, *14*, 9. [CrossRef]
29. Llana-Ruiz-Cabello, M.; Gutiérrez-Praena, D.; Pichardo, S.; Moreno, F.J.; Bermúdez, J.M.; Aucejo, S.; Cameán, A.M. Cytotoxicity and Morphological Effects Induced by Carvacrol and Thymol on the Human Cell Line Caco-2. *Food Chem. Toxicol.* **2014**, *64*, 281–290. [CrossRef]
30. Kozlowska, J.; Prus, W.; Stachowiak, N. Microparticles Based on Natural and Synthetic Polymers for Cosmetic Applications. *Int. J. Biol. Macromol.* **2019**, *129*, 952–956. [CrossRef]
31. Kielkopf, C.L.; Bauer, W.; Urbatsch, I.L. Bradford Assay for Determining Protein Concentration. *Cold Spring Harb. Protoc.* **2020**, *2020*, 102269. [CrossRef]
32. Goldring, J.P.D. Measuring Protein Concentration with Absorbance, Lowry, Bradford Coomassie Blue, or the Smith Bicinchoninic Acid Assay before Electrophoresis. In *Electrophoretic Separation of Proteins*; Humana Press: New York, NY, USA, 2019; pp. 31–39.
33. Somo, S.I.; Langert, K.; Yang, C.-Y.; Vaicik, M.K.; Ibarra, V.; Appel, A.A.; Akar, B.; Cheng, M.-H.; Brey, E.M. Synthesis and Evaluation of Dual Crosslinked Alginate Microbeads. *Acta Biomater.* **2018**, *65*, 53–65. [CrossRef]
34. Martins, S.; Sarmento, B.; Souto, E.B.; Ferreira, D.C. Insulin-Loaded Alginate Microspheres for Oral Delivery—Effect of Polysaccharide Reinforcement on Physicochemical Properties and Release Profile. *Carbohydr. Polym.* **2007**, *69*, 725–731. [CrossRef]
35. Frent, O.D.; Duteanu, N.; Teusdea, A.C.; Ciocan, S.; Vicaș, L.; Jurca, T.; Muresan, M.; Pallag, A.; Ianasi, P.; Marian, E. Preparation and Characterization of Chitosan-Alginate Microspheres Loaded with Quercetin. *Polymers* **2022**, *14*, 490. [CrossRef] [PubMed]
36. Zhang, F.; Pei, X.; Peng, X.; Gou, D.; Fan, X.; Zheng, X.; Song, C.; Zhou, Y.; Cui, S. Dual Crosslinking of Folic Acid-Modified Pectin Nanoparticles for Enhanced Oral Insulin Delivery. *Biomater. Adv.* **2022**, *135*, 212746. [CrossRef] [PubMed]
37. Sambuy, Y.; De Angelis, I.; Ranaldi, G.; Scarino, M.L.; Stammati, A.; Zucco, F. The Caco-2 Cell Line as a Model of the Intestinal Barrier: Influence of Cell and Culture-Related Factors on Caco-2 Cell Functional Characteristics. *Cell Biol. Toxicol.* **2005**, *21*, 1–26. [CrossRef] [PubMed]
38. Pető, Á.; Kósa, D.; Haimhoffer, Á.; Fehér, P.; Ujhelyi, Z.; Sinka, D.; Fenyvesi, F.; Váradi, J.; Vecsernyés, M.; Gyöngyösi, A.; et al. Nicotinic Amidoxime Derivate BGP-15, Topical Dosage Formulation and Anti-Inflammatory Effect. *Pharmaceutics* **2021**, *13*, 2037. [CrossRef] [PubMed]
39. Konsoula, R.; Barile, F.A. Correlation of in Vitro Cytotoxicity with Paracellular Permeability in Caco-2 Cells. *Toxicol. Vitr.* **2005**, *19*, 675–684. [CrossRef]
40. Józsa, L.; Nemes, D.; Pető, Á.; Kósa, D.; Révész, R.; Bácskay, I.; Haimhoffer, Á.; Vasvári, G. Recent Options and Techniques to Assess Improved Bioavailability: In Vitro and Ex Vivo Methods. *Pharmaceutics* **2023**, *15*, 1146. [CrossRef]
41. Lopez-Escalera, S.; Wellejus, A. Evaluation of Caco-2 and Human Intestinal Epithelial Cells as In Vitro Models of Colonic and Small Intestinal Integrity. *Biochem. Biophys. Rep.* **2022**, *31*, 101314. [CrossRef]

42. *ISO 10993-5*; Biological Evaluation of Medical Devices. ISO: Geneva, Switzerland, 2009.
43. Yuan, H.; Guo, C.; Liu, L.; Zhao, L.; Zhang, Y.; Yin, T.; He, H.; Gou, J.; Pan, B.; Tang, X. Progress and Prospects of Polysaccharide-Based Nanocarriers for Oral Delivery of Proteins/Peptides. *Carbohydr. Polym.* **2023**, *312*, 120838. [CrossRef]
44. Holler, S.; Porcelli, C.; Ieropoulos, I.A.; Hanczyc, M.M. Transport of Live Cells Under Sterile Conditions Using a Chemotactic Droplet. *Sci. Rep.* **2018**, *8*, 8408. [CrossRef]
45. Lavrič, G.; Oberlintner, A.; Filipova, I.; Novak, U.; Likozar, B.; Vrabič-Brodnjak, U. Functional Nanocellulose, Alginate and Chitosan Nanocomposites Designed as Active Film Packaging Materials. *Polymers* **2021**, *13*, 2523. [CrossRef]
46. Sermkaew, N.; Wiwattanapatapee, R. Effect of Alginate and Surfactant on Physical Properties of Oil Entrapped Alginate Bead Formulation of Curcumin. *Int. J. Med. Pharm. Sci. Eng.* **2013**, *7*, 479–483.
47. Phan, V.H.G.; Mathiyalagan, R.; Nguyen, M.-T.; Tran, T.-T.; Murugesan, M.; Ho, T.-N.; Huong, H.; Yang, D.C.; Li, Y.; Thambi, T. Ionically Cross-Linked Alginate-Chitosan Core-Shell Hydrogel Beads for Oral Delivery of Insulin. *Int. J. Biol. Macromol.* **2022**, *222*, 262–271. [CrossRef] [PubMed]
48. Chuang, J.-J.; Huang, Y.-Y.; Lo, S.-H.; Hsu, T.-F.; Huang, W.-Y.; Huang, S.-L.; Lin, Y.-S. Effects of pH on the Shape of Alginate Particles and Its Release Behavior. *Int. J. Polym. Sci.* **2017**, *2017*, 3902704. [CrossRef]
49. Salehi, T.; Raeisi Estabragh, M.A.; Salarpour, S.; Ohadi, M.; Dehghannoudeh, G. Absorption Enhancer Approach for Protein Delivery by Various Routes of Administration: A Rapid Review. *J. Drug Target.* **2023**, *31*, 950–961. [CrossRef] [PubMed]
50. Yamamoto, A.; Ukai, H.; Morishita, M.; Katsumi, H. Approaches to Improve Intestinal and Transmucosal Absorption of Peptide and Protein Drugs. *Pharmacol. Ther.* **2020**, *211*, 107537. [CrossRef]
51. Maher, S.; Heade, J.; McCartney, F.; Waters, S.; Bleiel, S.B.; Brayden, D.J. Effects of Surfactant-Based Permeation Enhancers on Mannitol Permeability, Histology, and Electrogenic Ion Transport Responses in Excised Rat Colonic Mucosae. *Int. J. Pharm.* **2018**, *539*, 11–22. [CrossRef]
52. Déat-Lainé, E.; Hoffart, V.; Garrait, G.; Beyssac, E. Whey Protein and Alginate Hydrogel Microparticles for Insulin Intestinal Absorption: Evaluation of Permeability Enhancement Properties on Caco-2 Cells. *Int. J. Pharm.* **2013**, *453*, 336–342. [CrossRef]
53. Kumar, P.; Nagarajan, A.; Uchil, P.D. Analysis of Cell Viability by the MTT Assay. *Cold Spring Harb. Protoc.* **2018**, *2018*, 95505. [CrossRef]

Disclaimer/Publisher's Note: The statements, opinions and data contained in all publications are solely those of the individual author(s) and contributor(s) and not of MDPI and/or the editor(s). MDPI and/or the editor(s) disclaim responsibility for any injury to people or property resulting from any ideas, methods, instructions or products referred to in the content.

Article

Formulation and Evaluation of Transdermal Patches Containing BGP-15

Ildikó Bácskay [1,2,†], Zsolt Hosszú [1,†], István Budai [3], Zoltán Ujhelyi [1], Pálma Fehér [1], Dóra Kósa [1,2], Ádám Haimhoffer [1,2] and Ágota Pető [1,2,*]

1. Department of Pharmaceutical Technology, Faculty of Pharmacy, University of Debrecen, Nagyerdei körút 98, 4032 Debrecen, Hungary
2. Institute of Healthcare Industry, University of Debrecen, Nagyerdei körút 98, 4032 Debrecen, Hungary
3. Faculty of Engineering, University of Debrecen, Ótemető Utca 2-4, 4028 Debrecen, Hungary
* Correspondence: peto.agota@pharm.unideb.hu
† These authors contributed equally to this work.

Abstract: BGP-15 is an active ingredient with many advantages, e.g., beneficial cardiovascular and anti-inflammatory effects. The transdermal administration of BGP-15 has great potential, which has not been investigated yet, despite the fact that it is a non-invasive and safe form of treatment. The aim of our study was to formulate transdermal patches containing BGP-15 and optimize the production with the Box–Behnken design of experiment. The most optimal formulation was further combined with penetration enhancers to improve bioavailability of the active ingredient, and the in vitro drug release and in vitro permeation of BGP-15 from the patches were investigated. FTIR spectra of BGP-15, the formulations and the components were also studied. The most optimal formulation based on the tested parameters was dried for 24 h, with 67% polyvinyl alcohol (PVA) content and low ethanol content. The selected penetration enhancer excipients were not cytotoxic on HaCaT cells. The FTIR measurements and SEM photography proved the compatibility of the active substance and the vehicle; BGP-15 was present in the polymer matrix in dissolved form. The bioavailability of BGP-15 was most significantly enhanced by the combination of Transcutol and Labrasol. The in vitro permeation study confirmed that the formulated patches successfully enabled the transdermal administration of BGP-15.

Keywords: BGP-15; Box–Behnken design of experiment; penetration enhancers; bioavailability; transdermal patches; PVA; PVP; in vitro permeation; porcine skin

1. Introduction

In modern pharmacotherapy, there is an increasing demand to develop new pharmaceutical forms that can be safely administered with adequate bioavailability and patient compliance in order to achieve successful therapeutic responses [1]. Transdermal drug delivery (TDD) is an innovative and appealing alternative form of oral and parenteral drug administration as it uses the skin as its drug-absorbing medium [2]. Although several types of transdermal therapeutic systems (TTSs) can be distinguished, the most common and frequently used forms are transdermal patches [3,4].

These patches are designed to be applied to the skin while delivering a therapeutically effective dose of one or more active ingredients into the systemic circulation through the layers of the skin [4–6]. The most basic and important components of transdermal patches are the polymers as they provide numerous functions such as forming the matrix, controlling the rate of drug delivery, providing protection, adhesion, flexibility and permeation [1,7–9].

These matrices can be formulated by the dispersion of an active pharmaceutical ingredient in a solid state or liquid polymer base [1,7]. An ideal polymer should meet some requirements such as proper stability and good compatibility with the chemical agent and the other elements that were used; moreover, they should contribute to a predictable drug release [10].

The ingredients incorporated into the formulation, the selected polymers and excipients have a significant influence on the physical properties of the patches, as well as their drug release and applicability. During the development of the composition, the properties of the active substance(s) must be considered as an important influencing factor as well [1,11]. The most commonly used polymers in patches are cellulosic derivates (e.g., hydroxypropyl methylcellulose (HPMC)), polyvinyl pyrrolidone (PVP), PVA, polyacrylates and acrylate derivates, as well as chitosan, but of course there are several other options available [10–12].

PVA is a copolymer of vinyl acetate and vinyl alcohol that is widely utilized in pharmaceutical formulations for its biocompatible, non-toxic and hydrophilic properties [13–15]. The extensive use of PVA is dictated by its beneficial properties, such as outstanding film-forming capability, impressive adhesive and emulsifying characteristics, chemical resistance and mechanical stability. However, PVA-based formulations present some shortcomings as well, which may restrict their use, e.g., insufficient lubrication properties in hydrogels because of the strong action of the intermolecular hydrogen bonds. To overcome these difficulties, some methods have been introduced, among which mixing with PVP showed quite promising results. PVP is a synthetic polymer of N-vinyl pyrrolidone and can be used in the formulation of several drug delivery forms including transdermal patches. PVP has advantageous properties like water solubility, biocompatibility, non-toxicity, inertness, biodegradability and inherent matrix-forming characteristics. Adding PVP to PVA can improve the surface lubrication, and synergistic effects were observed on the structure via the combination of the two polymers [16,17]. The combination of the two polymers has many advantages. However, their ideal ratio differs for each composition and dosage form, thus, it is important to determine the optimal manufacturing conditions and the ratio of solvents and polymers, as these have a significant impact on the physical properties and drug release as well.

In transdermal formulations, sufficient drug penetration is a critical factor. Carefully selected penetration enhancer excipients can support this factor [18,19], and they are able to alter bioavailability and drug penetration as well. Excipients should be selected according to their ability to permeate into different skin layers, considering toxicity and compatibility with all the other components of the formulation [20,21]. There are widespread penetration enhancer excipients and combinations thereof which are preferentially used in external formulations because they can enhance the effect of the active substance by ensuring good drug delivery through the skin [22].

BGP-15 is an active substance currently in the clinical trial stage. It is a solid, yellowish material. BGP-15 is a small molecule, and its molar weight is 351.272 g/mol. Its water solubility is 28 mg/mL at room temperature. BGP-15 is usually administered orally, in the form of capsules. However, the topical administration of the drug also has advantages; in some studies, ointments were formulated as well. Recently, numerous beneficial pharmacological effects of the drug were studied [23]. It is highly effective in the prevention and treatment of diabetes type 2 due to its insulin sensitizing effect [24]. Moreover, BGP-15 has beneficial cardioprotective effects; it is proven to be effective in the treatment of heart failure [25]. In the last few years, the topical administration of the drug was investigated as well. In those studies, photoprotective and anti-inflammatory effects were observed [26,27]. The mechanism of the effect is still not completely understood, but some of the key mechanisms have been identified. BGP-15 is a PARP inhibitor. It increases heat shock protein synthesis, and it is able to increase membrane fluidity as well.

The purpose of our study was to formulate transdermal patches containing BGP-15 as the transdermal administration of the active substance has never been studied before in spite of its great potential in the abovementioned therapeutic indications. In the formulation process, our aim was to prepare PVA- and PVP-based transdermal patches and determine the most suitable proportion of these two polymers, the solvent proportion and the drying time to optimize the process with the help of the Box–Behnken design of experiment. After finding the most optimal composition, our aim was to combine it with different penetration enhancer excipients to improve the bioavailability of BGP-15 and investigate in vitro drug release and the modified permeation test from the patches.

2. Materials and Methods

2.1. Materials

Transcutol and Labrasol were kind gifts from Gattefossé (Lyon, France). 3-(4,5-Dimethylthiazol-2-yl)-2,5-diphenyltetrazolium bromide (MTT paint), Dulbecco's modified Eagle's medium (DMEM), phosphate-buffered saline (PBS), trypsin–EDTA, heat-inactivated fetal bovine serum (FBS), L-glutamine, non-essential amino acids solution, penicillin–streptomycin, polyethylene glycol 400 (PEG 400), PVA and PVP were purchased from Sigma Aldrich. Twelve-well plates were purchased from Corning (Corning, NY, USA). HaCaT cells were supplied from Cell Lines Service (CLS, Heidelberg, Germany). BGP-15 was purchased from SONEAS Chemicals Ltd. (formerly known as Ubichem Pharma Services), Budapest, Hungary. Propylene glycol was obtained from Hungaropharma Ltd. (Budapest, Hungary).

2.2. Formulation of Transdermal Patches

Drug-loaded transdermal patches of BGP-15 were formulated by using the solvent casting method [28]. For this purpose, 12-well plates (diameter 2 cm) were chosen. Polymers (PVA and PVP) were weighed accurately and dissolved in 10 mL of the mixture of water and in ethanol solution of various percentages by volume, diluted from 70% ethyl alcohol and put aside to form a clear solution. The active ingredient (10 $w/w\%$) was dissolved in the abovementioned solution and mixed until a clear solution was obtained. PEG 400 and propylene glycol were used as plasticizers. The resulting homogeneous solution was cast in the plates and dried at 40 °C for predetermined time intervals. The dried patches were further studied from different aspects. The steps of the formulation are presented in Figure 1.

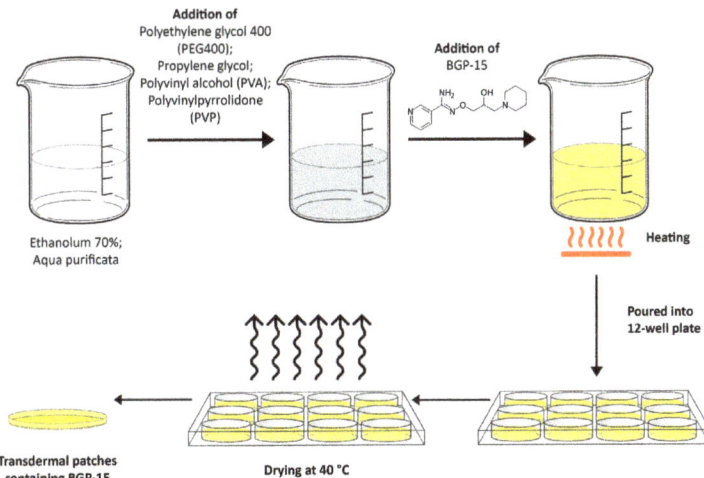

Figure 1. Formulation process of the transdermal patches via the solvent casting method. The polymers (PVA, PVP) and the plasticizers (PEG 400 and propylene glycol) were measured into the mixture of ethanol and purified water. In the next step, the active substance was incorporated into the composition, and then this mixture was heated until we obtained a viscous but clear solution, which was poured into a 12-well plate and dried at 40 °C.

2.3. Design of Experiment

Production of the patches was optimized by using a Box–Behnken design of experiment. During the process, 3 independent and 3 dependent factors were evaluated. Independent variables were the amount of PVA ($w/v\%$), ethanol content ($w/w\%$) and drying time (h); these were considered the critical parameters in the production process with an effect on product quality. The experimental factors were varied in the design, at 3 levels in 15 runs/compositions, which are presented in Table 1. The design of experiments considered the reproducibility and the significant effect of each factor on the observed variables. Tensile strength, moisture content and moisture uptake were taken as dependent variables. The quadratic response surface was used to construct a second-order polynomial model using TIBCO Statistica® 13.4 (StatSoft Hungary, Budapest, Hungary). The 3D response surface plots for dependent factors were plotted according to the regression model by keeping one variable at the center level [29].

Table 1. Compositions of the formulated transdermal patches. Each composition was prepared using the solvent casting method and dried for predetermined time intervals.

Composition	Solvent ($w/w\%$)	PVA ($w/v\%$)	Drying Time (h)
1	50	33	24
2	20	33	24
3	50	67	24
4	20	67	24
5	50	50	12
6	20	50	12
7	50	50	36
8	20	50	36
9	35	33	12
10	35	67	12
11	35	33	36
12	35	67	36
13	35	50	24
14	35	50	24
15	35	50	24

The solvent was the mixture of purified water and ethanol (70 $v/v\%$). In the table, the quantity of ethanol is represented in the solvent mixture. The selected polymers for the films were PVA and PVP. In the table, the quantity of PVA is displayed from the mixture of the polymers. The center point formulations are marked with gray color.

Preformulation studies were carried out to establish the criteria for the optimization, and the relevant scientific literature was also studied. PVA content of the patches under 30% proved to be extremely sticky, rupturing too easily. Over 70% PVA patches were rigid and difficult to tear, with little elasticity. Scientific literature suggests that PVA should be in the majority when using a mixture of PVA and PVP [17]. Drying time was determined by preformulation studies. Under 12 h, the patches had too high moisture content, that made them too sticky and ruptured too easily, while over 36 h, the patches were overdried, the moisture content was too low, and the patches could not be removed from the plate, so these values were taken as the extreme values during production. Ethanol content provides sufficient solubility of PVA and PVP in the range of 20–50%.

2.3.1. Tensile Strength

Tensile strength and tear characteristics of the polymer films were evaluated using a Brookfield CT3 texture analyzer instrument. It contained two load cell grips, of which the lower one was secured and the upper one was mobile. Film strips with dimensions of 1 × 1 cm were fixed between the cell grips, and force was increasingly applied until the film broke. Tensile strength was measured in mN [30].

2.3.2. Moisture Content

Moisture content of the patches was investigated with a KERN DAB moisture analyzer instrument. The initial weights of the patches were accurately weighed, and they were heated by the instrument to 120 °C. Water content was measured with the instrument, and the moisture content of the films was calculated by taking into account the initial weights and expressed as a percentage [31]:

$$\text{Moisture content} = \frac{\text{Water content}}{\text{Initial weight}} \times 100 \quad (1)$$

2.3.3. Moisture Uptake

Moisture uptake of the patches was studied with the help of a climate chamber. The patches were kept in the chamber at room temperature and 80% humidity for 48 h. The initial weights of the patches were previously weighed, and after 48 h they were weighed again [32]. Moisture uptake was calculated based on the weight increase and expressed as a percentage according to the following equation:

$$\text{Moisture uptake} = \frac{\text{Final weight} - \text{Initial weight}}{\text{Initial weight}} \times 100 \quad (2)$$

2.4. Penetration Enhancement

After finding the most optimal formulation, composition 4 was further combined with penetration enhancer excipients to improve the bioavailability of BGP-15. The selected excipients were Transcutol and Labrasol, following the suggestions of Gattefossé. Labrasol or Transcutol or a 1:1 mixture of the two excipients was added to the patches at 0.1% during the formulation process.

2.5. MTT Assay

To assess the toxicity of the selected excipients, an MTT assay was performed. This procedure was carried out on the HaCaT cell line. The cells were maintained by weekly passages in Dulbecco's DMEM culture media. For the assay, the keratinocyte cells were seeded on a 96-well plate with the density of 10.000 cells/well. When the cells had completely grown over the well's membrane, the experiment was ready to perform. First, culture media was removed, then the samples were applied, and the cells were incubated with them for 30 min. After half an hour, the test solutions were removed, and the MTT paint solution was added at a 5 mg/mL concentration to the cells. Then, a 3 h long incubation followed. The viable cells transformed the water-soluble tetrazolium–bromide into formazan precipitate. When the incubation was finished, formazan precipitate was dissolved with the help of isopropanol/hydrochloride acid at a 25:1 proportion. After that, the absorbance of the solutions was measured using a spectrophotometer (Fluostar Optima), and it was directly proportional to the number of viable cells [33].

2.6. Fourier-Transform Infrared Spectroscopy (FTIR)

The infrared spectra of:

- The active substance (solid BGP-15);
- Transdermal patches with BGP-15, without penetration enhancers;
- The transdermal patches with BGP-15 and the penetration enhancers (Labrasol or Transcutol or the mixture of Labrasol and Transcutol);
- Transdermal patches without penetration enhancers and BGP-15 were obtained by using a JASCO FT/IR-4600 spectrometer with an ATR accessory (Zn/Se ATR PRO ONE Single-Reflection, ABL&E-JASCO, Hungary, Budapest). All the samples were directly placed on the diamond crystal of the equipment. Scanning was run in the wavelength range of 500–4000 cm^{-1}. The spectra were collected from 32 scans to obtain

smooth spectra at the spectral resolution of 1 cm^{-1}. Corrections of environmental CO_2 and H_2O were carried out using the software's built-in method [34].

2.7. Scanning Electron Microscopy (SEM)

The morphology of the patches was studied with a Hitachi tabletop microscope (TM3030 Plus, Hitachi High-Technologies Corporation, Tokyo, Japan) in high-resolution mode. The samples were attached to a fixture with a double-sided adhesive tape containing graphite. A low accelerating voltage (15 kV) and vacuum were used to investigate the structure of the cut patches at 500× magnification [13].

2.8. In Vitro Release of the Active Ingredient

In vitro drug release was investigated using Franz diffusion chamber apparatus. During the experiment, an artificial cellulose–acetate membrane was placed between the donor and the acceptor phase. Samples were taken from the acceptor phase at predetermined times. The patches were placed on the membrane (0.45 μm pore size) as the donor phase, and as the acceptor phase, a pH = 5.5 buffer was chosen to imitate the skin's pH with 7 mL/cell volume. The surface area of the cell was 1766 cm^2. The solubility of BGP-15 is 28 mg/mL in this media [23], thus, theoretically it would be able to dissolve 196 mg BGP-15. The transdermal patches contained 50 mg BGP-15, so the media could dissolve more than triple the amount of the active substance. Prior to the experiment, the membrane was impregnated with isopropyl myristate to match the lipophilic character of the skin. The acceptor phase was set to 32 °C to imitate the temperature of the skin [35].

The diffused amount of BGP-15 was measured with the following HPLC method [36]. The samples were filtered on 0.2 μm polyethersulfone membrane. The sample solutions were analyzed using a HPLC system (Merck-Hitachi, Tokyo, Japan ELITE with photodiode array detector (DAD)). The column was an Aquasil C18 (5 μm 100 × 2.1 mm) with a C18 guard column (5 μm, 4 × 3 mm) and kept at 40 °C, and the DAD was set to 254 nm. The mobile phase was an acetonitrile and water solution at a ratio of 1:9 (containing 0.1% acetic acid), and a 1.0 mL flow rate was used. The analyses were performed with EZChrom Elite software^{TM} 3.2.0. (Hitachi, Tokyo, Japan), which was also used for collecting and processing the data. Standard solution (10 μL) and purified samples were injected.

Dissolution profiles were characterized in several ways. *Flux* was calculated using the following equation:

$$Flux = \frac{Q}{t} \quad (3)$$

where Q is the amount of drug released per unit area (mg/cm^2) and diffusion time (t).

Dissolution curves were fitted to the zero-order, first-order, Korsmeyer–Peppas, Higuchi and Weibull models using a graphical technique.

In order to compare the release values of BGP-15 transdermal patches, difference factors were calculated via a model-independent approach [37]:

$$f_1 = \frac{\sum_{j=1}^{n} |R_j - T_j|}{\sum_{j=1}^{n} R_j} \times 100 \quad (4)$$

here, n is the sampling number, and R_j and T_j are the percent dissolved of the reference and the test products at each time point j, respectively.

$$f_2 = 50 \times \log \left\{ \left[1 + (1/n) \sum_{j=1}^{n} w_j |R_j - T_j|^2 \right]^{-0.5} \times 100 \right\} \quad (5)$$

here, w_j is an optional weight factor.

2.9. In Vitro Permeation Studies

In vitro permeation studies were performed in Franz diffusion cell apparatus with a modification whereby the artificial cellulose acetate membrane was replaced by previously prepared pieces of pig ear skin. As acceptor phase, pH = 5.5 phosphate buffer was chosen, with 7 mL/cell volume. The pig ear was obtained from a slaughterhouse. Skin slices of 1 mm thickness were isolated from the inner, thinner, intact side of pig ears and were then frozen at $-18\ °C$ until the experiment. The isolated skin samples were defrosted and rehydrated in physiological saline solution with sodium azide (0.01 $w/v\%$) at 25 °C for 30 min to preserve functionality. After washing with azide-free saline solution, the skin layer was used instead of the membrane used in the in vitro experiment (Section 2.8, In Vitro Release of the Active Ingredient). The stratum corneum faced upwards in the donor phase [38].

2.10. Determination of BGP-15 in Skin Samples

The amounts of BGP-15 that accumulated in the skin and in the acceptor phase were determined at the end of the in vitro permeation studies. The used porcine skin underwent solvent extraction to determine the distribution of BGP-15 between the stratum corneum and the dermis with epidermis. At the end of the permeation test, the application surface of the ear skin was washed with physiological washing saline solution to remove the sticky formulation. Then, the skin was dried with the help of cotton wool, and adhesive cellophane tapes were used to remove the stratum corneum by tape-stripping 25 times. The BGP-15 content was washed from the stripping tapes with 5 mL of methanol into glass vials. The remaining stripped skin (epidermis without stratum corneum plus dermis) was then cut into small pieces that were placed in 5 mL of methanol for solvent extraction. Extractions were carried out in an ultrasonic bath at 40 °C for 15 min and repeated three times. The samples were then evaporated under a stream of N_2 gas at 45 °C and dissolved back into the mobile phase with the help of an ultrasonic bath (5 min). The samples were then centrifuged (4000 rpm, 15 min), and the supernatants were filtered in a 0.2 µm PES membrane [38].

2.11. Statistical Analysis

Data were analyzed with GraphPad Prism 6 and presented as means ± SD. Comparison of the groups in MTT assays was performed with one-way ANOVA test and the t-test. Significant differences in the figures are indicated with asterisks. Differences were regarded as significant at $p < 0.05$. All experiments were performed at least in triplicate.

3. Results

3.1. Design of Experiment

3.1.1. Tensile Strength

The drying time did not show any significant difference in the tensile strength, therefore, only the correlation between PVA and the solvent was investigated. The curve in Figure 2 shows that increasing the concentration of PVA increased the tensile strength of the patch linearly, and the 3D surface displays that PVA rundown was linear. As for the solvent, a non-linear correlation was observed, and the plot could be well described by an exponential trend. At 20–40 $w/w\%$, a slower increase in the tensile strength was observed, while further increasing the ethanol concentration in the solvent mixture resulted in a faster ascending section.

3.1.2. Moisture Content

The moisture content of the formulated patches was not significantly affected by the solvent; however, PVA concentration and drying time significantly influenced it. Figure 3 represents the results. Increasing the concentration of PVA resulted in an increase in the moisture content, which no longer increased linearly after a certain polymer concentration.

Increasing the drying time decreased the moisture content up to 24–30 h; afterwards, there was no significant difference in the curve.

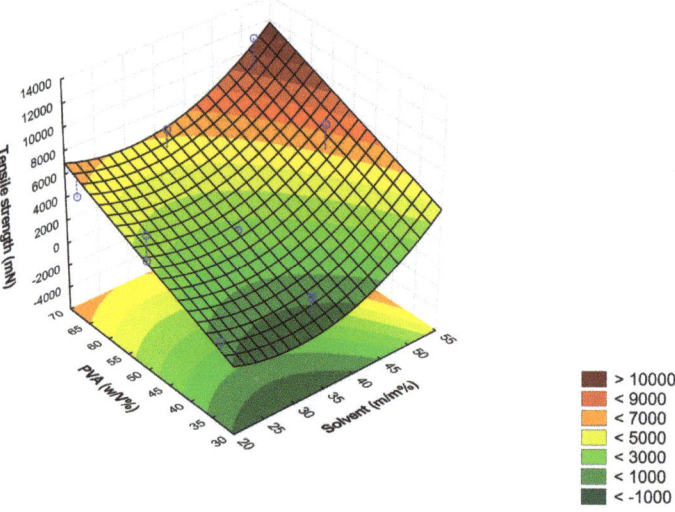

Figure 2. Increasing the concentration of PVA in the composition increased the tensile strength of the transdermal patches. As for the solvent, ethanol in 20–40 w/w% concentration slowly increased the tensile strength, while the further increase in ethanol content resulted in a faster ascending section.

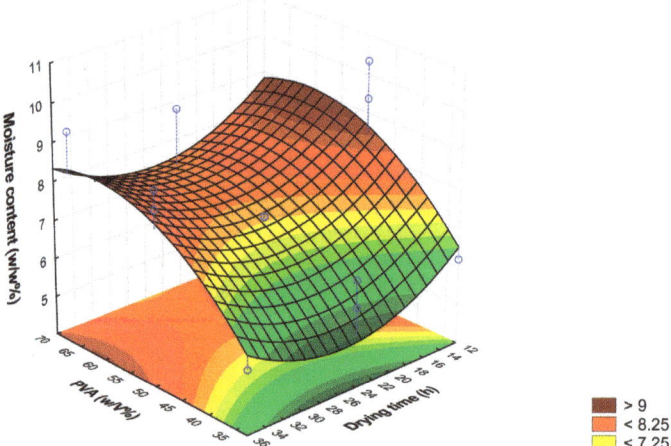

Figure 3. The correlation of PVA concentration and moisture content shows that increasing PVA content resulted in an increase in moisture content, while the increase in drying time decreased moisture content.

3.1.3. Moisture Uptake

Moisture uptake was not affected by the investigated factors (PVA concentration, ethanol concentration and drying time) during the formulation. No significant differences were detected. The average moisture uptake of the patches was $22.05 \pm 4.06\ w/w\%$.

3.1.4. Incorporating Penetration Enhancers into the Formulation

Based on the result of the Box–Behnken design of experiment, composition 4 was proved to be the most optimal formulation with 67% PVA, 20% ethanol content and 24 h of drying time. Thus, it was further combined with penetration enhancer excipients to improve the bioavailability of BGP-15. Transcutol and Labrasol were chosen as the penetration enhancers. The formulations are listed in Table 2.

Table 2. The composition of the transdermal formulations in combination with penetration enhancers.

Formulation	
W.P.	Transdermal patch without any penetration enhancer excipient
T	Transdermal patch with 0.1% Transcutol
L	Transdermal patch with 0.1% Labrasol
T + L	Transdermal patch with 0.1% Transcutol and Labrasol

3.2. MTT Assay

The results of the MTT assays are represented in Figure 4a,b. The two penetration enhancer excipients, Labrasol and Transcutol, were dissolved in PBS prior to the experiment, and different concentrations of these materials were tested on HaCaT cells. PBS was selected as a negative control and Triton-X 100 as a positive control. The values of cell viability were compared with those in PBS, and they are indicated as a percentage. In the experiment, both Labrasol and Transcutol proved to be safe and well tolerated by the cells in the tested concentration range, since cell viability values were above 70%.

3.3. FTIR Measurements

The characteristic chemical groups of BGP-15 (N'-[2-hydroxy-3-(1-piperidinyl) propoxy] pyridine-3-carboximidamide) were studied using the FTIR method. The IR spectra showed the location of the characteristic groups. A broad region in the 3200–3400 range was observed, characteristic of the OH group. The characteristic peaks for the amine group were 3375, 3279 and 1634 cm^{-1}, respectively. Characteristic peaks for the ether group were found at 2991 and 2929 cm^{-1}. The FTIR spectrum of BGP-15 is presented in Figure 5.

During the formulation of the patches, BGP-15 formed secondary bonds with the polymers used as the base for the patch. This was indicated by the band shift of BGP-15 amine groups from 1634 to 1641. No further band shifts were found when penetration enhancers were incorporated into the composition. The results confirmed that BGP-15 was in a soluble form in the formulation and did not degrade chemically during the preparation. FTIR spectra are summarized in Figure 6.

3.4. SEM

The morphology of the patches was studied via scanning electron microscopy. The photographs confirmed the compatibility of BGP-15 with the polymer matrix as it showed homogeneous films. The thickness of the patches was measured as well; it was between 120 and 190 μm. The scans of the transdermal patches are demonstrated in Figure 7.

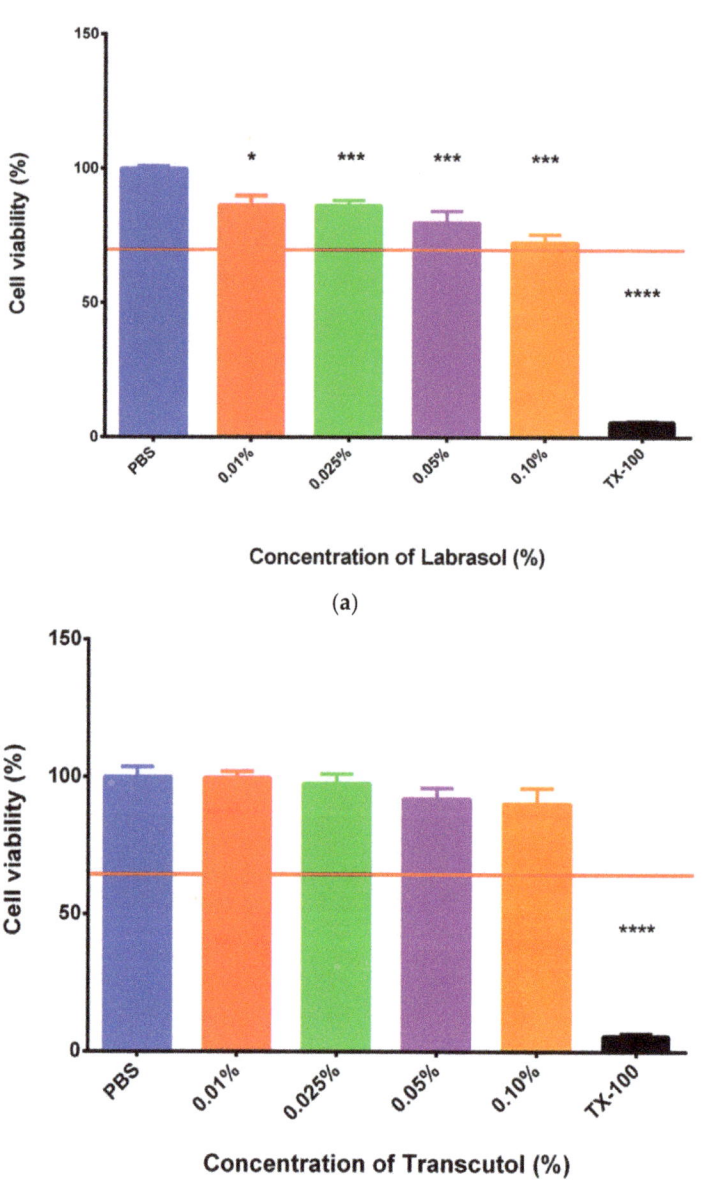

Figure 4. Cytotoxicity of Labrasol (**a**); cytotoxicity of Transcutol (**b**). Cell viability was determined as the percentage of PBS. The concentrations used in the formulations proved to be safe in all cases, and cell viability values were above 70% (marked with a red line) in every case. Data represent the mean of 6 wells ± SD. For statistical analysis, the t-test and one-way ANOVA test were carried out. Significant difference is marked with asterisks. *, *** and **** show statistically significant difference at $p < 0.05$; $p < 0.001$ and $p < 0.0001$.

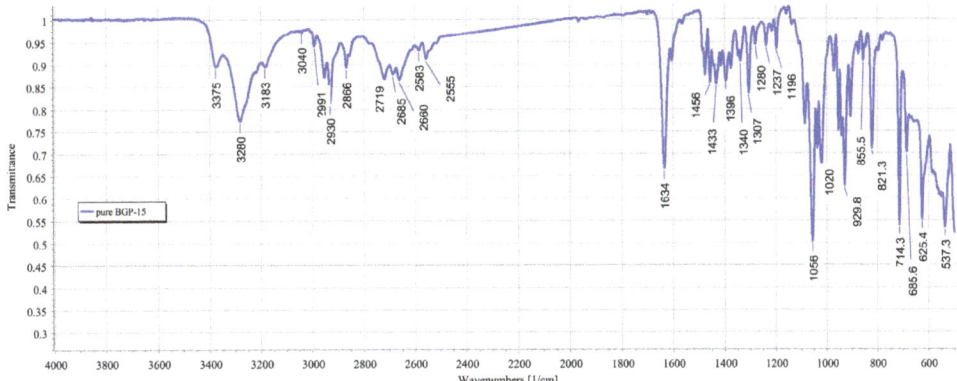

Figure 5. FTIR spectrum of BGP-15. A broad region in the 3200–3400 range was observed, characteristic of the OH group. The characteristic peaks of the amine group were 3375, 3279 and 1634 cm^{-1}, respectively. Characteristic peaks of the ether group were found at 2991 and 2929 cm^{-1}.

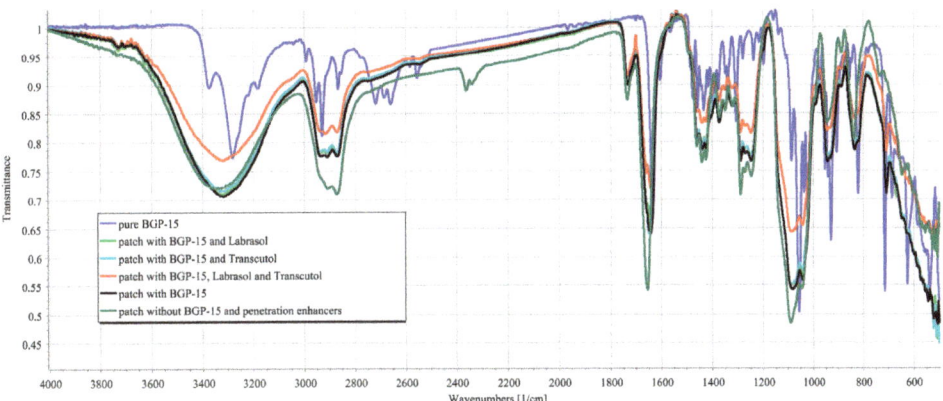

Figure 6. FTIR-spectra of the active substance (solid BGP-15), transdermal patches with BGP-15, without penetration enhancers, the transdermal patches with BGP-15 and the penetration enhancers (Labrasol or Transcutol, or the mixture of Labrasol and Transcutol), transdermal patches without penetration enhancers and BGP-15.

3.5. In Vitro Drug Release

Figure 8 represents the diffused amount of BGP-15 across the isopropyl myristate-impregnated cellulose acetate membrane from the different transdermal patches with or without penetration enhancers. Those compositions, which contained Labrasol or the combination of Labrasol and Transcutol achieved higher drug release values. The best result was achieved by using the combination of Transcutol and Labrasol, where the diffused drug amount was 37.19%. The second-best result was obtained by the patch formulated with Labrasol, where the diffused drug amount was 29.58%. The lowest release rates were achieved by the patches prepared with Transcutol or without any penetration enhancer excipient.

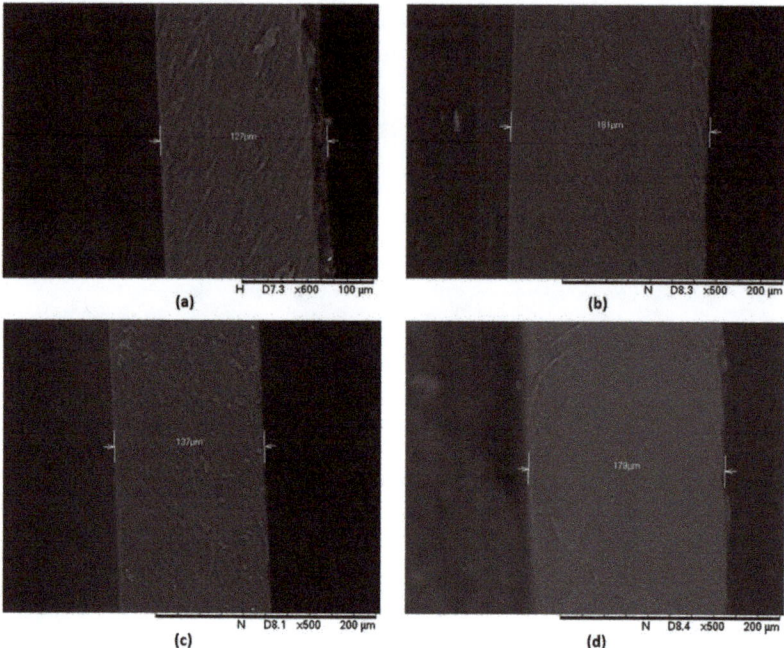

Figure 7. SEM photography of BGP-15 containing transdermal patches without penetration enhancers (**a**), with Labrasol (**b**), with Transcutol (**c**) and with the combination of Labrasol and Transcutol (**d**).

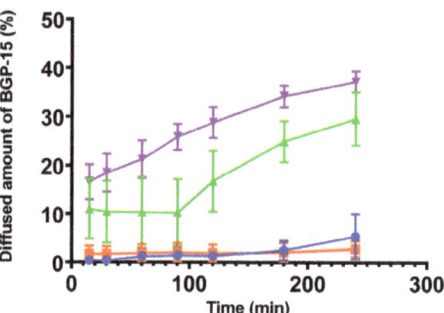

- Transdermal patch without penetration enhancers
- Transdermal patch with Transcutol
- Transdermal patch with Labrasol
- Transdermal patch with Transcutol and Labrasol

Figure 8. Release profiles of BGP-15 across the cellulose acetate membrane from the transdermal patches. The best result was obtained by the formulation which contained the combination of Transcutol and Labrasol, while the lowest release values belonged to the patches containing Transcutol or no penetration enhancer excipient at all.

Comparing the flux of the compositions (Table 3), the patch with Transcutol and Labrasol showed a nearly tenfold higher value than the patch without enhancers. The Transcutol sample alone showed no significant difference from the composition without enhancers.

Table 3. Summary of the dissolution kinetic model.

	Transdermal Patches			
	Without Penetration Enhancers	With Transcutol	With Labrasol	With Transcutol and Labrasol
Flux (mg/cm^2 × h^{-1})	0.3843	0.2007	2.0940	2.6324

Kinetic model fitting showed the difference between the formulations in Table 4. The Weibull model best described the drug release of patches without penetration enhancers. In the case of penetration enhancers, drug release was better described by different modeling. Transcutol showed zero-order kinetics, while Labrasol showed first-order kinetics. When the penetration enhancers were used together, first-order kinetics showed the best correlation.

Table 4. Summary of the dissolution kinetic model.

Kinetic Model [1]	Transdermal Patches			
	Without Penetration Enhancers	With Transcutol	With Labrasol	With Transcutol and Labrasol
Zero	0.8780	0.8107	0.8977	0.9772
First	0.8741	0.8100	0.8984	0.9857
Korsmeyer–Peppas	0.8871	0.6630	0.6253	0.9636
Higuchi	0.7494	0.7600	0.8668	0.9597
Weibull	0.9097	0.6624	0.6251	0.9578

[1] The table contains the correlation coefficient value of the fitting line.

Release profiles of the transdermal formulations were compared. The calculated similarity and difference factors are listed in Table 5. Two formulations were recognized as similar if their similarity factor (f_2) was between 50 and 100, and different if their difference factor (f_1) was between 0 and 15. According to the calculated values, a great similarity was confirmed between the patches, which were formulated without penetration enhancers or with Transcutol. Transdermal patches prepared without penetration enhancers or Labrasol were significantly different. Patches without penetration enhancers compared with the combination of Transcutol and Labrasol turned out to be significantly different, as did the Labrasol-containing patch versus the combined one.

Table 5. Difference and similarity factors to compare the release profiles of the formulations (W.P.: transdermal patch without penetration enhancer; T.: transdermal patch formulated with Transcutol; L.: transdermal patch formulated with Labrasol; T and L.: transdermal patch formulated with the combination of Transcutol and Labrasol).

Formulation	f_1 [1]	f_2 [2]
W.P. vs. T.	9.45	89.48
W.P. vs. L.	88.53	40.39
W.P. vs. T and L.	92.88	30.17
L. vs. T and L.	37.91	49.17

[1] Two formulations are recognized as similar if their similarity factor (f_2) is between 50 and 100. [2] Two formulations are recognized as similar if their difference factor (f_1) is higher than 15.

3.6. In Vitro Permeation

In Figure 9, the results of the in vitro permeation study are presented. In this experiment, the permeation of the patch formulated with the combination of Transcutol and Labrasol was studied across pig's ear skin. According to the results, 39.3% (19.69 mg) of BGP-15 was able to permeate to the acceptor phase through the skin. In the skin (dermis plus epidermis), 9.2% of the initial BGP-15 was detected. In the case of skin, the flux of BGP-15 was 0.4647 mg/cm^2 × h^{-1}.

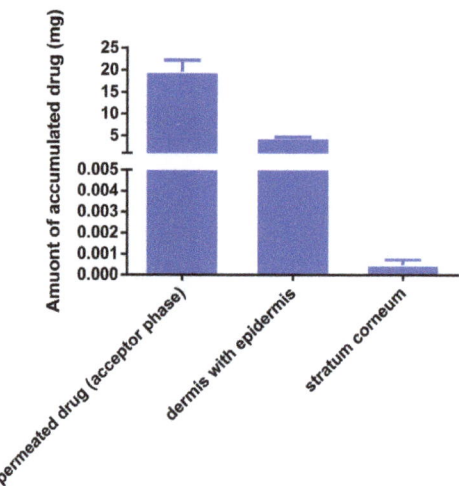

Figure 9. In vitro permeation of BGP-15 across porcine skin; 39.3% (19.69 mg) of the initial BGP-15 quantity was able to permeate to the acceptor phase.

4. Discussion

BGP-15 has been intensively studied in recent years, and many favorable effects of the drug candidate have been identified throughout this period. Beside the insulin sensitizing effect [39], advantageous cardioprotective [40,41] and anti-inflammatory effects [36] were observed. Transdermal administration is an under-investigated research area of BGP-15, as is topical application, since few studies on its utilization in ointment form are available. In our previous work, we investigated the topical application and the anti-inflammatory effect of the active ingredient [36]. The possibility of applying BGP-15 transdermally counts as a novelty as it has never been investigated before, although it could be particularly advantageous in the abovementioned indications.

In the present study, transdermal patches were formulated to promote the transdermal delivery of the active substance. Some of the most commonly used polymers in transdermal patches are PVA and PVP. The combination of these two polymers can be especially beneficial. However, very little information is available in the scientific literature about their ideal proportion in transdermal patches, the proper solvents and the circumstances of an optimal production. In our series of experiments, we aimed to determine the optimal production conditions of transdermal patches with the two polymers PVA and PVP to ensure the suitable transdermal dosage form for BGP-15. To optimize the production, the Box–Behnken design of experiment was used. In the factorial design, PVA content proved to be a key factor, as it increased the tensile strength and the moisture uptake as well, which are important characteristics of transdermal patches. The ethanol content was also important; at a 20–40% concentration it resulted in an increase in tensile strength. Based on these results, composition 4 was selected as the most optimal formulation with 67% PVA, 20% ethanol content and 24 h of drying time. The PVA content of the transdermal patches has key importance, as it determines the tensile strength. Lee et al. studied different transdermal patches and found that the larger the PVP proportion was in the formulation, the worse mechanical strength the composition had [17]. This complies with our experiences and results, as a PVP content above 50% resulted in patches that tore too easily. Gao et al. formulated transdermal patches with a PVA and PVP base. They used different ratios of polymers. They found that the larger PVA proportion worked the best; according to their results, a 7:1 PVA/PVP proportion was the most ideal as it determined the drug release and the quality of the transdermal patches [42]. The alcohol content influences the polymer expansion and the formation of secondary interactions [43].

Due to the solubilities of PVA and PVP [44], it is important to determine the ideal alcohol content where both molecules can unfold and interact to form a stable matrix after drying, which serves as the basis for our patch. Due to the PVA or PVP content of the films, the drying time at a given temperature is an important parameter. The drying time affects the recrystallisation of the polymers and the physical changes in their structure. As drying time increases, the hydration decreases, which can lead to loss of secondary interactions and crystallization [45].

To increase the bioavailability of BGP-15, different penetration enhancer excipients were incorporated into composition 4, namely, 0.1% Transcutol or 0.1% Labrasol or the combination of these two at 0.1%. Since safety is an important aspect of pharmaceutical formulations, cytotoxicity of these excipients was investigated using MTT assay on the HaCaT cell line. Based on the results, the selected excipients in the used concentration were safe and well tolerated, and cell viability was above 70%, which is the recommendation of ISO 10993-5 [46].

FTIR spectra of BGP-15 were first described by our research group. Besides BGP-15 itself, all the transdermal patches were studied using the FTIR method. The results confirmed the compatibility of the vehicle and the active substance; BGP-15 was dissolved in the polymer matrix. Taher et al. studied isonicotinic acid in PVA blend, and according to their FTIR measurements, the active substance was in dissolved form, similar to our case [47]. The results of SEM confirmed this as well since no crystals or other particles were found in the SEM photography. This also confirmed the theory that PVP inhibits the crystallization of substances.

In vitro drug release from the patches was investigated using Franz diffusion chamber apparatus. The active ingredient is present in a dissolved form, so penetration was expected to be faster than in crystalline form, which was confirmed by the in vitro drug release test. In this study, the best results were achieved by those formulations which contained both penetration enhancers Labrasol and Transcutol in combination. The second-best results were obtained by the Labrasol-containing patches, and those which contained Transcutol or no penetration enhancer at all achieved lower release values. Even though Transcutol is a well-known and powerful penetration enhancer, in some cases it is not able to enhance drug release and permeation [48]. Labrasol is a widespread and excellent penetration enhancer as well. In combination with Transcutol, the highest drug release was observed in our in vitro experiment, which can be explained by the synergistic penetration enhancer effect of the two excipients. Transcutol is often used in combination with other penetration enhancers; Amitkumar et al. found that oleic acid and Transcutol in combination significantly improved the transdermal drug delivery of oxcarbazepine [49]. The dissolution from the patches without penetration enhancers was well described with the Weibull model. The model is useful for determining the release profiles of matrix-type drug delivery. The correlation was obtained with slightly lower values for the Korsmeyer–Peppas model, which is suitable for predicting the release mechanism from a polymeric system [50]. The Higuchi relationship is used in the case of modified transdermal systems [51], nevertheless, it resulted in the worst match to the dissolution of patches as in other articles [52]. Penetration enhancers have already been described to affect drug delivery differently depending on the solubility or pKa value of the active substance [53,54]. Preparations containing a penetration enhancer can be described better with first- or zero-order kinetics.

The in vitro permeation study was carried out with composition 4 combined with the mixture of Labrasol and Transcutol, as this formulation achieved the best results through the synthetic membrane. A total of 39.3% of the initial BGP-15 was able to permeate to the acceptor phase, and only 9.2% BGP-15 was detected in the skin. This leads to the conclusion that BGP-15 does not accumulate in the skin but rather in the acceptor phase, so the formulated transdermal patch is suitable for transdermal delivery of the active ingredient. BGP-15 was present in a semi-dissociated form at pH 5.5, which facilitated its permeation through biological membranes; thus, a fast and efficient permeation was observed, as expected. Minor BGP-15 accumulation was measured in the skin. Drug flux across the biological membrane was reduced, as expected, due to the more complex system. According to the results, the formulated transdermal patch enables BGP-15 delivery to the systemic circulation; thus, the formulation provides a new therapeutic option and improved patient compliance.

The novelty of our work is the transdermal application of BGP-15, the development of an optimal transdermal dosage form for the active substance and the improvement of bioavailability with penetration enhancers. FTIR spectra of the active substance were characterized for the first time in the scientific literature.

5. Conclusions

In our series of experiments, we aimed to complete the currently available knowledge about BGP-15 by developing a suitable transdermal formulation for it and improving its bioavailability with penetration enhancers. Our study highlights the relevance of choosing appropriate excipients as it highly affects the formulation in many aspects. In the research, the ideal proportion of the selected polymers was determined, as well as the solvent ratio and the circumstances of the production. By further combining the most optimal composition, we were able to enhance the bioavailability of BGP-15. In the in vitro tests of drug release and permeation, we confirmed that the formulation is suitable for transdermal delivery of the active substance. This research enables and supports the transdermal administration of BGP-15, which is an important and promising perspective considering its indication field.

Author Contributions: Conceptualization, Á.P. and I.B. (Ildikó Bácskay); methodology, Á.H. and D.K.; software, Á.H. and D.K.; validation, Z.H., formal analysis, P.F.; investigation, Á.P. and Z.H.; resources, I.B. (Ildikó Bácskay); data curation, Á.H. and I.B. (Ildikó Bácskay); writing—original draft preparation, Á.P. and Z.H.; writing—review and editing, Á.P.; visualization, Z.U.; supervision, Á.P.; project administration, I.B. (István Budai); funding acquisition, I.B. (Ildikó Bácskay). All authors have read and agreed to the published version of the manuscript.

Funding: This research was supported by the ÚNKP-22-4-I National Excellence Program of the Ministry for Innovation and Technology from the source of the National Research, Development and Innovation Fund. Project no. TKP2021-EGA-19 was implemented with the support provided by the Ministry of Culture and Innovation of Hungary from the National Research, Development and Innovation Fund, financed under the TKP2021-EGA funding scheme. The publication was supported by the GINOP-2.3.1-20-2020-00004 and GINOP-2.3.4-15-2016-00002 projects. The project was co-financed by the European Union and the European Regional Development Fund.

Institutional Review Board Statement: Not applicable.

Informed Consent Statement: Not applicable.

Data Availability Statement: Data are available from the corresponding author with the permission of the head of the department. The data that support the findings of this study are available from the corresponding author (peto.agota@pharm.unideb.hu) upon reasonable request.

Conflicts of Interest: The authors declare no conflicts of interest.

References

1. Al Hanbali, O.A.; Khan, H.M.S.; Sarfraz, M.; Arafat, M.; Ijaz, S.; Hameed, A. Transdermal patches: Design and current approaches to painless drug delivery. *Acta Pharm.* **2019**, *69*, 197–215. [CrossRef] [PubMed]
2. Alkilani, A.; McCrudden, M.T.; Donnelly, R. Transdermal Drug Delivery: Innovative Pharmaceutical Developments Based on Disruption of the Barrier Properties of the Stratum Corneum. *Pharmaceutics* **2015**, *7*, 438–470. [CrossRef] [PubMed]
3. Prausnitz, M.R.; Langer, R. Transdermal drug delivery. *Nat. Biotechnol.* **2008**, *26*, 1261–1268. [CrossRef] [PubMed]
4. Peddapalli, H.; Ganta, R.P.; Boggula, N. Formulation and evaluation of transdermal patches for antianxiety drug. *Asian J. Pharm.* **2018**, *12*, 127–136.
5. Wokovich, A.; Prodduturi, S.; Doub, W.; Hussain, A.; Buhse, L. Transdermal drug delivery system (TDDS) adhesion as a critical safety, efficacy and quality attribute. *Eur. J. Pharm. Biopharm.* **2006**, *64*, 1–8. [CrossRef]

6. Hadžiabdić, J.; Šejto, L.; Rahić, O.; Tucak, A.; Hindija, L.; Sirbubalo, M. Transdermal Patches as Noninvasive Drug Delivery Systems. In Proceedings of the International Conference on Medical and Biological Engineering, Mostar, Bosnia and Herzegovina, 21–24 April 2021; pp. 395–402.
7. Das, S.; Sarkar, P.; Majee, S.B. Polymers in Matrix Type Transdermal Patch. *Int. J. Pharm. Sci. Rev. Res.* **2022**, *73*, 77–86. [CrossRef]
8. Latif, M.S.; Al-Harbi, F.F.; Nawaz, A.; Rashid, S.A.; Farid, A.; Al Mohaini, M.; Alsalman, A.J.; Al Hawaj, M.A.; Alhashem, Y.N. Formulation and Evaluation of Hydrophilic Polymer Based Methotrexate Patches: In Vitro and In Vivo Characterization. *Polymers* **2022**, *14*, 1310. [CrossRef]
9. Bhatt, P.; Trehan, S.; Inamdar, N.; Mourya, V.K.; Misra, A. Polymers in Drug Delivery: An Update. In *Applications of Polymers in Drug Delivery*; Elsevier: Amsterdam, The Netherlands, 2021; pp. 1–42.
10. Valenta, C.; Auner, B.G. The use of polymers for dermal and transdermal delivery. *Eur. J. Pharm. Biopharm.* **2004**, *58*, 279–289. [CrossRef]
11. Yewale, C.; Tandel, H.; Patel, A.; Misra, A. Polymers in Transdermal Drug Delivery. In *Applications of Polymers in Drug Delivery*; Elsevier: Amsterdam, The Netherlands, 2021; pp. 131–158.
12. Santos, L.F.; Correia, I.J.; Silva, A.S.; Mano, J.F. Biomaterials for drug delivery patches. *Eur. J. Pharm. Sci.* **2018**, *118*, 49–66. [CrossRef]
13. Sa'adon, S.; Abd Razak, S.I.; Ismail, A.E.; Fakhruddin, K. Fabrication of Dual Layer Polyvinyl Alcohol Transdermal Patch: Effect of Freezing-Thawing Cycles on Morphological and Swelling Ability. *Procedia Comput. Sci.* **2019**, *158*, 51–57. [CrossRef]
14. Zahra, F.T.; Quick, Q.; Mu, R. Electrospun PVA Fibers for Drug Delivery: A Review. *Polymers* **2023**, *15*, 3837. [CrossRef] [PubMed]
15. DeMerlis, C.; Schoneker, D. Review of the oral toxicity of polyvinyl alcohol (PVA). *Food Chem. Toxicol.* **2003**, *41*, 319–326. [CrossRef] [PubMed]
16. Teodorescu, M.; Bercea, M.; Morariu, S. Biomaterials of PVA and PVP in medical and pharmaceutical applications: Perspectives and challenges. *Biotechnol. Adv.* **2019**, *37*, 109–131. [CrossRef] [PubMed]
17. Lee, I.-C.; He, J.-S.; Tsai, M.-T.; Lin, K.-C. Fabrication of a novel partially dissolving polymer microneedle patch for transdermal drug delivery. *J. Mater. Chem. B* **2015**, *3*, 276–285. [CrossRef] [PubMed]
18. Nokhodchi, A.; Shokri, J.; Dashbolaghi, A.; Hassan-Zadeh, D.; Ghafourian, T.; Barzegar-Jalali, M. The enhancement effect of surfactants on the penetration of lorazepam through rat skin. *Int. J. Pharm.* **2003**, *250*, 359–369. [CrossRef] [PubMed]
19. Hagen, M.; Baker, M. Skin penetration and tissue permeation after topical administration of diclofenac. *Curr. Med. Res. Opin.* **2017**, *33*, 1623–1634. [CrossRef]
20. Som, I.; Bhatia, K.; Yasir, M. Status of surfactants as penetration enhancers in transdermal drug delivery. *J. Pharm. Bioallied Sci.* **2012**, *4*, 2–9. [CrossRef]
21. Korhonen, O.; Pajula, K.; Laitinen, R. Rational excipient selection for co-amorphous formulations. *Expert Opin. Drug Deliv.* **2017**, *14*, 551–569. [CrossRef]
22. Bando, H.; Yamashita, F.; Takakura, Y.; Hashida, M. Skin Penetration Enhancement of Acyclovir by Prodrug-Enhancer Combination. *Biol. Pharm. Bull.* **1994**, *17*, 1141–1143. [CrossRef]
23. Pető, Á.; Kósa, D.; Fehér, P.; Ujhelyi, Z.; Sinka, D.; Vecsernyés, M.; Szilvássy, Z.; Juhász, B.; Csanádi, Z.; Vígh, L.; et al. Pharmacological overview of the BGP-15 chemical agent as a new drug candidate for the treatment of symptoms of metabolic syndrome. *Molecules* **2020**, *25*, 429. [CrossRef]
24. Literati-Nagy, Z.; Tory, K.; Literáti-Nagy, B.; Kolonics, A.; Vígh, L., Jr.; Vígh, L.; Mandl, J.; Szilvássy, Z. A Novel Insulin Sensitizer Drug Candidate—BGP-15—Can Prevent Metabolic Side Effects of Atypical Antipsychotics. *Pathol. Oncol. Res.* **2012**, *18*, 1071–1076. [CrossRef] [PubMed]
25. Horvath, O.; Ordog, K.; Bruszt, K.; Deres, L.; Gallyas, F.; Sumegi, B.; Toth, K.; Halmosi, R. BGP-15 Protects against Heart Failure by Enhanced Mitochondrial Biogenesis and Decreased Fibrotic Remodelling in Spontaneously Hypertensive Rats. *Oxid. Med. Cell. Longev.* **2021**, *2021*, 1250858. [CrossRef] [PubMed]
26. Farkas, B.; Magyarlaki, M.; Csete, B.; Nemeth, J.; Rabloczky, G.; Bernath, S.; Nagy, P.L.; Sümegi, B. Reduction of acute photodamage in skin by topical application of a novel PARP inhibitor. *Biochem. Pharmacol.* **2002**, *63*, 921–932. [CrossRef] [PubMed]
27. Rodriguez, B.; Larsson, L.; Z'Graggen, W.J. Critical Illness Myopathy: Diagnostic Approach and Resulting Therapeutic Implications. *Curr. Treat. Options Neurol.* **2022**, *24*, 173–182. [CrossRef]
28. Prajapati, S.T.; Patel, C.G.; Patel, C.N. Formulation and Evaluation of Transdermal Patch of Repaglinide. *ISRN Pharm.* **2011**, *2011*, 651909. [CrossRef]
29. Haimhoffer, Á.; Vasvári, G.; Trencsényi, G.; Béresová, M.; Budai, I.; Czomba, Z.; Rusznyák, Á.; Váradi, J.; Bácskay, I.; Ujhelyi, Z.; et al. Process Optimization for the Continuous Production of a Gastroretentive Dosage Form Based on Melt Foaming. *AAPS PharmSciTech* **2021**, *22*, 187. [CrossRef]
30. Głąb, M.; Drabczyk, A.; Kudłacik-Kramarczyk, S.; Guigou, M.D.; Makara, A.; Gajda, P.; Jampilek, J.; Tyliszczak, B. Starch Solutions Prepared under Different Conditions as Modifiers of Chitosan/Poly(aspartic acid)-Based Hydrogels. *Materials* **2021**, *14*, 4443. [CrossRef]
31. Thakur, N.; Goswami, M.; Deka Dey, A.; Kaur, B.; Sharma, C.; Kumar, A. Fabrication and Synthesis of Thiococlchicoside Loaded Matrix Type Transdermal Patch. *Pharm. Nanotechnol.* **2023**, *11*. [CrossRef]
32. Suksaeree, J.; Prasomkij, J.; Panrat, K.; Pichayakorn, W. Comparison of Pectin Layers for Nicotine Transdermal Patch Preparation. *Adv. Pharm. Bull.* **2018**, *8*, 401–410. [CrossRef]

33. Kósa, D.; Pető, Á.; Fenyvesi, F.; Váradi, J.; Vecsernyés, M.; Gonda, S.; Vasas, G.; Fehér, P.; Bácskay, I.; Ujhelyi, Z. Formulation of Novel Liquid Crystal (LC) Formulations with Skin-Permeation-Enhancing Abilities of Plantago lanceolata (PL) Extract and Their Assessment on HaCaT Cells. *Molecules* **2021**, *26*, 1023. [CrossRef]
34. Sabir, F.; Qindeel, M.; Rehman, A.U.; Ahmad, N.M.; Khan, G.M.; Csoka, I.; Ahmed, N. An efficient approach for development and optimisation of curcumin-loaded solid lipid nanoparticles' patch for transdermal delivery. *J. Microencapsul.* **2021**, *38*, 233–248. [CrossRef] [PubMed]
35. Khalid, A.; Sarwar, H.S.; Sarfraz, M.; Sohail, M.F.; Jalil, A.; Bin Jardan, Y.A.; Arshad, R.; Tahir, I.; Ahmad, Z. Formulation and characterization of thiolated chitosan/polyvinyl acetate based microneedle patch for transdermal delivery of dydrogesterone. *Saudi Pharm. J.* **2023**, *31*, 669–677. [CrossRef] [PubMed]
36. Pető, Á.; Kósa, D.; Haimhoffer, Á.; Fehér, P.; Ujhelyi, Z.; Sinka, D.; Fenyvesi, F.; Váradi, J.; Vecsernyés, M.; Gyöngyösi, A.; et al. Nicotinic amidoxime derivate bgp-15, topical dosage formulation and anti-inflammatory effect. *Pharmaceutics* **2021**, *13*, 2037. [CrossRef] [PubMed]
37. Costa, P.; Lobo, J.M.S. Modeling and comparison of dissolution profiles. *Eur. J. Pharm. Sci.* **2001**, *13*, 123–133. [CrossRef] [PubMed]
38. Argenziano, M.; Haimhoffer, A.; Bastiancich, C.; Jicsinszky, L.; Caldera, F.; Trotta, F.; Scutera, S.; Alotto, D.; Fumagalli, M.; Musso, T.; et al. In Vitro Enhanced Skin Permeation and Retention of Imiquimod Loaded in β-Cyclodextrin Nanosponge Hydrogel. *Pharmaceutics* **2019**, *11*, 138. [CrossRef] [PubMed]
39. Literáti-Nagy, B.; Tory, K.; Peitl, B.; Bajza, Á.; Korányi, L.; Literáti-Nagy, Z.; Hooper, P.L.; Vígh, L.; Szilvássy, Z. Improvement of Insulin Sensitivity by a Novel Drug Candidate, BGP-15, in Different Animal Studies. *Metab. Syndr. Relat. Disord.* **2014**, *12*, 125–131. [CrossRef]
40. Kozma, M.; Bombicz, M.; Varga, B.; Priksz, D.; Gesztelyi, R.; Tarjanyi, V.; Kiss, R.; Szekeres, R.; Takacs, B.; Menes, A.; et al. Cardio-protective Role of BGP-15 in Ageing Zucker Diabetic Fatty Rat (ZDF) Model: Extended Mitochondrial Longevity. *Pharmaceutics* **2022**, *14*, 226. [CrossRef]
41. Priksz, D.; Lampe, N.; Kovacs, A.; Herwig, M.; Bombicz, M.; Varga, B.; Wilisicz, T.; Szilvassy, J.; Posa, A.; Kiss, R.; et al. Nicotinic-acid derivative BGP-15 improves diastolic function in a rabbit model of atherosclerotic cardiomyopathy. *Br. J. Pharmacol.* **2022**, *179*, 2240–2258. [CrossRef]
42. Gao, Y.; Liang, J.; Liu, J.; Xiao, Y. Double-layer weekly sustained release transdermal patch containing gestodene and ethinylestradiol. *Int. J. Pharm.* **2009**, *377*, 128–134. [CrossRef]
43. Kamli, M.; Guettari, M.; Tajouri, T. Structure of polyvinylpyrrolidone in water/ethanol mixture in dilute and semi-dilute regimes: Roles of solvents mixture composition and polymer concentration. *J. Mol. Liq.* **2023**, *382*, 122014. [CrossRef]
44. Lopes, J.F.A.; Simoneau, C. Solubility of Polyvinyl Alcohol in Ethanol. *EFSA Support. Publ.* **2014**, *11*, 660E. [CrossRef]
45. Xiang, A.; Lv, C.; Zhou, H. Changes in Crystallization Behaviors of Poly(Vinyl Alcohol) Induced by Water Content. *J. Vinyl Addit. Technol.* **2020**, *26*, 613–622. [CrossRef]
46. ISO 10993-5; Biological Evaluation of Medical Devices. ISO: Geneva, Switzerland, 2009.
47. Taher, M.A.; Elsherbiny, E.A. Impact of Isonicotinic Acid Blending in Chitosan/Polyvinyl Alcohol on Ripening-Dependent Changes of Green Stage Tomato. *Polymers* **2023**, *15*, 825. [CrossRef]
48. Csizmazia, E.; Erős, G.; Berkesi, O.; Berkó, S.; Szabó-Révész, P.; Csányi, E. Pénétration enhancer effect of sucrose laurate and Transcutol on ibuprofen. *J. Drug Deliv. Sci. Technol.* **2011**, *21*, 411–415. [CrossRef]
49. Virani, A.; Puri, V.; Mohd, H.; Michniak-Kohn, B. Effect of Penetration Enhancers on Transdermal Delivery of Oxcarbazepine, an Antiepileptic Drug Using Microemulsions. *Pharmaceutics* **2023**, *15*, 183. [CrossRef] [PubMed]
50. Dash, S.; Murthy, P.N.; Nath, L.; Chowdhury, P. Kinetic modeling on drug release from controlled drug delivery systems. *Acta Pol. Pharm.-Drug Res.* **2010**, *67*, 217–223.
51. Altun, E.; Yuca, E.; Ekren, N.; Kalaskar, D.M.; Ficai, D.; Dolete, G.; Ficai, A.; Gunduz, O. Kinetic Release Studies of Antibiotic Patches for Local Transdermal Delivery. *Pharmaceutics* **2021**, *13*, 613. [CrossRef]
52. Bom, S.; Santos, C.; Barros, R.; Martins, A.M.; Paradiso, P.; Cláudio, R.; Pinto, P.C.; Ribeiro, H.M.; Marto, J. Effects of Starch Incorporation on the Physicochemical Properties and Release Kinetics of Alginate-Based 3D Hydrogel Patches for Topical Delivery. *Pharmaceutics* **2020**, *12*, 719. [CrossRef]
53. Ruan, J.; Liu, C.; Song, H.; Zhong, T.; Quan, P.; Fang, L. Sustainable and efficient skin absorption behaviour of transdermal drug: The effect of the release kinetics of permeation enhancer. *Int. J. Pharm.* **2022**, *612*, 121377. [CrossRef]
54. Jafri, I.; Shoaib, M.H.; Yousuf, R.I.; Ali, F.R. Effect of permeation enhancers on in vitro release and transdermal delivery of lamotrigine from Eudragit®RS100 polymer matrix-type drug in adhesive patches. *Prog. Biomater.* **2019**, *8*, 91–100. [CrossRef]

Disclaimer/Publisher's Note: The statements, opinions and data contained in all publications are solely those of the individual author(s) and contributor(s) and not of MDPI and/or the editor(s). MDPI and/or the editor(s) disclaim responsibility for any injury to people or property resulting from any ideas, methods, instructions or products referred to in the content.

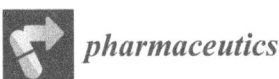

Article

Formulation and Investigation of CK2 Inhibitor-Loaded Alginate Microbeads with Different Excipients

Boglárka Papp [1,2], Marc Le Borgne [3], Florent Perret [4], Christelle Marminon [3], Liza Józsa [1,2], Ágota Pető [1,2], Dóra Kósa [1,2], Lajos Nagy [5], Sándor Kéki [5], Zoltán Ujhelyi [1,6], Ádám Pallér [1], István Budai [7], Ildikó Bácskay [1,2,6] and Pálma Fehér [1,6,*]

1. Department of Pharmaceutical Technology, Faculty of Pharmacy, University of Debrecen, Nagyerdei Körút 98, H-4032 Debrecen, Hungary; papp.boglarka@pharm.unideb.hu (B.P.); jozsa.liza@pharm.unideb.hu (L.J.); peto.agota@pharm.unideb.hu (Á.P.); kosa.dora@pharm.unideb.hu (D.K.); ujhelyi.zoltan@pharm.unideb.hu (Z.U.); adampaller@gmail.com (Á.P.); bacskay.ildiko@pharm.unideb.hu (I.B.)
2. Institute of Healthcare Industry, University of Debrecen, Nagyerdei Körút 98, H-4032 Debrecen, Hungary
3. Small Molecules for Biological Targets Team, Centre de Recherche en Cancérologie de Lyon, Centre Léon Bérard, CNRS 5286, INSERM 1052, Université Claude Bernard Lyon 1, Univ Lyon, 69373 Lyon, France; marc.le-borgne@univ-lyon1.fr (M.L.B.); christelle.marminon-davoust@univ-lyon1.fr (C.M.)
4. Univ Lyon, Université Lyon 1, CNRS, INSA, CPE, ICBMS, 69622 Lyon, France; florent.perret@univ-lyon1.fr
5. Department of Applied Chemistry, Faculty of Science and Technology, Institute of Chemistry, University of Debrecen, Egyetem Tér 1, H-4032 Debrecen, Hungary; nagy.lajos@science.unideb.hu (L.N.); keki.sandor@science.unideb.hu (S.K.)
6. Doctoral School of Pharmaceutical Sciences, University of Debrecen, Nagyerdei Körút 98, H-4032 Debrecen, Hungary
7. Faculty of Engineering, University of Debrecen, Ótemető Utca 2–4, H-4028 Debrecen, Hungary; budai.istvan@eng.unideb.hu
* Correspondence: feher.palma@pharm.unideb.hu

Abstract: The aim of this study was to formulate and characterize CK2 inhibitor-loaded alginate microbeads via the polymerization method. Different excipients were used in the formulation to improve the penetration of an active agent and to stabilize our preparations. Transcutol® HP was added to the drug–sodium alginate mixture and polyvinylpyrrolidone (PVP) was added to the hardening solution, alone and in combination. To characterize the formulations, mean particle size, scanning electron microscopy analysis, encapsulation efficiency, swelling behavior, an enzymatic stability test and an in vitro dissolution study were performed. The cell viability assay and permeability test were also carried out on the Caco-2 cell line. The anti-oxidant and anti-inflammatory effects of the formulations were finally evaluated. The combination of Transcutol® HP and PVP in the formulation of sodium alginate microbeads could improve the stability, in vitro permeability, anti-oxidant and anti-inflammatory effects of the CK2 inhibitor.

Keywords: protein kinase CK2; CK2 inhibitor DMAT; alginate microbeads; Transcutol® HP; polyvinylpyrrolidone

1. Introduction

Protein kinase CK2, also known as casein kinase 2, is a serine/threonine kinase with two catalytic subunits (α) and/or (α') and two regulatory subunits [1]. CK2 regulates multiple signaling pathways involved in tumor cell survival, proliferation, migration, and invasion [2,3]. The expression and kinase activity of CK2 is elevated in various types of cancers, and increases tumor aggressiveness through the phosphorylation of numerous cytosolic substrates [2,4,5].

Elevated CK2 kinase activity is frequently observed in many types of human tumors [6]. The downregulation of CK2 by chemical inhibitors or via genetic approaches promotes cell apoptosis and inhibits tumor cell migration and tumor growth [6].

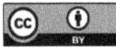

Protein kinase CK2 has been also suggested as a possible target in inflammatory processes and is proposed to have some complex and important roles in the pathogenesis of inflammatory diseases [7,8]. CK2 activity promotes the activation of the NF-kB, PI3K–Akt–mTOR, and JAK–STAT pathways [8]. The protein kinase CK2 is therefore a target for the development of new anti-cancer and anti-inflammatory therapies [7].

CK2 activation was also reported to enhance reactive oxygen species production [9]. CK2 plays an important role in the oxidative stress signaling pathway. The anti-oxidant-activated transcription factor, nuclear erythroid factor 2 (Nrf2), regulates the induction of cytoprotective genes against oxidative injuries. Treatment with CK2 inhibitor can block the induction of these endogenous nuclear genes in cells, preventing oxidative damage [10,11].

Pagano et al. demonstrated that substituted benzimidazole derivatives are potent inhibitors of CK2 [12]. The substituted heterocyclic structure designed to address the ATP-binding pocket of CK2 allows a diverse derivatization of the ring system. Therefore, numerous benzimidazole derivatives inhibiting CK2 have already been described [13,14]. Due to the poor solubility of the molecule, the development of an efficient drug delivery system was a challenging task. The active ingredient selected for our study was 2-dimethylamino-4,5,6,7-tetrabromo-1*H*-benzimidazole (DMAT).

Among various natural polysaccharides, alginates have been widely used in the formulation of drug delivery systems for last three decades [15]. Alginate is a copolymer of (1,4)-linked β-D-mannuronate and α-L-guluronate. Alginate-based microparticles as drug delivery systems are biocompatible and biodegradable, and protect the drug from the harsh environmental conditions of the GI tract [16]. Furthermore, they have targeting efficiency, sustainability, and controllable release [17–19]. During the formulation of alginate-based microbeads, the active substance is entrapped in a gel of alginate that is crosslinked with divalent cations such as Ca^{2+}, Ba^{2+}, and Sr^{2+}, with uronic acid residues in alginate [20–23].

Transcutol® HP (TC) is a diethylene glycol monomethyl ether that is widely used as a solvent/solubilizer and can improve the solubility of various poorly water-soluble drugs. It is also used as a penetration enhancer in various dosage forms and several authors demonstrated that it could improve in vivo drug absorption, the in vitro dissolution rate and drug release, leading to the improved oral bioavailability of the drug [24–26].

Polyvinylpyrrolidone (PVP) is a bulky, non-toxic, non-ionic polymer of an amphiphilic nature that is widely used for the formulation of microparticles (MP). It prevents the aggregation of MPs, may serve as a surface stabilizer, and may provide solubility in diverse solvents [27]. The safe use of PVP in pharmaceutical dosage forms has been demonstrated in several articles [28].

The aim of our present study was to prepare CK2 inhibitor-loaded alginate microbeads to enhance the bioavailability of the active ingredient. A potent and selective CK2 inhibitor, DMAT, was selected as an active ingredient, and two different excipients alone and in combination were used in our formulations. TC was chosen to improve the solubility, in vitro drug release and permeability of DMAT. PVP was added to the compositions to prevent drug leaching during preparation and to stabilize our formulations.

In order to characterize the formulations, mean particle size, encapsulation efficiency, and swelling behavior were determined, and scanning electron scanning (SEM) analysis was conducted. The biocompatibility and permeability of our formulations were tested on the Caco-2 adenocarcinoma cell line. In vitro dissolution and enzymatic stability tests were also performed. Finally, the anti-oxidant and anti-inflammatory effects of our formulations were also tested.

2. Materials and Methods

2.1. Materials

DMAT (CAS# 749234-11-5) was obtained from Sigma-Aldrich Buchs (St. Gallen, Switzerland). The in silico physicochemical characterization of DMAT was carried out using SwissADME [29]. Low-viscosity-grade sodium alginate was obtained from BÜCHI Labortechnik AG (Flawil, Switzerland). Transcutol® HP (diethylene glycol monoethyl ether) was obtained from Gattefossé (Saint-Priest, France). The human adenocarcinoma cancer cell line (Caco-2) originated from the European Collection of Authenticated Cell Cultures (ECACC, Public Health England, Salisbury, UK). TrypLE™ Express Enzyme (no phenol red) was bought from Thermo Fisher Scientific (Waltham, MA, USA). Calcium chloride dihydrate, 96-well cell culture plates, and culturing flasks were purchased from VWR International (Debrecen, Hungary). Transwell® 24-well cell culture inserts were supplied by Greiner Bio-One Hungary Kft. (Mosonmagyaróvár, Hungary). All other products were purchased from Sigma-Aldrich (St. Louis, MI, USA).

2.2. Formulation of CK2 Inhibitor-Loaded Alginate Beads

In order to obtain alginate microparticles, 3.30 g of sodium alginate powder was previously dissolved in 200 mL of distilled water to obtain a 1.5% alginate solution. Due to the hygroscopicity of sodium alginate, a 10–15% excess of the powder should be measured based on the manufacturer's description. To prepare a 100 mM solution of $CaCl_2$, 14.701 g of calcium chloride dihydrate was dissolved in 1000 mL of distilled water. Four compositions containing DMAT (0.5 mg/mL) were prepared (Table 1). In the case of composition 1, DMAT was dissolved in the alginate solution, transferred to a syringe and applied to the appropriate part of the BÜCHI encapsulator B-395 Pro apparat. For composition 2, TC was added, and for composition 3, PVP was added. In the case of composition 4, both excipients were used. According to the manufacturer, the use of highly purified TC is recommended for oral dosage forms. In the production of the microbeads, PVP was dissolved in the hardening solution and TC was dissolved in the alginate solution.

Table 1. Diverse formulations of CK2 inhibitor-loaded alginate beads.

Entry	Composition	Excipient
1	CK2 inhib. beads	-
2	CK2 inhib. beads + TC	Transcutol® HP (0.01% v/v)
3	CK2 inhib. beads + PVP	PVP (2% w/v)
4	CK2 inhib. beads + TC + PVP	Transcutol® HP (0.01% v/v)PVP (2% w/v)

According to the diameter of the nozzle, the parameters of the encapsulator (liquid flow, vibration frequency, and electrostatic voltage) were set to obtain the correct microparticle chain in the light of a stroboscope lamp (Table 2). A large flat beaker filled with calcium chloride solution (100 mM) was placed under a nozzle on a magnetic stirrer. The alginate beads were left to harden for 15 min in calcium chloride solution. The finely divided particles were washed with distilled water and filtered on a 0.4 μm pore size membrane using a vacuum pump and lyophilized with Scanvac CoolSafe Touch 110-4 Freeze Dryer for 24 h at −110 °C.

Table 2. The applied parameters of the encapsulator.

Diameter of the Nozzle [μm]	Vibration Frequency [Hz]	Electrostatic Voltage [V]	Flow Rate (mL/min)
200	1800	1000–1200	5.06

2.3. Mean Particle Size and SEM

The particle size of the microbeads was determined using a HoribaPartica LA-950V2 laser diffraction particle size analyzer (Horiba, Ltd., Kyoto, Japan). Samples were first diluted 1000×, and then measurements were performed in wet mode. At least five parallel measurements were performed with each sample.

To determine the morphology of particles, SEM analysis was performed on a Hitachi desktop microscope (TM3030 Plus) (Hitachi High-Technologies Corporation, Tokyo, Japan).

The instrument is suitable for the direct investigation of the specimens without any surface pre-treatments. Samples were placed on a specific plate with double-sided adhesive and examined using an accelerating voltage of 5 kV [30].

2.4. Encapsulation Efficiency

To determine the encapsulated drug content in the beads, a 1 mL sample was taken from the hardening solution (calcium chloride 100 mM) right after formulation. Drug concentration was determined using a UV-VIS spectrophotometer at 420 nm. The amount of entrapped drug was determined from the amount of DMAT remaining free in the hardening solution relative to the amount of the initial drug [31]. The amount of the encapsulated DMAT was calculated using the following formula:

$$\text{Encapsulation efficiency}(EE\%) = \frac{\text{amount of initial drug} - \text{amount of free(not formulated)drug(mg)}}{\text{amount of initial drug (mg)}} \times 100 \quad (1)$$

2.5. Swelling Behavior

The water sorption behavior of each composition was determined via swelling. The swelling capacity of beads containing DMAT was determined in purified water. One gram from the beads was added to 50 mL of purified water and the dispersions were mixed at 37 °C using a Radelkis OP-912 magnetic stirrer (Radelkis, Budapest, Hungary). For the swelling study, beads were carefully taken out from the water after 24 h, drained with filter paper to remove excess water, and weighed. Weight changes were calculated using the following equation:

$$EWU = \left(\frac{Ws - Wd}{Ws}\right) \times 100 \quad (2)$$

where Ws is the weight of swollen beads and Wd is the initial weight of the dry beads [32].

2.6. Enzymatic Stability Test

The study focused on enzymatic degradation using proteolytic enzymes, namely pepsin and pancreatin. An amount of 20 mg of DMAT-loaded particles was introduced into 100 mL of simulated gastric fluid (SGF) containing pepsin or simulated intestinal fluid (SIF) containing pancreatin. The samples were incubated at 37 °C with constant stirring at 100 rpm. The preparation of SGF and SIF followed European Pharmacopoeia specifications. Samples of 1000 µL were collected at predetermined intervals over 120 min, and to stop the enzymatic reaction, an equivalent volume of ice-cold reagent (0.10 M NaOH for SGF and 0.10 M HCl for SIF) was added. Spectrophotometric analysis was then performed at a wavelength of 420 nm [33].

2.7. In Vitro Dissolution Study

To investigate the dissolution profile of DMAT-containing microbeads, a USP dissolution apparatus (Erweka, DT 800, Langen, Germany) was used at a 100 rpm paddle speed with 900 mL of dissolution medium at 37 °C. Freshly prepared simulated intestinal fluid (SIF) without pancreatin (pH 6.8) was used as the dissolution medium. During the assay, the dissolution medium (5 mL) was continuously sampled at defined intervals (0, 8 and 24 h) using a syringe. Samples were previously filtered through a 0.45 µm membrane filter and the amount of DMAT was determined using a standard calibration curve. The absorbance of the samples was measured at 420 nm using UV/VIS [34].

2.8. MTT Assay

To measure cell viability, an MTT assay was performed on the Caco-2 cell line. Cells were seeded at a density of 10^4 cells/well in Dulbecco's DMEM culture media within 96-well plates until complete confluence was achieved. The medium was removed from cells and washed with PBS. Beads containing no active substance and beads containing DMAT were incubated for 1 h at 37 °C with 5% CO_2. An amount of 100 mg of the samples was dissolved in 10 mL of PBS. After 1 h, the samples were removed from the cells and MTT paint solution (5 mg/mL) was added. The cells were incubated with the solution for 3 h at 37 °C under 5% CO_2. The paint was then removed from the samples and the resulting formazan crystals were dissolved in a 25:1 mixture of 2-propanol:hydrochloric acid. The yellow tetrazonium salt was converted into purple insoluble formazan crystals by mitochondrial enzymes due to the metabolic activity of the cells. The absorbance of the solutions was measured with a spectrophotometer at a 570 nm wavelength (Thermo-Fisher Multiskan Go (Thermo-Fisher, Waltham, MA, USA), from which the percentage of surviving cells could be calculated. PBS was used as positive control and Triton-X 100 (10% w/v) was used as a negative control.

2.9. Transepithelial Electrical Resistance Measurement

To determine the membrane integrity of adenocarcinoma cells, transepithelial electrical resistance (TEER) was measured. Cells were seeded at a density of 40^4 cell/well to form a confluent layer. As a negative control, PBS was used, and as a positive control, Triton X-100 (10% w/v) was used. Measurement was carried out when Caco-2 cell line monolayers presented TEER values between 1000 and 1200 Ω cm^2. The cells were incubated with the samples for 1 h with continuous measuring at given intervals during the assay. TEER was measured using a pair of electrodes with Millipore Millicell-ERS 00001 equipment (Merck, Waltham, MA, USA). As a follow-up, measurements were continued in the following 12 h to investigate recovery [35].

2.10. In Vitro Permeability Studies

Specific transport studies of all compositions have been performed on the Caco-2 cell line. For the permeability assay, Caco-2 cells were seeded on Transwell® 24-well polycarbonate filter inserts (area: 1.12 cm^2; pore size: 0.4 µm) at a concentration of 40^4 cells/insert. TEER was measured before the experiment.

In transport experiments, we studied the permeability of four formulations containing DMAT via sampling at different intervals. In total, 100 mg of the samples was dissolved in 10 mL of PBS buffer.

The permeability assay was commenced with the addition of 400 µL of the sample solution to the apical chambers of the inserts. A 50 µL aliquot was taken from the apical and basal chamber containing PBS immediately, after 4 h and 24 h. The samples were measured with high-performance liquid chromatography (HPLC) [30].

2.11. HPLC Measurements

The HPLC determination of DMAT was performed using the Waters 2695 Separations module equipped with a thermostable autosampler (5 °C), a column module (35 °C), and a Waters 2996 diode array detector (DAD). The separation of the compounds was achieved using a VDSphere PUR C18-M-SE (4.6 × 150 mm, 5 µm) (Agilent technologies, Palo Alto, CA, USA) column. For HPLC-MS measurements, the HPLC instrument was coupled with a MicroTOF-Q-type Qq-TOF MS instrument equipped with an ESI source from Bruker (Bruker Daltoniks, Bremen, Germany). The flow rate and run time were 1.0 mL/min and 12 min, respectively. The active component DMAT was detected with DAD at 260 nm and MS. For the separation of the compounds, isocratic eluent composed of 25% methanol, 40% AcN/water (9/1) containing 0.1% trifluoroacetic acid (TFA), and 35% water was used.

2.12. DPPH Anti-Oxidant Test

The DPPH assay is a colorimetric method based on the ability of 2,2-diphenyl-1-picrylhydrazyl (DPPH) to change its dark purple color to yellow in the presence of an anti-oxidant due to its scavenging property. The anti-oxidant scavenging properties of the four formulations containing the CK2 inhibitor were investigated. The test solution was made using DPPH powder (M = 394.33 g/mol) diluted with 96% ethanol. Briefly, 100 µL of each sample diluted in PBS was added to 2 mL of the DPPH test solution (0.06 mM). The reaction mixtures were incubated for 30 min and sheltered from light. As a positive control, Trolox dissolved in PBS (10.0 µM) was used, and as a negative control, 2.0 mL of DPPH solution was used. The quantitative measurement of the remaining DPPH was carried out using the UV spectrophotometer at a wavelength of 517 nm. The anti-oxidant activity percentage (AA%) was determined using the following equation [36]:

$$AA\% = 100 - \frac{(\text{Abs sample} - \text{Abs blank}) \times 100}{\text{Abs control}} \quad (3)$$

2.13. Examination of Anti-Inflammatory Effect

The anti-inflammatory effect of the microbeads was investigated on the Caco-2 cell line. Cells were seeded at a density of 10^4 cells/well on 96-well plates until complete confluency was achieved and the culture medium was removed. The cells were washed with PBS and incubated with the test solutions for 1 h. Briefly, 100 mg of each microbead diluted with PBS was used to perform the test. To induce inflammation, 50 µL of IL-4 (30 ng/mL) was added to the cells and incubated overnight. After incubation, the supernatant was removed from the cells and human TNF-α ELISA Kit (Sigma—RAB0476) was used in accordance with the manufacturer's instructions. The absorbance of these solutions was measured using Thermo Scientific Multiskan GO microplate spectrophotometer (Thermo-Fisher, Waltham, MA, USA) and was directly proportional to the inflammatory effect of the samples.

2.14. Statistical Analysis

All data were analyzed using GraphPad Prism (version 6; GraphPad Software, San Diego, CA, USA) and are herein presented as means ± SD. A comparison of the results of the swelling behavior, in vitro dissolution test, enzymatic stability assessment, permeability test, TEER measurement, DPPH anti-oxidant test, in vitro anti-inflammatory effect test and MTT cell viability assay was performed with a one-way ANOVA and repeated measures ANOVA followed by Tukey or Dunnett post-testing. The difference in means was considered significant in the case of $p < 0.05$. All experiments were carried out in quintuplicates and repeated at least five times.

3. Results

3.1. In Silico Physicochemical Characterization of DMAT

The physicochemical characterization of DMAT (476.79 g/mol) was performed using SwissADME [29]. DMAT has low water solubility and high penetration through the GI tract, but poor penetration through the BBB. Skin penetration occurred at −5.86 cm/s. The Log $P_{o/w}$ for DMAT was calculated and the consensus value was equal to 4.12 (the average of five predictions). This consensus value corresponds, for example, to the Log $P_{o/w}$ value of the CK2 inhibitor **4p** (5-isopropyl-4-(3-methylbut-2-enyloxy)-5,6,7,8-tetrahydroindeno[1,2-b]indole-9,10-dione, consensus Log $P_{o/w}$ = 3.91) [37]. Figure 1 shows the structure of DMAT.

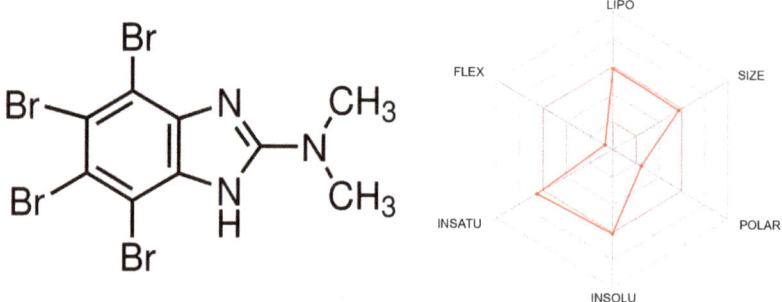

Figure 1. Structure and physicochemical properties of DMAT.

3.2. Mean Particle Size and SEM

The size of microparticles was calculated using a laser diffraction particle size analyzer and was between 273 (DMAT beads) and 295 µm (beads with both excipients TC and PVP) (Table 3). As shown in Table 3, for each entry, PDI values were between 0.24 and 0.40. Entry 3 (CK2 inhib. beads + PVP) yielded the narrowest size distribution value (PDI = 0.24)

Table 3. Mean particle size and polydispersity index (PDI) values of the different DMAT-loaded alginate beads. Values are expressed as mean ± S.D., $n = 5$.

Entry	Composition	Particle Size (µm)	PDI
1	CK2 inhib. (DMAT) beads	272.62 ± 10.03	0.40 ± 0.03
2	CK2 inhib. beads+ TC	279.67 ± 10.49	0.38 ± 0.02
3	CK2 inhib. beads + PVP	288.91 ± 5.28	0.24 ± 0.01
4	CK2 inhib. beads + TC + PVP	294.83 ± 8.46	0.33 ± 0.04

Figure 2 shows the image of different dry formulations containing DMAT obtained via SEM. The round morphology of the microparticles was preserved in all four samples; however, the bead structure was damaged in the case of beads containing excipients, presumably due to the high surfactant content. A significant morphological variation was observed when samples containing TC, PVP, or both were compared to the microparticles without excipients. For samples containing the PVP excipient, the difference was clearly visible, and calcium chloride crystals remaining from the hardening solution could be detected in the images.

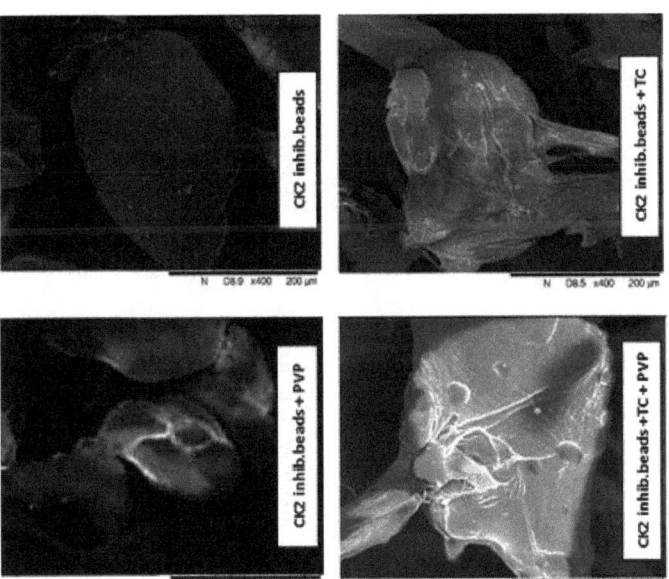

Figure 2. SEM images of the different beads containing DMAT.

3.3. Encapsulation Efficiency

The encapsulated DMAT content in the alginate beads was calculated from the equation described in Section 2.4. According to our investigation, the encapsulation efficiency (EE) was in the range of 64 to 84%, as presented in Table 4. There was no significant difference between the DMAT concentrations in composition 2 and 3, which indicated uniform drug dispersion in these formulations. It was justified that there were significant differences in the drug content of the formulation with or without solubilizing excipients. It was observed that composition 4, which contained both TC and PVP, had the highest DMAT content. Comparing the effect of TC and PVP, it can be concluded that the usage of PVP resulted in a higher DMAT content in the beads.

Table 4. Encapsulation efficiency of the different compositions containing DMAT.

Entry	Composition [a]	EE (%) [b]
1	CK2 inhib. (DMAT) beads	64.32 ± 0.72
2	CK2 inhib. beads + TC	70.12 ± 0.81
3	CK2 inhib. beads + PVP	72.35 ± 0.66
4	CK2 inhib. beads + TC+ PVP	84.07 ± 1.02

[a] Microbeads containing both TC and PVP showed the highest EE% of all the formulations. [b] Each data point represents the mean ± SD; $n = 5$.

3.4. Swelling Behavior

The equilibrium water uptake of the different compositions was calculated from the equation described in Section 2.5. Figure 3 shows the change in the beads' weight due to water uptake after 24 h. Alginate (entry 1) and TC excipient + alginate (entry 2) beads showed very similar swelling rates within 24 h (79 and 81%). The water uptake of the PVP excipient containing beads (entry 3) did not significantly increase, as it was 84%. For entry 4, which contained both TC and PVP excipients, the equilibrium water uptake was 89%, which was significantly higher than that for the other compositions. Alginate was mainly responsible for water uptake since, at pH 7, this polymer has the property of swelling, thus increasing its weight.

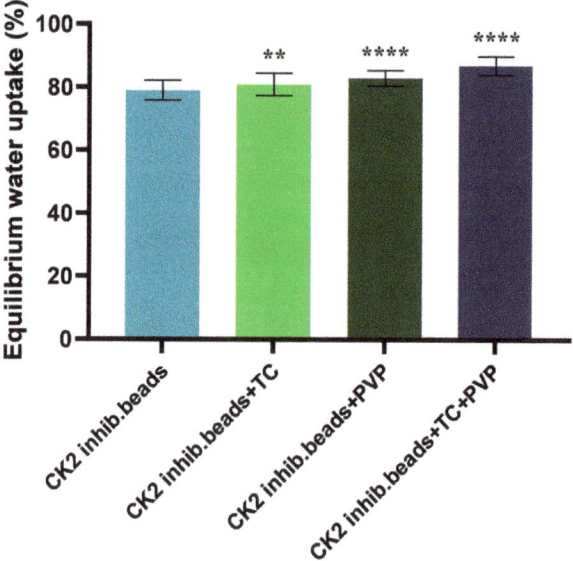

Figure 3. The swelling capacity of the CK2 inhibitor containing beads in distilled water. One gram from the beads was added to 50 mL of distilled water. All of the compositions are represented by the water equilibrium value. Each data point represents the mean ± SD ($n = 5$). An ordinary one-way ANOVA with Dunett's multiple comparison test was performed to compare the different formulations with excipients with the formulation with DMAT alone. ** and **** indicate statistically significant differences at $p < 0.05$ and $p < 0.0001$.

3.5. Result of Enzymatic Stability Test

According to the results, from the free DMAT samples (not formulated), only 2% could be measured in SGF, while 7% could be measured in SIF after 60 min of incubation. The active compound was nearly degraded after 60 min of incubation in SGF, and after 120 min of incubation in SIF. Our experiments revealed that bead formulations are able to protect the active substance. For each formulation, at least 50% of DMAT was protected against degradation by SGF and SIF. Figure 4 depicts the results of this experiment.

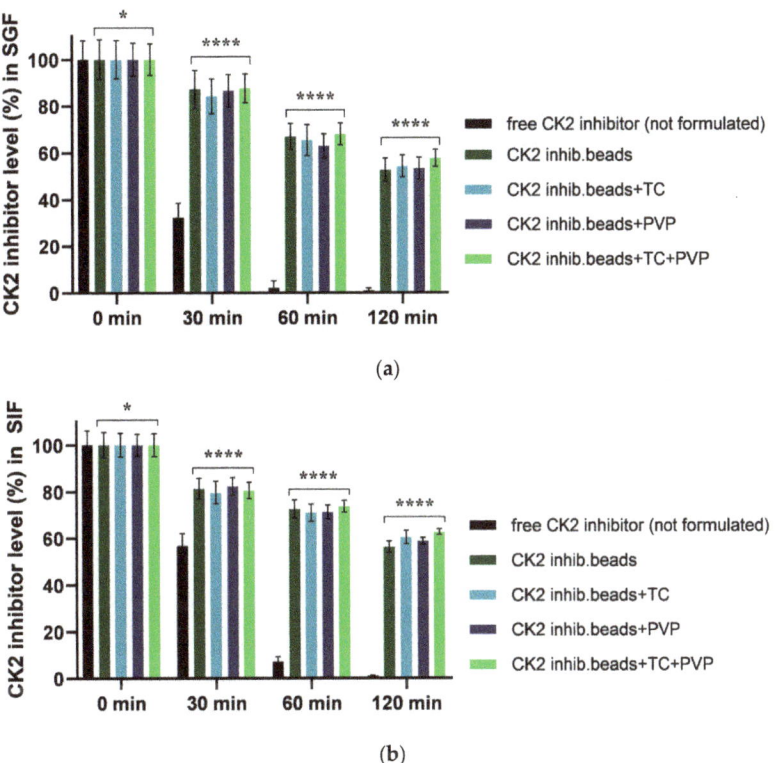

Figure 4. Enzymatic stability of CK2 inhibitor (DMAT)-loaded alginate microbeads in SGF (**a**) and in SIF medium (**b**). Free DMAT (not formulated) was used as a control. Each data point represents the mean ± SD, $n = 5$. Ordinary one-way ANOVA with Dunett's multiple comparison test was performed to compare the different formulations with excipients with the free (not formulated) DMAT. * and **** indicate statistically significant differences at $p < 0.01$ and $p < 0.0001$.

3.6. In Vitro Dissolution Study

The CK2 inhibitor release from the different microbeads at pH 6.8 is presented in Figure 5. Our results show that compositions with PVP (entries 3 and 4) had better drug release and dissolution than did compositions without PVP (entries 1 and 2). It was also detected that adding TC to the formulations resulted in better drug release compared with that when adding the formulation that contained only the active agent, DMAT, without excipients. The highest diffused amount of the active substance was from composition 4, which contained both excipients, and DMAT release achieved a value of more than 60% after 24 h.

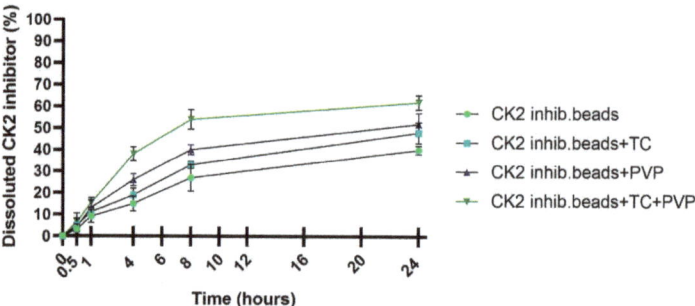

Figure 5. In vitro dissolution profile of CK2 inhibitor form sodium alginate beads in simulated intestinal fluid (SIF) without pancreatin (pH = 6.8). Each data point represents the mean ± SD, n = 5.

3.7. MTT Assay

The results of the MTT test are presented in Figure 6. In the experiment, PBS was used as a negative control and Triton X-100 was used as a positive control. Cell viability values were compared to those for PBS and expressed as a percentage of the negative control. For the blank sodium alginate beads, the preparations were found to be safe and well tolerated by the cells, with cell viability consistently exceeding 70% in all cases, which is in accordance with the ISO 10993-5:2009 recommendation [38]. The added excipients were also well tolerated. However, in the case of beads containing DMAT, cell viability was reduced. This reduction in cell viability could be attributed to the presence of the active substance, as empty beads did not show any cytotoxic effect.

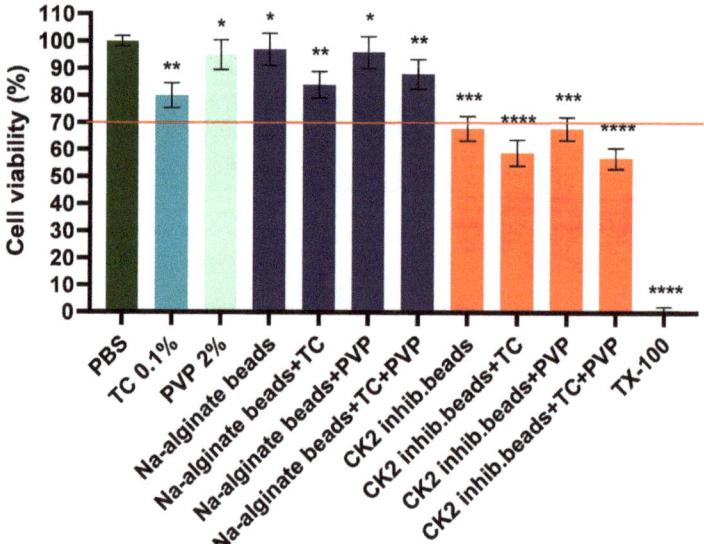

Figure 6. Cell viability test with the MTT assay on Caco-2 cells after incubation with the formulations for 1 h. Cell viability is expressed as the percentage of the negative control (PBS). Each datapoint represents the mean ± SD and n = 6. An ordinary one-way ANOVA with Dunett's multiple comparison test was performed to compare the different formulations with PBS. *, **, *** and **** indicate statistically significant differences at $p < 0.05$, $p < 0.01$, $p < 0.001$ and $p < 0.0001$.

3.8. In Vitro Permeability Test

The permeability test was performed on the Caco-2 cell line when TEER values reached 800–1000 Ω cm². The amount of permeated components as a function of time is shown in Figure 7. Sampling was performed at 4 and 24 h from both the apical and basolateral parts. Comparing the results to those of the bead without excipients, the highest penetration was obtained for the formulation containing TC and PVP excipients.

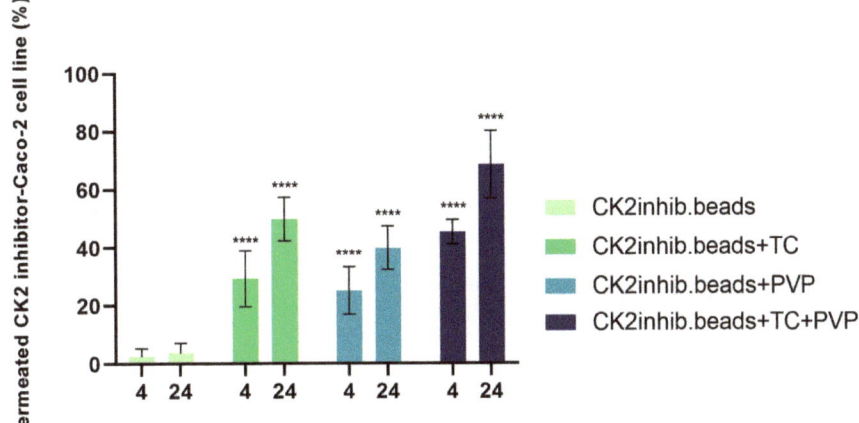

Figure 7. The permeability test of DMAT-loaded alginate microbeads without excipients and with TC and PVP alone and in combination on the Caco-2 cell line. Statistical analysis was performed; **** indicates statistically significant differences at $p < 0.0001$.

3.9. Transepithelial Electrical Resistance Measurements

The membrane integrity of adenocarcinoma cells was determined by TEER measurement. The samples showed a decrease in integrity 15 min after the start of the assay and a steady decrease up to 60 min. After 1 h of treatment, culture medium was added to the cells again, and after 12 h of incubation, the cell integrity had increased to above 90% of the baseline value at the end of the experiment. PBS was used as negative control and (10% w/v) Triton X-100 as positive control. The sample containing TC and PVP excipients was able to disrupt cell integrity to the greatest extent. Results are shown in Figure 8.

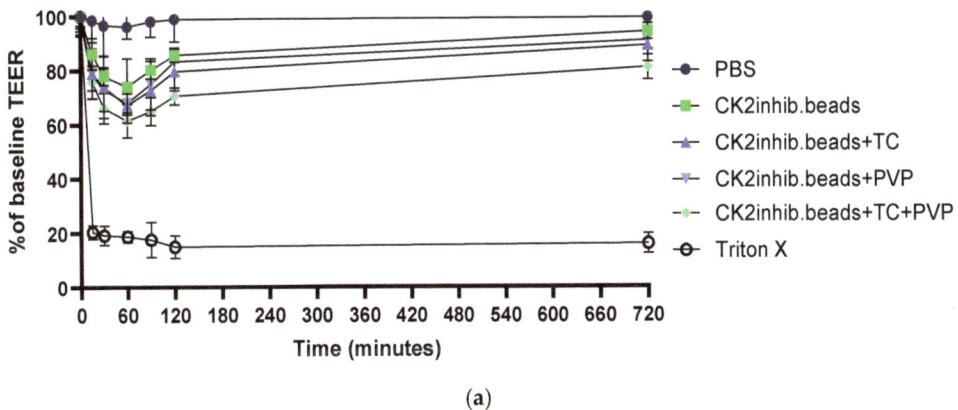

(a)

Figure 8. *Cont.*

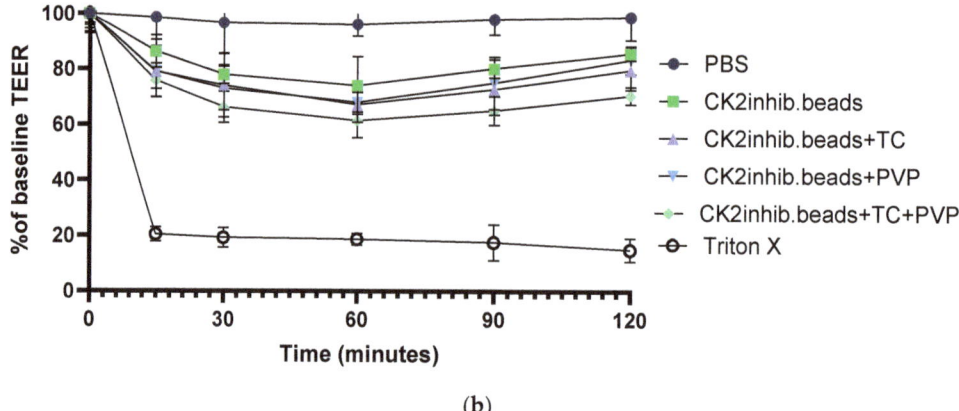

(b)

Figure 8. Evaluation of the transepithelial electrical resistance of Caco-2 cells in two contexts: (**a**) across the entire experiment, and (**b**) with a specific emphasis on the initial 120 min. Each data point represents the mean ± SD, $n = 5$.

3.10. DPPH Scavenging Activity Test

The percentage of the anti-oxidant activity (AA%) of the four formulations was determined using a DPPH test solution. Comparing the four formulations, the microbeads without TC and PVP excipients showed less radical scavenging activity. According to the results, the microbeads containing TC and PVP excipients showed more effective anti-oxidant activity than did the others. The results indicated that DMAT has more effective anti-oxidant activity in the case when microbeads formulated with TC and PVP excipients are used. Figure 9 depicts the results of this experiment.

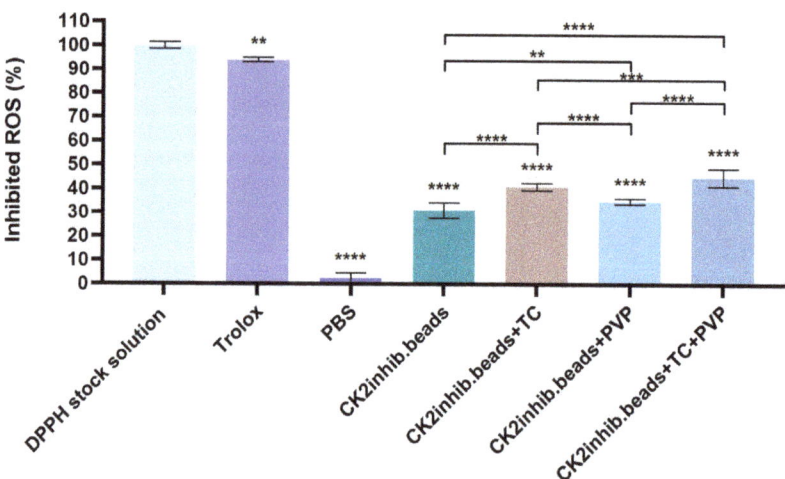

Figure 9. DPPH-scavenging activity of the composition. Data are presented as mean ± SD ($n = 6$). An ordinary one-way ANOVA with Dunett's multiple comparison test was performed to compare the different formulations with PBS and to compare the formulations with each other. **, *** and **** indicate statistically significant differences at $p < 0.01$, $p < 0.05$ and $p < 0.0001$.

3.11. Examination of In Vitro Anti-Inflammatory Effect

The anti-inflammatory effect of the DMAT-loaded microbeads diluted in PBS were conducted by ELISA test on Caco-2 cell line. The negative control was PBS and the mean of the absorbance values was considered as 100% to which the test substances were compared and expressed as a percentage. Figure 10 presents the final results of the anti-inflammatory test on Caco-2 cell line as a percentage of TNF-α level. The results of the study showed that all products were effective in reducing inflammation. The microbeads formulated with TC excipient and the combination of PVP and TC excipients showed the most potent anti-inflammatory effect. The results showed that treatment with DMAT-loaded microbeads resulted in a significant reduction in TNF-α levels on Caco-2 cell line.

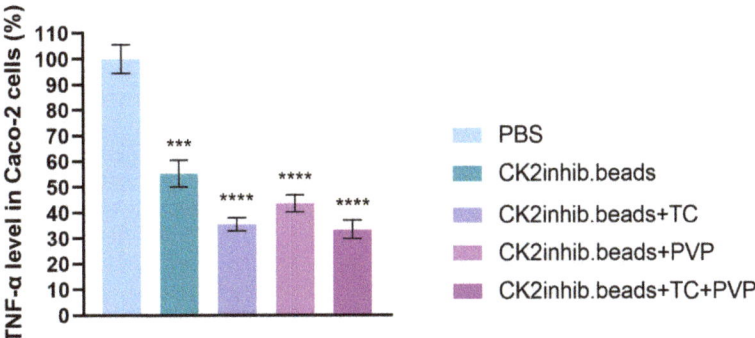

Figure 10. Results of the TNF-α level in the Caco-2 cell line. An ordinary one-way ANOVA with Dunnett's multiple comparison test was performed to compare the different formulations with PBS. ***, and **** indicate statistically significant differences at $p < 0.001$, and $p < 0.0001$.

4. Discussion

The overexpression and important roles of CK2 in several cancers including kidney, lung, head and neck, and prostate, and even in glioblastoma (GBM) have been already reported [2,39]. For instance, CK2 inhibitors induced apoptosis, inhibited tumor cell migration and reduced tumor growth in mouse xenograft models of human GBMs [40,41]. Zheng et al. stated that the CK2α gene is amplified in a large percentage of GBM, and the inhibition of CK2 with CX-4945 (*per os* CK2 inhibitor) inhibits GBM growth in mice.

In our study, we selected the tetrahalogenated CK2 inhibitor DMAT, in order to obtain a proof of concept for the preparation of alginate microbeads. Formulation can be effective for CK2 inhibitors based on an indeniindole scaffold [42]. Then, DMAT-loaded alginate microbeads were formulated via the controlled polymerization method with the Büchi Encapsulator B-395 Pro apparatus. TC was added to the polymer solution in order to improve drug release and to enhance the penetration of DMAT, and PVP was added to the hardening solution to stabilize the formulations [42]. In order to characterize the physical parameters of our microbead formulations, mean particle size was determined.

The size of droplets plays a crucial role in microformulations, as it has the potential to impact both drug release and absorption.

The shape and morphology of the beads were examined via SEM. Among the four formulations, the formulation containing no surfactants retained a regular bead shape, while the formulations containing excipients showed a tailing effect of the beads. According to the literature, this phenomenon often occurs when the amount of surfactants in the formulation is high [43,44]. In order to achieve beneficial properties and adequate toxicity values, slight changes in the bead shape of the surfactant amount were not considered. In light of the cytotoxicity data and with the knowledge of the results of the drug stability studies, the use of high levels of surfactants was indicated.

The microbead formulation containing both TC and PVP excipients showed the highest equilibrium water uptake (89%) compared to that of the other compositions. During formulation, the swelling property is an important factor as swelling behavior influences applicability [45].

The encapsulation efficiency was 64% in the formulation where the CK2 inhibitor was without excipients. Adding PVP to our formulations resulted in a higher CK2 inhibitor content in the beads; the highest value (84%) resulted from those preparations where both TC and PVP were added. PVP improves encapsulation efficiency by preventing the leaching of the drug during preparation. This may be due to PVP increasing the viscosity of the cross-linking solution, so that it can block the pores of the alginate beads and thus prevent the drug's release into the cross-linking solution [46].

According to our in vitro dissolution test, the excipients TC and PVP improved the release profile of the CK2 inhibitor from that in the microbead formulation. The best release value was from the composition containing both excipients as CK2 inhibitor release was more than 60% after 24 h. This greater release of dissolved CK2 inhibitor from the composition could lead to higher bioavailability and absorption [47].

The development of a polymeric and biodegradable matrix prevents active substances from conditions during transit through the gastrointestinal tract [48]. According to our enzyme stability tests, our formulations could successfully shelter the CK2 inhibitor from the harsh environment of the stimulated conditions of the gastrointestinal tract.

The in vitro permeation tests were performed on the Caco-2 cell line. The Caco-2 cell line is derived from colon adenocarcinoma and is widely used as a model of the intestinal epithelial barrier as these cells express similar drug transporters to those in the human intestine [49,50].

Our results showed that sodium alginate microbeads as a carrier system alone could deliver the CK2 inhibitor active agent through the Caco-2 cell line. A study has demonstrated that microcapsules made of alginate could successfully encapsulate and deliver endostatin, an angiogenic inhibitor, to tumor cells [51]. TC improved the permeation of the active substance but the combination of TC and PVP resulted in the highest permeated amount of DMAT through the cell line. Kósa et al. reported that the combination of alginate carriers with amphiphilic surfactants TC and Labrasol improved the absorption of the active substance via the reversible alteration of barrier functions [45].

This study demonstrated that peptide-loaded alginate beads with penetration enhancers play a key role in the bioavailability improvement of the active substance [45]. Mangla et al. formulated nanostructured lipid carriers to enhance the oral delivery of tamoxifen and sulforaphene [52]. Those formulations that contained TC resulted in a better in vitro and ex vivo drug release profile as well as better intestinal permeability [52]. To select the appropriate concentrations of the used excipients, a preliminary viability study was carried out. The concentrations used proved to be the highest that were still tolerable by Caco-2 cells.

TC may improve the bioavailability of active substances in formulations. Hashemzadeh et al. revealed that the efficiency of diethylene glycol monoethyl ether as a solubilizer/penetration enhancer depends on its performed concentration alone or in combination with other excipients [24].

PVP in drug delivery systems has been shown to enhance the drug circulatory time in plasma. Several studies showed that PVP has the longest circulation lifetime among various polymers and its tissue distribution was extremely restricted [53].

The cytotoxic effect of the excipients is a crucial point in the formulations. In order to see the biocompatibility of our formulations, an MTT assay on the Caco-2 cell line was performed. The results showed that the empty sodium alginate beads with and without the excipients TC and PVP were safe and well tolerated by the cells as the cell viability was over 70% in each case. For beads containing DMAT, the cytotoxicity values remained below 70%, which was expected considering the effect of the compound.

DPPH scavenging activity of the four compositions was determined in order to see the anti-oxidant effect of our formulations. DMAT-loaded microbead formulation without excipients showed that DPPH scavenging activity was at 31%; however, those formulations that contained the excipients TC or PVP alone or in combination had a better anti-oxidant effect (41%, 35% and 45%). These results are in accordance with the in vitro dissolution studies, as the excipients could improve the dissolution of DMAT, and a higher amount of the active ingredient resulted in a higher anti-oxidant effect. Thus, the anti-oxidant effect of the formulation depended on the amount of active ingredient dissolved. Several authors demonstrated that TC can improve in vivo drug absorption, the in vitro dissolution rate and drug release, leading to the improved oral bioavailability of the drug [24–26]. Spaglova et al. reported that TC improved the solubility and the drug release properties of indomethacin, for example [54].

Several diseases—in which an inflammatory response plays an important role—have been reported to be associated with aberrant CK2 signaling (e.g., breast cancer, glomerulonephritis, and T cell lymphoma) [7,55]; thus, CK2 has been proposed as a target in inflammatory diseases [7].

Wang et al. demonstrated that the CK2 inhibitor (PD144795) inhibited TNF-α-induced p65 phosphorylation on HeLa cells [56]. The anti-inflammatory effect of the DMAT-loaded microbeads were studied using an ELISA test on the Caco-2 cell line. The level of TNF-α, a classic pleiotropic pro-inflammatory cytokine, was determined in anti-inflammatory experiments [57]. CK2 microbead formulation without excipients slightly reduced the level of TNF-α (55%). After adding the excipients TC and PVP to the formulations, higher anti-inflammatory effects were detected (36% and 44%, respectively). The microbeads with both excipients showed the highest anti-inflammatory effect (33%). According to our previous study, using the TC excipient in SNEDDS formulations containing curcumin could improve the anti-inflammatory effect of formulations [58]. Also, these results demonstrated that the excipients influenced in vitro drug release from the formulations, and then modulated the anti-inflammatory effect.

Our results showed that we developed and optimized the formulation of DMAT-loaded alginate microbeads with the efficient help of TC and PVP excipients. Sodium alginate microbeads as a carrier system were proven to prevent the active substance from enzymatic degradation and could improve the permeation of DMAT through the Caco-2 cell-line. The excipient PVP stabilized our formulations and the excipient TC could improve the permeation of active substance through the Caco-2 monolayer. Our formulations also showed good anti-oxidant and anti-inflammatory effects, which were also influenced by the excipients.

5. Conclusions

In the present study, alginate microbeads loaded with DMAT were designed with different excipients. The combination of TC and PVP in the formulations improved enzymatic stability and the in vitro dissolution of active ingredient, and also enhanced the permeability of the CK2 inhibitor on the Caco-2 cell line. The in vitro anti-oxidant and anti-inflammatory effect of our formulations were also proven. These results demonstrate that alginate beads may be a promising delivery system for CK2 inhibitors but also point out that choosing the appropriate excipients is a crucial point in formulation.

The role of CK2 and its overexpression is already demonstrated in different types of solid tumors. Furthermore, several CK2 inhibitors are now available and have been shown to be effective against cancers in vitro, in vivo and also in pre-clinical studies. In the future, in vivo animal experiments should be planned, with our formulations, that would prove the relevance of these preparations in cancer therapy.

Author Contributions: P.F., I.B. (Ildikó Bácskay), and M.L.B. designed the experiments. F.P. and C.M. conducted physicochemical evaluations of CK2 inhibitors. B.P. conducted formulation and characterization of CK2 microbeads. B.P. performed statistical analysis. D.K. performed the enzymatic stability test. Á.P. (Ágota Pető) carried out MTT assays on the CaCo-2 cell line. Z.U. and Á.P.(Ádám Pallér) conducted the in vitro permeability tests. L.J. and B.P. conducted anti-inflammatory and anti-oxidant experiments. L.N. and S.K. performed analytical measurements of DMAT. I.B.(István Budai) performed SEM analysis. P.F. and I.B. (Ildikó Bácskay) wrote the manuscript. P.F. and M.L.B. edited the manuscript. All authors have read and agreed to the published version of the manuscript.

Funding: The work was supported by 2019-2.1.11-TÉT-2020-00098, titled 'Formulation of kinase-inhibitor microparticles in glioblastoma brain tumor therapy'. Project no. TKP2021-EGA-18 has been implemented with the support provided by the Ministry of Culture and Innovation of Hungary from the National Research, Development and Innovation Fund, financed under the TKP2021-EGA funding scheme. This research was also funded by "Institut Convergence PLAsCAN", ANR-17-CONV-0002.

Institutional Review Board Statement: Not applicable.

Informed Consent Statement: Not applicable.

Data Availability Statement: The data that support the findings of this study are available from the corresponding author (feher.palma@pharm.unideb.hu) with the permission of the head of the department, upon reasonable request.

Acknowledgments: Marc Le Borgne would like to thank Christine Janssen for editing the manuscript.

Conflicts of Interest: The authors declare no conflict of interest.

Sample Availability: Samples of the compounds are available from the authors.

References

1. Silva-Pavez, E.; Tapia, J.C. Protein Kinase CK2 in Cancer Energetics. *Front. Oncol.* **2020**, *10*, 893. [CrossRef] [PubMed]
2. Rowse, A.L.; Gibson, S.A.; Meares, G.P.; Rajbhandari, R.; Nozell, S.E.; Dees, K.J.; Hjelmeland, A.B.; McFarland, B.C.; Benveniste, E.N. Protein Kinase CK2 Is Important for the Function of Glioblastoma Brain Tumor Initiating Cells. *J. Neurooncol.* **2017**, *132*, 219–229. [CrossRef] [PubMed]
3. Fakhoury, M. Drug Delivery Approaches for the Treatment of Glioblastoma Multiforme. *Artif. Cells Nanomed. Biotechnol.* **2016**, *44*, 1365–1373. [CrossRef] [PubMed]
4. Michael, J.S.; Lee, B.-S.; Zhang, M.; Yu, J.S. Nanotechnology for Treatment of Glioblastoma Multiforme. *J. Transl. Int. Med.* **2018**, *6*, 128–133. [CrossRef] [PubMed]
5. Borgo, C.; D'Amore, C.; Sarno, S.; Salvi, M.; Ruzzene, M. Protein Kinase CK2: A Potential Therapeutic Target for Diverse Human Diseases. *Signal Transduct. Target. Ther.* **2021**, *6*, 183. [CrossRef]
6. Ji, H.; Lu, Z. The Role of Protein Kinase CK2 in Glioblastoma Development. *Clin. Cancer Res.* **2013**, *19*, 6335–6337. [CrossRef]
7. Singh, N.N.; Ramji, D.P. Protein Kinase CK2, an Important Regulator of the Inflammatory Response? *J. Mol. Med.* **2008**, *86*, 887–897. [CrossRef]
8. Gibson, S.A.; Benveniste, E.N. Protein Kinase CK2: An Emerging Regulator of Immunity. *Trends Immunol.* **2018**, *39*, 82–85. [CrossRef]
9. Ka, S.-O.; Hwang, H.P.; Jang, J.-H.; Hyuk Bang, I.; Bae, U.-J.; Yu, H.C.; Cho, B.H.; Park, B.-H. The Protein Kinase 2 Inhibitor Tetrabromobenzotriazole Protects against Renal Ischemia Reperfusion Injury. *Sci. Rep.* **2015**, *5*, 14816. [CrossRef]
10. Apopa, P.L.; He, X.; Ma, Q. Phosphorylation of Nrf2 in the Transcription Activation Domain by Casein Kinase 2 (CK2) Is Critical for the Nuclear Translocation and Transcription Activation Function of Nrf2 in IMR-32 Neuroblastoma Cells. *J. Biochem. Mol. Toxicol* **2008**, *22*, 63–76. [CrossRef]
11. Pi, J.; Bai, Y.; Reece, J.M.; Williams, J.; Liu, D.; Freeman, M.L.; Fahl, W.E.; Shugar, D.; Liu, J.; Qu, W. Molecular Mechanism of Human Nrf2 Activation and Degradation: Role of Sequential Phosphorylation by Protein Kinase CK2. *Free Radic. Biol. Med.* **2007**, *42*, 1797–1806. [CrossRef] [PubMed]
12. Pagano, M.A.; Meggio, F.; Ruzzene, M.; Andrzejewska, M.; Kazimierczuk, Z.; Pinna, L.A. 2-Dimethylamino-4,5,6,7-Tetrabromo-1H-Benzimidazole: A Novel Powerful and Selective Inhibitor of Protein Kinase CK2. *Biochem. Biophys. Res. Commun.* **2004**, *321*, 1040–1044. [CrossRef] [PubMed]
13. Battistutta, R.; Mazzorana, M.; Sarno, S.; Kazimierczuk, Z.; Zanotti, G.; Pinna, L.A. Inspecting the Structure-Activity Relationship of Protein Kinase CK2 Inhibitors Derived from Tetrabromo-Benzimidazole. *Chem. Biol.* **2005**, *12*, 1211–1219. [CrossRef] [PubMed]
14. Łukowska-Chojnacka, E.; Wińska, P.; Wielechowska, M.; Poprzeczko, M.; Bretner, M. Synthesis of Novel Polybrominated Benzimidazole Derivatives—Potential CK2 Inhibitors with Anticancer and Proapoptotic Activity. *Bioorg. Med. Chem.* **2016**, *24*, 735–741. [CrossRef] [PubMed]
15. Dodero, A.; Alberti, S.; Gaggero, G.; Ferretti, M.; Botter, R.; Vicini, S.; Castellano, M. An Up-to-Date Review on Alginate Nanoparticles and Nanofibers for Biomedical and Pharmaceutical Applications. *Adv. Mater. Interfaces* **2021**, *8*, 2100809. [CrossRef]
16. Nayak, A.K.; Das, B.; Maji, R. Calcium Alginate/Gum Arabic Beads Containing Glibenclamide: Development and In Vitro Characterization. *Int. J. Biol. Macromol.* **2012**, *51*, 1070–1078. [CrossRef]
17. Bhujbal, S.V.; Paredes-Juarez, G.A.; Niclou, S.P.; de Vos, P. Factors Influencing the Mechanical Stability of Alginate Beads Applicable for Immunoisolation of Mammalian Cells. *J. Mech. Behav. Biomed. Mater.* **2014**, *37*, 196–208. [CrossRef]
18. Moradhaseli, S.; Sarzaeem, A.; Mirakabadi, A.Z.; Mohammadpour Dounighi, N.; Soheily, S.; Borumand, M.R. Preparation and Characterization of Sodium Alginate Nanoparticles Containing ICD-85 (Venom Derived Peptides). *Int. J. Innov. Appl. Stud.* **2013**, *4*, 534–542.

19. Dounighi, N.; Zolfagharian, H.; Khaki, P.; Bidhendi, S.; Sarei, F. Alginate Nanoparticles as a Promising Adjuvant and Vaccine Delivery System. *Indian J. Pharm. Sci.* **2013**, *75*, 442. [CrossRef]
20. Venkatesan, J.; Anil, S.; Singh, S.K.; Kim, S.-K. Preparations and Applications of Alginate Nanoparticles. In *Seaweed Polysaccharides*; Elsevier: Amsterdam, The Netherlands, 2017; pp. 251–268.
21. Thai, H.; Thuy Nguyen, C.; Thi Thach, L.; Thi Tran, M.; Duc Mai, H.; Thi Thu Nguyen, T.; Duc Le, G.; Van Can, M.; Dai Tran, L.; Long Bach, G.; et al. Characterization of Chitosan/Alginate/Lovastatin Nanoparticles and Investigation of Their Toxic Effects In Vitro and In Vivo. *Sci. Rep.* **2020**, *10*, 909. [CrossRef]
22. Daemi, H.; Barikani, M. Synthesis and Characterization of Calcium Alginate Nanoparticles, Sodium Homopolymannuronate Salt and Its Calcium Nanoparticles. *Sci. Iran.* **2012**, *19*, 2023–2028. [CrossRef]
23. Adrian, E.; Treľová, D.; Filová, E.; Kumorek, M.; Lobaz, V.; Poreba, R.; Janoušková, O.; Pop-Georgievski, O.; Lacík, I.; Kubies, D. Complexation of CXCL12, FGF-2 and VEGF with Heparin Modulates the Protein Release from Alginate Microbeads. *Int. J. Mol. Sci.* **2021**, *22*, 11666. [CrossRef] [PubMed]
24. Hashemzadeh, N.; Jouyban, A. Review of Pharmaceutical Applications of Diethylene Glycol Monoethyl Ether. *J. Pharm. Pharm. Sci.* **2022**, *25*, 340–353. [CrossRef] [PubMed]
25. Singh, D.; Tiwary, A.K.; Bedi, N. Canagliflozin Loaded SMEDDS: Formulation Optimization for Improved Solubility, Permeability and Pharmacokinetic Performance. *J. Pharm. Investig.* **2019**, *49*, 67–85. [CrossRef]
26. Alvi, M.M.; Chatterjee, P. A Prospective Analysis of Co-Processed Non-Ionic Surfactants in Enhancing Permeability of a Model Hydrophilic Drug. *AAPS PharmSciTech* **2014**, *15*, 339–353. [CrossRef]
27. Luo, Y.; Hong, Y.; Shen, L.; Wu, F.; Lin, X. Multifunctional Role of Polyvinylpyrrolidone in Pharmaceutical Formulations. *AAPS PharmSciTech* **2021**, *22*, 34. [CrossRef]
28. Koczkur, K.M.; Mourdikoudis, S.; Polavarapu, L.; Skrabalak, S.E. Polyvinylpyrrolidone (PVP) in Nanoparticle Synthesis. *Dalton Trans.* **2015**, *44*, 17883–17905. [CrossRef]
29. Daina, A.; Michielin, O.; Zoete, V. SwissADME: A Free Web Tool to Evaluate Pharmacokinetics, Drug-Likeness and Medicinal Chemistry Friendliness of Small Molecules. *Sci. Rep.* **2017**, *7*, 42717. [CrossRef]
30. Haimhoffer, Á.; Vas, A.; Árvai, G.; Fenyvesi, É.; Jicsinszky, L.; Budai, I.; Bényei, A.; Regdon, G.; Rusznyák, Á.; Vasvári, G.; et al. Investigation of the Drug Carrier Properties of Insoluble Cyclodextrin Polymer Microspheres. *Biomolecules* **2022**, *12*, 931. [CrossRef]
31. Amini, Y.; Amel Jamehdar, S.; Sadri, K.; Zare, S.; Musavi, D.; Tafaghodi, M. Different Methods to Determine the Encapsulation Efficiency of Protein in PLGA Nanoparticles. *Biomed. Mater. Eng.* **2017**, *28*, 613–620. [CrossRef]
32. Manjanna, K.M.; Pramod Kumar, T.M.; Shivakumar, B. Calcium Alginate Cross-Linked Polymeric Microbeads for Oral Sustained Drug Delivery in Arthritis. *Drug Discov. Ther.* **2010**, *4*, 109–122. [PubMed]
33. Mallikarjuna Setty, C.; Sahoo, S.; Sa, B. Alginate-Coated Alginate-Polyethyleneimine Beads for Prolonged Release of Furosemide in Simulated Intestinal Fluid. *Drug Dev. Ind. Pharm.* **2005**, *31*, 435–446. [CrossRef] [PubMed]
34. Medina, J.R.; Aguilar, E.; Hurtado, M. Dissolution behavior of carbamazepine suspensions using the usp dissolution apparatus 2 and the flow-through cell method with simulated gi fluids. *Int. J. Pharm. Pharm. Sci.* **2017**, *9*, 111. [CrossRef]
35. Srinivasan, B.; Kolli, A.R.; Esch, M.B.; Abaci, H.E.; Shuler, M.L.; Hickman, J.J. TEER Measurement Techniques for In Vitro Barrier Model Systems. *SLAS Technol.* **2015**, *20*, 107–126. [CrossRef] [PubMed]
36. Baliyan, S.; Mukherjee, R.; Priyadarshini, A.; Vibhuti, A.; Gupta, A.; Pandey, R.P.; Chang, C.-M. Determination of Antioxidants by DPPH Radical Scavenging Activity and Quantitative Phytochemical Analysis of Ficus Religiosa. *Molecules* **2022**, *27*, 1326. [CrossRef]
37. Jabor Gozzi, G.; Bouaziz, Z.; Winter, E.; Daflon-Yunes, N.; Aichele, D.; Nacereddine, A.; Marminon, C.; Valdameri, G.; Zeinyeh, W.; Bollacke, A.; et al. Converting Potent Indeno [1,2-b]Indole Inhibitors of Protein Kinase CK2 into Selective Inhibitors of the Breast Cancer Resistance Protein ABCG2. *J. Med. Chem.* **2015**, *58*, 265–277. [CrossRef] [PubMed]
38. *ISO 10993-5:2009*; Biological Evaluation of Medical Devices—Part 5: Tests for In Vitro Cytotoxicity, German version EN ISO 10993-5:2009. ISO: Geneva, Switzerland, 2009.
39. Pagano, M.A.; Bain, J.; Kazimierczuk, Z.; Sarno, S.; Ruzzene, M.; Di Maira, G.; Elliott, M.; Orzeszko, A.; Cozza, G.; Meggio, F.; et al. The Selectivity of Inhibitors of Protein Kinase CK2: An Update. *Biochem. J.* **2008**, *415*, 353–365. [CrossRef]
40. Prudent, R.; Moucadel, V.; Nguyen, C.-H.; Barette, C.; Schmidt, F.; Florent, J.-C.; Lafanechère, L.; Sautel, C.F.; Duchemin-Pelletier, E.; Spreux, E.; et al. Antitumor Activity of Pyridocarbazole and Benzopyridoindole Derivatives That Inhibit Protein Kinase CK2. *Cancer Res.* **2010**, *70*, 9865–9874. [CrossRef]
41. Zheng, Y.; McFarland, B.C.; Drygin, D.; Yu, H.; Bellis, S.L.; Kim, H.; Bredel, M.; Benveniste, E.N. Targeting Protein Kinase CK2 Suppresses Prosurvival Signaling Pathways and Growth of Glioblastoma. *Clin. Cancer Res.* **2013**, *19*, 6484–6494. [CrossRef]
42. Zhao, Y.; Liu, D.; Yan, Z.; Zhang, Z.; Zheng, Y.; Zhang, Y.; Xue, C. Preparation and Characterization of the Ag2Se Flexible Films Tuned by PVP for Wearable Thermoelectric Generator. *J. Mater. Sci. Mater. Electron.* **2021**, *32*, 20295–20305. [CrossRef]
43. McDonald, B.F.; Coulter, I.S.; Marison, I.W. Microbeads: A Novel Multiparticulate Drug Delivery Technology for Increasing the Solubility and Dissolution of Celecoxib. *Pharm. Dev. Technol.* **2015**, *20*, 211–218. [CrossRef] [PubMed]
44. Cerea, M.; Pattarino, F.; Foglio Bonda, A.; Palugan, L.; Segale, L.; Vecchio, C. Preparation of Multiparticulate Systems for Oral Delivery of a Micronized or Nanosized Poorly Soluble Drug. *Drug Dev. Ind. Pharm.* **2016**, *42*, 1466–1475. [CrossRef] [PubMed]

45. Kósa, D.; Pető, Á.; Fenyvesi, F.; Váradi, J.; Vecsernyés, M.; Budai, I.; Németh, J.; Fehér, P.; Bácskay, I.; Ujhelyi, Z. Oral Bioavailability Enhancement of Melanin Concentrating Hormone, Development and In Vitro Pharmaceutical Assessment of Novel Delivery Systems. *Pharmaceutics* **2021**, *14*, 9. [CrossRef] [PubMed]
46. Nayak, A.K.; Pal, D. Development of PH-Sensitive Tamarind Seed Polysaccharide–Alginate Composite Beads for Controlled Diclofenac Sodium Delivery Using Response Surface Methodology. *Int. J. Biol. Macromol.* **2011**, *49*, 784–793. [CrossRef] [PubMed]
47. Nasr, A.; Gardouh, A.; Ghorab, M. Novel Solid Self-Nanoemulsifying Drug Delivery System (S-SNEDDS) for Oral Delivery of Olmesartan Medoxomil: Design, Formulation, Pharmacokinetic and Bioavailability Evaluation. *Pharmaceutics* **2016**, *8*, 20. [CrossRef] [PubMed]
48. Lee, K.Y.; Mooney, D.J. Alginate: Properties and Biomedical Applications. *Prog. Polym. Sci.* **2012**, *37*, 106–126. [CrossRef] [PubMed]
49. Hidalgo, I.J.; Raub, T.J.; Borchardt, R.T. Characterization of the Human Colon Carcinoma Cell Line (Caco-2) as a Model System for Intestinal Epithelial Permeability. *Gastroenterology* **1989**, *96*, 736–749. [CrossRef]
50. Seithel, A.; Karlsson, J.; Hilgendorf, C.; Björquist, A.; Ungell, A.-L. Variability in MRNA Expression of ABC- and SLC-Transporters in Human Intestinal Cells: Comparison between Human Segments and Caco-2 Cells. *Eur. J. Pharm. Sci.* **2006**, *28*, 291–299. [CrossRef]
51. Joki, T.; Machluf, M.; Atala, A.; Zhu, J.; Seyfried, N.T.; Dunn, I.F.; Abe, T.; Carroll, R.S.; Black, P.M. Continuous Release of Endostatin from Microencapsulated Engineered Cells for Tumor Therapy. *Nat. Biotechnol.* **2001**, *19*, 35–39. [CrossRef]
52. Mangla, B.; Neupane, Y.R.; Singh, A.; Kumar, P.; Shafi, S.; Kohli, K. Lipid-Nanopotentiated Combinatorial Delivery of Tamoxifen and Sulforaphane: Ex Vivo, In Vivo and Toxicity Studies. *Nanomedicine* **2020**, *15*, 2563–2583. [CrossRef]
53. Kaneda, Y.; Tsutsumi, Y.; Yoshioka, Y.; Kamada, H.; Yamamoto, Y.; Kodaira, H.; Tsunoda, S.; Okamoto, T.; Mukai, Y.; Shibata, H.; et al. The Use of PVP as a Polymeric Carrier to Improve the Plasma Half-Life of Drugs. *Biomaterials* **2004**, *25*, 3259–3266. [CrossRef] [PubMed]
54. Špaglová, M.; Čuchorová, M.; Šimunková, V.; Matúšová, D.; Čierna, M.; Starýchová, L.; Bauerová, K. Possibilities of the Microemulsion Use as Indomethacin Solubilizer and Its Effect on In Vitro and Ex Vivo Drug Permeation from Dermal Gels in Comparison with Transcutol®. *Drug Dev. Ind. Pharm.* **2020**, *46*, 1468–1476. [CrossRef] [PubMed]
55. Yamada, M.; Katsuma, S.; Adachi, T.; Hirasawa, A.; Shiojima, S.; Kadowaki, T.; Okuno, Y.; Koshimizu, T.-A.; Fujii, S.; Sekiya, Y.; et al. Inhibition of Protein Kinase CK2 Prevents the Progression of Glomerulonephritis. *Proc. Natl. Acad. Sci. USA* **2005**, *102*, 7736–7741. [CrossRef] [PubMed]
56. Wang, D.; Westerheide, S.D.; Hanson, J.L.; Baldwin, A.S. Tumor Necrosis Factor α-Induced Phosphorylation of RelA/P65 on Ser529 Is Controlled by Casein Kinase II. *J. Biol. Chem.* **2000**, *275*, 32592–32597. [CrossRef]
57. Sethi, J.K.; Hotamisligil, G.S. Metabolic Messengers: Tumour Necrosis Factor. *Nat. Metab.* **2021**, *3*, 1302–1312. [CrossRef]
58. Józsa, L.; Vasvári, G.; Sinka, D.; Nemes, D.; Ujhelyi, Z.; Vecsernyés, M.; Váradi, J.; Fenyvesi, F.; Lekli, I.; Gyöngyösi, A.; et al. Enhanced Antioxidant and Anti-Inflammatory Effects of Self-Nano and Microemulsifying Drug Delivery Systems Containing Curcumin. *Molecules* **2022**, *27*, 6652. [CrossRef]

Disclaimer/Publisher's Note: The statements, opinions and data contained in all publications are solely those of the individual author(s) and contributor(s) and not of MDPI and/or the editor(s). MDPI and/or the editor(s) disclaim responsibility for any injury to people or property resulting from any ideas, methods, instructions or products referred to in the content.

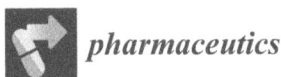 *pharmaceutics*

Article

The Development of Lipid-Based Sorafenib Granules to Enhance the Oral Absorption of Sorafenib

Jaylen C. Mans and Xiaowei Dong *

Department of Pharmaceutical Sciences, University of North Texas Health Science Center, Fort Worth, TX 76107, USA
* Correspondence: xiaowei.dong@unthsc.edu; Tel.: +1-(817)-735-2785; Fax:+1-(817)-735-2603

Abstract: Sorafenib (SFN) is an anticancer multi-kinase inhibitor with great therapeutic potential. However, SFN has low aqueous solubility, which limits its oral absorption. Lipids and surfactants have the potential to improve the solubility of water-insoluble drugs. The aim of this study is thus to develop novel lipid-based SFN granules that can improve the oral absorption of SFN. SFN powder was coated with a stable binary lipid mixture and then absorbed on Aeroperl 300 to form dry SFN granules with 10% drug loading. SFN granules were stable at room temperature for at least three months. Compared to SFN powder, SFN granules significantly increased SFN release in simulated gastric fluid and simulated intestinal fluid with pancreatin. Pharmacokinetics and tissue distribution of SFN granules and SFN powder were measured following oral administration to Sprague Dawley rats. SFN granules significantly increased SFN absorption compared to SFN powder. Overall, the lipid-based SFN granules provide a promising approach to enhancing the oral absorption of SFN.

Keywords: oral formulation; lipid-based formulations; poorly water-soluble drug; bioavailability enhancement; anticancer

1. Introduction

Sorafenib (SFN) is a promising anticancer therapeutic agent approved by the Food and Drug Administration (FDA) for the treatment of patients with advanced hepatocellular carcinoma, advanced renal cell carcinoma, and differentiated thyroid cancer. SFN works as a multi-kinase tyrosine inhibitor, with activity disrupting RAF, vascular endothelial growth factor receptor (VEGFR), and platelet-derived growth factor receptor (PDGFR) kinases [1,2]. The broad pharmacodynamic activity against RAF, VEGFR, and PDGFR kinases provides SFN with extensive antiangiogenic and antitumor proliferative activity against a range of cancers [1,2]. However, SFN is highly lipophilic (LogP 3.8) and insoluble in water (<25 ng/mL). The commercially available sorafenib oral tablet, Nexavar, contains crystalline sorafenib tosylate, a salt form to improve solubility; however, sorafenib tosylate is still insoluble (only 60 μg/mL in water). As a biopharmaceutical classification system class II compound, SFN exhibits poor water solubility, which restricts its absorption into the systemic circulation [3,4]. In addition to poor water solubility, SFN undergoes extensive first-pass metabolism, further reducing its bioavailability [5–7]. Clinicians must use frequent high-dosage administration of SFN (400 mg per day) to overcome the low solubility and extensive first-pass metabolism of SFN. The usage of a high dose of SFN could contribute to toxicity observed in patients such as hand–foot skin reactions, hypertension, and gastrointestinal issues, as well as lesser reported issues [8–11]. These toxicities can be poorly tolerated by patients, often leading to clinical dose management or complete treatment discontinuation [12–14]. With poor oral bioavailability and low tissue exposure levels, SFN is restricted in terms of its therapeutic potential as an oral anti-cancer agent [3,15,16]. Consequently, researchers have been investigating alternative formulation strategies to overcome the poor water solubility of SFN, thereby increasing the oral bioavailability and improving the therapeutic outcome. Improved SFN formulations could produce the same therapeutic effect at lower doses, thereby reducing the associated toxicity risk and presumably increasing patient satisfaction.

Lipid-based formulations such as solid lipid nanoparticles, microemulsions, and liposomes have the potential to solve the solubility issues of poorly water-soluble drugs. They are prepared from biodegradable and biocompatible lipids and surfactants, reducing likelihood of excipient-safety concerns. However, nanoparticles commonly are made in aqueous phases. Nanoparticles naturally tend to aggregate together over time during storage to decrease their free energy, which can lead to erratic changes in particle behavior and stability [17]. Other lipid-based formulations such as microemulsions and emulsions are also prepared as liquids, leading to issues with stability, the manufacturing process, and costs. Conversion of liquid lipid-based formulations to solid dosage forms is desirable; however, low drug loading (DL) in final solid forms, complex drying procedures, and size increase after drying have hindered such conversion for oral medication formulations. To overcome these issues and use lipid-based formulations in solid dosage forms for oral administration, our lab discovered a new approach to preparing lipid-based solid drug granules with high DL [18–21]. Recently, we confirmed that the binary lipid mixture of Miglyol 812 and D-α-tocopheryl polyethylene glycol 1000 succinate (TPGS) we used in the granules formed stable particles that were not impacted by water dilution in a pseudo-ternary phase diagram [20].

In this study, we aimed to prepare novel lipid-based SFN granules to enhance the oral absorption of SFN. We investigated if coating SFN with the stable binary lipid mixture of Miglyol 812 and TPGS will increase oral absorption. The novel SFN granules were characterized by stability in simulated fluids, two-step biorelevant dissolution, physical state, long-term stability, and in vivo studies, including pharmacokinetics and tissue distribution.

2. Methods

2.1. Materials

Research-grade SFN free base was purchased from LC Laboratories (Woburn, MA, USA). TPGS was provided as a gift from BASF (Ludwigshafen, Germany). Miglyol 812 (middle-chain triglycerides) was obtained as gifts from Cremer (Eatontown, NJ, USA). Aeroperl 300 (colloidal silicon dioxide) was provided as a gift from Evonik (Parsippany, NJ, USA). Amicon Ultra-0.5 centrifugal filter unit with a molecular weight cutoff of 100 kDa was purchased from Millipore (Bedford, MA, USA). HPLC-grade methanol was purchased from Fisher Scientific (Fair Lawn, NJ, USA).

2.2. Animals

Sprague Dawley rats (males, 276–300 g) were purchased from Charles River Laboratories (Wilmington, MA, USA). All animal experiments were carried out under an approved protocol by the Institutional Animal Care and Use Committee at the University of North Texas Health Science Center on 27 March 2020. Rats were housed in groups of 2 under a 12 h light/dark cycle with free access to food and water for one week before use.

2.3. Preparation of SFN Granules

SFN granules were prepared at 10% DL. Briefly, 16.8 mg of SFN free base, 50 mg of Miglyol 812, and 50 mg of TPGS were weighed into a glass vial. The mixture was stirred at 50 °C for 15 min. Next, 50 mg of Aeroperl 300 was incrementally added to the vial. After the mixture was thoroughly homogenized, the mixture was cooled to room temperature to form SFN granules.

2.4. Characterization of SFN Granules

2.4.1. Differential Scanning Calorimetry and Fourier Transform Infrared Spectroscopy Analysis of SFN Granules

The physical state of SFN within SFN granules was evaluated by using differential scanning calorimetry (DSC) and Fourier transform infrared spectroscopy (FTIR) analysis.

DSC analysis of SFN granules was performed using a PerkinElmer DSC 4000. Briefly, samples were sealed inside an aluminum DSC pan and equilibrated to 20 °C for 1 min. Next, samples were heated along a heat curve of 10 °C/min from 20 °C to 240 °C. Relative heat flow was recorded for comparative analysis. SFN granules were also analyzed via Thermo Scientific Nicolet iS5 FTIR spectrometer to measure infrared transmittance from 500 cm^{-1} to 3700 cm^{-1}. The fingerprint FTIR spectra of SFN granules, blank granules, unprocessed physical mixtures, and SFN free base were compared for analysis. Blank granules were prepared by following the procedure in Section 2.3 without SFN.

2.4.2. Measurement of Drug Loading in SFN Granules

DL in SFN granules was measured by HPLC. Briefly, SFN granules were dissolved in methanol and then centrifuged for 5 min at 15,000 rpm. Following centrifugation, 200 µL of supernatant was collected for HPLC analysis as previously reported [22]. The experiments were conducted in triplicate. DL was calculated as follows:

% DL = [(drug in the granules)/(total weight of drug granules)] × 100% (w/w)

2.5. Characterization of Particles Released from SFN Granules

2.5.1. Determination of Particle Size and Size Distribution

SFN granules were suspended in Milliq water. The mixture was vortexed for 30 s and centrifuged for 5 min at 15,000 rpm at room temperature. The supernatant was measured for particle size and size distribution by a dynamic light scattering system (Malvern Zetasizer Ultra Particle Analyzer).

2.5.2. Determination of the Percentage of SFN Entrapped in Particles

After SFN-loaded particles (the supernatant as described above) were collected, the total drug content in the particles was measured by HPLC. To measure how much SFN was entrapped in the particles, free SFN in the SFN-loaded particles was separated using an Amicon Ultra-0.5 centrifugal filter unit with a molecular weight cutoff of 100 KD. The filter was pretreated with a solution containing 0.2% Tween 80 and 0.9% NaCl to prevent the binding of SFN to the filter membrane. The experiments were conducted in triplicate. The concentration of SFN in the filtrate was measured by HPLC. The percentage of SFN entrapped in the particles was calculated as follows:

% entrapped SFN = [1 − (free SFN/total SFN in the particles)] × 100% (w/w)

2.5.3. Evaluation of Morphology for SFN-Loaded Particles

SFN-loaded particles were imaged using an FEI Tecnai G^2 Spirit Transmission Electron Microscope (TEM) equipped with a LaB6 source at 120 kV using a Gatan ultrascan CCD camera. The SFN samples were prepared for imaging with the following procedure: Formvar carbon grids were placed on a glass slide and glow-discharged. Next, SFN-loaded particles were diluted with water (10:90, v/v), and 2.5 µL of diluted SFN-loaded particles was placed onto the grid and dried for 30 min. Then, 2.5 µL of uranyl acetate was applied to the grid and left to dry for 30 min. The mounted grids were loaded into TEM for imaging.

2.6. Short-Term Particle Size Stability of SFN-Loaded Particles at 37 °C in Physiologically Relevant Media

The two-step media including simulated gastric fluid (SGF, pH 1.2) and simulated intestinal fluid (SIF, pH 6.8) were prepared as previously reported [23]. A total of 12 mg of SFN granules were added into 11 mL of SGF, pH 1.2 at 37 °C, stirring at 150 rpm. At 0, 1, and 2 h, 1.5 mL media were withdrawn and centrifuged at 15,000 rpm for 10 min at room temperature. Following centrifugation, 1 mL of supernatant was collected into a cuvette for particle size analysis as described in Section 2.5.1. Immediately following the 2 h collection interval, the SGF medium was replenished to its initial volume and adjusted to pH 6.8 by adding 200 µL of 2 M KH_2PO_4 and 2.5 mL of 0.5 M NaOH to mimic SIF. Subsequently, at 4,

6, and 8 h, samples were withdrawn for particle size measurement as described above. The experiments were conducted in triplicate.

2.7. Long-Term Stability of SFN Granules

The long-term stability of SFN granules was assessed at room temperature. Parameters of particle size, DL, and entrapped SFN in the particles were measured as described above over three months. The degradation of SFN was monitored according to the appearance of extra peaks on HPLC chromatograms. Three independent batches of SFN granules were prepared and monitored for long-term stability.

2.8. In Vitro Dissolution Studies

The two-step dissolution of SFN granules and SFN powder was conducted as previously reported [23]. Briefly, 50 mg of SFN granules was added to 24 mL of SGF medium and stirred at 225 rpm at 37 °C. At 0, 15 min, 30 min, 1 h, 1.5 h, and 2 h, 1 mL of sample was withdrawn and centrifuged at 15,000 rm for 5 min at room temperature. After centrifugation, 200 µL of supernatant was diluted with methanol, vortexed for 1 min, and then centrifuged at 15,000 rpm for 5 min. After centrifugation, 200 µL of supernatant was collected for HPLC analysis as previously described. After withdrawing samples from SGF at 2 h, 0.3 mL 2M KH_2PO_4 and 16 mL of water were added to switch the media to SIF, and 2M NaOH was used to adjust pH to 6.8, and then 4 mL of pancreatin solution was added to the media. Sample collection was continued at 10 min, 20 min, 30 min, 45 min, 1 h, 2 h, 3 h, and 4 h. Drug concentrations were measured by HPLC as described above. SFN powder at an equivalent amount of SFN was tested as a control. The experiments were conducted in triplicate.

2.9. Pharmacokinetic Study

Sprague Dawley male rats (276–300 g, n = 3 per group) were randomly grouped and given SFN powder or SFN granules by oral gavage at 30 mg/kg of SFN. SFN powder and SFN granules were pre-mixed with water before dosing. After dose administration, blood samples were collected at 0, 0.5, 1, 2, 3, 4, 5, 6, 7, 8, 32, 48, and 72 h in EDTA-coated tubes. Blood samples were immediately centrifuged at 4000 rpm for 5 min at 4 °C to obtain plasma samples. Plasma samples were stored at −80 °C until further analysis within three months. SFN concentrations in plasma samples were measured by a previously reported LC-MS method [22].

2.10. Tissue Distribution Study

The tissue distribution of SFN granules and SFN powder was measured in Sprague Dawley male rats (276–300 g, n = 3 per group). Briefly, SFN powder and SFN granules, which were suspended in water, were orally administered to randomly divided rats at 30 mg/kg of SFN, respectively. After 2 h, rats were sacrificed to collect tissues including lung, mesenteric lymph node, liver, kidney, brain, heart, and spleen. Tissue samples were stored at −80 °C until further analysis within three months. SFN concentrations in tissue samples were measured by a previously reported LC-MS method [22].

2.11. Statistical Analysis

The results were expressed as mean ± standard deviation (SD). The data were compared using a Student t-test at a 95% confidence level, and p values < 0.05 were considered significantly different.

3. Results

3.1. Characterization of SFN Granules and SFN-Loaded Particles

SFN granules were successfully prepared with a binary lipid mixture of Miglyol 812 and TPGS. As demonstrated by the previous study, Miglyol 812 and TPGS at a 1:1 ratio (w/w) formed a stable binary system that is resistant to physical changes caused by water dilution [20]. Aeroperl 300 was used as a solid carrier to prepare dry granules with a good flow. When the amount of Aeroperl 300 reached 30% of the total amount of the granule, the flow of the granules was good. SFN granules had 10% DL and showed good flow properties. Upon contact with water, SFN granules spontaneously produced SFN-loaded particles. The particle size of SFN-loaded particles was 154 nm with a monodispersed size distribution indicated by a polydispersity index (P.I.) of 0.27 (Figure 1A). A TEM image further demonstrated the formation and size of SFN-loaded particles as well as their spherical morphology (Figure 1B). As shown in Table 1, about 99% of SFN was entrapped in the particles. SFN granules remained stable over a 3-month measurement period in terms of DL% and degradation %. During the storage period, SFN granules produced stable SFN-loaded particles. Although the particle size of SFN-loaded particles increased in the second and third month, they were still below 200 nm.

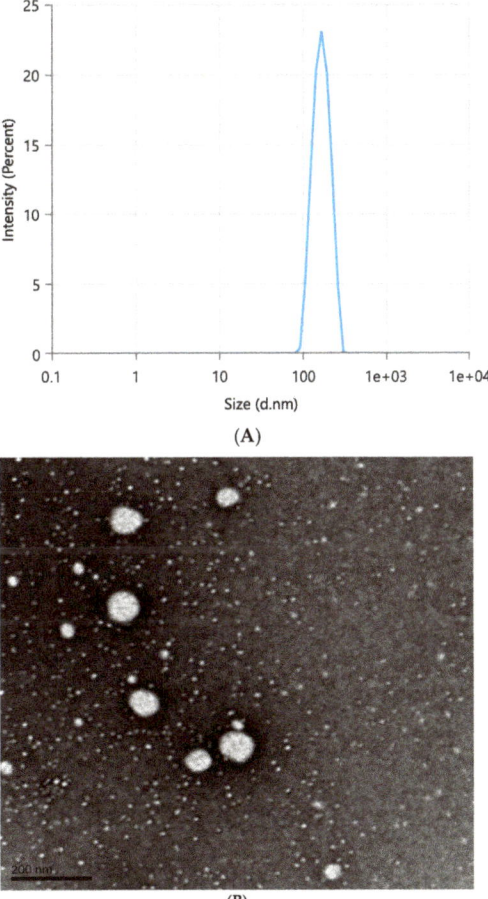

Figure 1. SFN granules produced SFN-loaded particles when introduced to contact with water. (**A**) Particle size and size distribution of SFN-loaded particles. (**B**) TEM image of SFN-loaded particles.

Table 1. Long-term stability of SFN granules and SFN-loaded particles (*n* = 3). Data are presented as mean ± SD. DL% and degradation% were measured for SFN granules. Entrapped SFN%, particle size and P.I. were measured for SFN-loaded particles that were produced once SFN granules mixed with water.

Parameters	Day 0	Two Weeks	One Month	Two Months	Three Months
Measured DL%	9.7 ± 0.1	9.5 ± 0.4	9.5 ± 0.3	9.2 ± 0.2	9.4 ± 0.2
Degradation%	0	0	0	0	0
Entrapped SFN%	99.9 ± 0.029	100 ± 0	100 ± 0	100 ± 0	99.9 ± 0.018
Particle size (nm)	145 ± 5	146 ± 1	147 ± 4	160 ± 8	162 ± 22
P.I.	0.266 ± 0.045	0.272 ± 0.028	0.29 ± 0.062	0.262 ± 0.05	0.268 ± 0.01

3.2. Physical state of SFN in SFN Granules

The physical state of SFN in SFN granules was evaluated by DSC and FTIR analysis. In the DSC analysis, SFN powder displays a heat flow peak at 211.6 °C that was correlated to the melting point of SFN crystals. The melting point of SFN did not appear in blank granules nor SFN granules (Figure 2). To further test the physical state of SFN in the granules, FTIR analysis served as an alternative measurement for crystallinity to validate the DSC analysis. In FTIR analysis, both SFN powder and the physical mixture showed sharp characteristic peaks at 3300–3340 cm^{-1}, 1550–1650 cm^{-1}, and 670–680 cm^{-1}, which were present, yet significantly reduced in SFN granules, and completely absent in the blank granules (Figure 3). Thus, according to the FTIR results, SFN was partially converted to an amorphous form in SFN granules. It is very likely, during the heating process in DSC measurement, that crystal SFN dissolved in the excipients, which resulted in the disappearance of the thermal peak in the physical mixture and SFN granules.

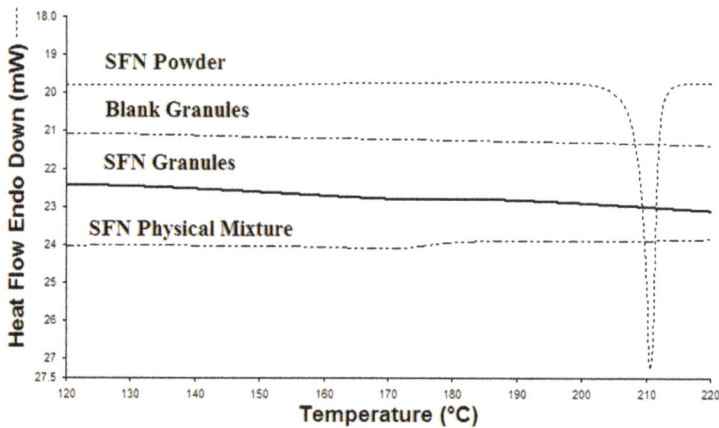

Figure 2. DSC differential thermograms of SFN powder, SFN granules, SFN physical mixture, and blank granules.

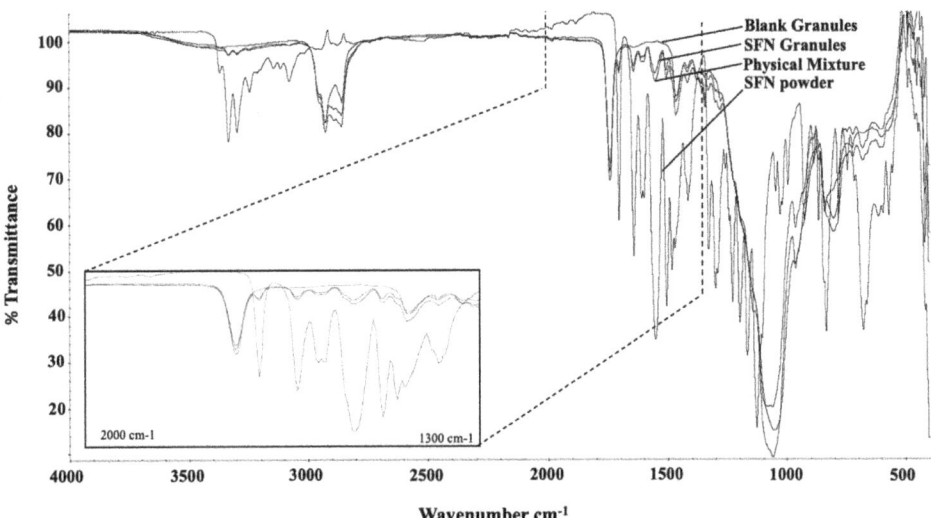

Figure 3. FTIR spectra of SFN powder, physical mixture, SFN granules, and blank granules. SFN was partially converted to an amorphous form.

3.3. Short-Term Particle Stability of SFN-Loaded Particles in Physiological Conditions

The stability of SFN-loaded particles produced from SFN granules was assessed in SGF for 2 h to mimic the transition time in the stomach, followed by SIF for 6 h to mimic the transition time in the small intestine. As shown in Figure 4, the SFN-loaded particles maintained a narrow average size range of 143–198 nm, while the blank particles maintained a similar 157–226 nm average particle size range. There were no significant changes in the tested time points, compared to the size at time 0 for each group (Figure 4), indicating that SFN-loaded particles were stable in the tested physiological conditions.

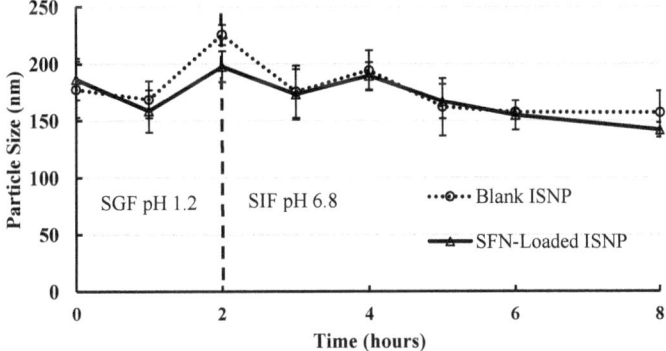

Figure 4. Short-term physical stability of SFN-loaded particles and blank particles in SGF for 2 h and SIF for following 6 h (n = 3). SFN-loaded particles were stable in SGF for 2 h and SIF for 6 h. Data are presented as mean ± SD.

3.4. Two-Step In Vitro Dissolution

Dissolution studies were conducted over 2 h in SGF solution and 4 h in SIF in the presence of pancreatin. The current clinical single dose of SFN is 400 mg. To mimic SFN concentration in the stomach, 50 mg of SFN granules was used in the dissolution study in 24 mL media. As shown in Figure 5, about 27% of SFN was released from SFN granules, whereas about ~1% of SFN was released from SFN powder in the first 90 min. After the media were adjusted to SIF with pancreatin, the dissolution of SFN granules increased to 91% while SFN powder reached 7.3% ($n = 3$). Comparing SFN granules with SFN powder, there was a significant difference in the dissolution profiles in both the SGF and SIF with pancreatin media ($p < 0.05$).

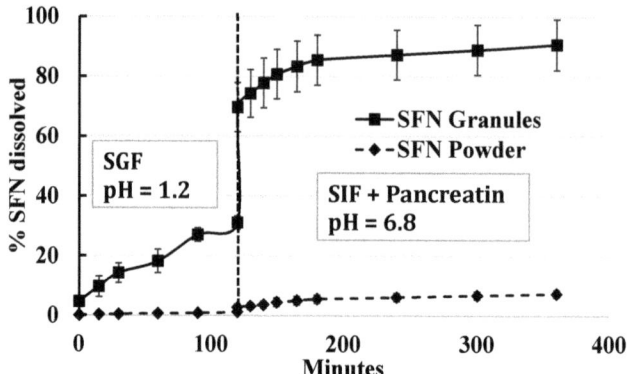

Figure 5. In vitro dissolution profile of SFN granules and SFN powder in SGF for 2 h, followed by SIF with the addition of pancreatin for 4 h ($n = 3$). SFN granules increased the dissolution of SFN compared to SFN powder. In SIF, about 90% of SFN was released from SFN granules. Data are presented as mean ± SD.

3.5. Pharmacokinetics and Tissue Distribution

The pharmacokinetic and biodistribution experiments were performed on Sprague Dawley rats. Pharmacokinetics measure drug concentrations in blood circulation, and biodistribution measures drug concentrations in each tissue. In the pharmacokinetic study, SFN granules demonstrated an over 4-fold increase in C_{max} compared to SFN powder ($p < 0.05$) (Figure 6). For tissue distribution, SFN granules significantly increased SFN uptake in all measured tissues by 6–10 fold, excluding brain tissue (Figure 7). Importantly, in mesenteric lymph nodes, SFN granules demonstrated a 20-fold increase in SFN concentration compared to SFN powder (Figure 7).

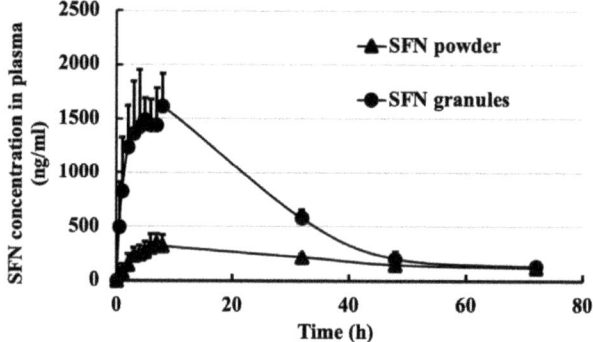

Figure 6. SFN plasma concentration in rats over 72 h following oral administration of SFN powder and SFN granules at 30 mg/kg ($n = 3$). SFN granules increased the SFN concentration in blood compared to SFN powder. Data are presented as mean ± SD.

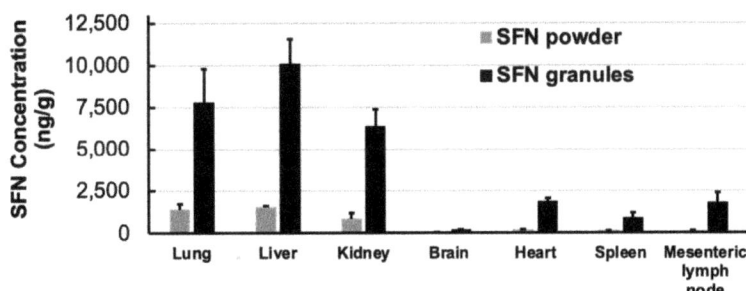

Figure 7. SFN concentrations in rat tissues following oral administration of SFN powder and SFN granules at 30 mg/kg at 2 h (n = 3). SFN granules increased SFN absorption over 6–10 fold except in brain. Particularly, SFN granules greatly increased drug concentration in mesenteric lymph node (over 20-fold) compared to SFN powder, suggesting the enhanced lymphatic uptake by SFN granules. Data are presented as mean ± SD.

4. Discussion

SFN was the first molecular-targeted agent to be licensed for metastatic renal cell carcinoma in 2005 and later for unresectable hepatocellular carcinoma and advanced thyroid carcinoma. SFN is hydrophobic and has poor water solubility. Lipid-based formulations present an emerging mechanism to enhance drug absorption. However, conventional lipid-based formulations are not in solid forms and are filled in soft gelatin capsules [19]. To prolong shelf-life and improve the manufacturing process, the conversion of lipid-based formulation to solid forms has been studied. However, low DL and complicated processes were problematic. Here, we prepared SFN granules by coating SFN with a stable binary mixture composed of Miglyol 812 and TPGS. The DL of SFN granules was 10%. To understand the behavior of SFN granules upon contact with water, the particles in the supernatant after SFN granules were dispersed into the water were tested. The particle size and TEM data showed that after mixing with water, SFN granules generated SFN-loaded particles with high entrapment (Table 1 and Figure 1). In the granule preparation, the surface of SFN powder was coated with Miglyol 812 and TPGS, and then the coated SFN was absorbed on Aeroperl 300 to form dry SFN granules. Since SFN is water-insoluble, when SFN granules were mixed with water, Miglyol 812 and TPGS were released from Aeroperl 300 and formed stable particles by self-assembly, while SFN dissolved and was entrapped into Miglyol 812-TPGS particles. In this study, SFN granules were stable for three months in measured parameters without significant degradation. During the stability testing, SFN granules produced SFN-loaded particles without changes in particle size, size distribution, or the percentage of entrapped SFN (Table 1). The FTIR studies demonstrated that the crystal SFN was partially converted to an amorphous form in SFN granules, which could be caused by the interaction of the binary lipid mixture with the crystal SFN during the preparation.

One of the features of the binary lipid mixture of Miglyol 812 and TPGS is that they form stable particles in different physiological conditions. As demonstrated by the previous pseudo-ternary phase diagram, Miglyol 812 and TPGS formed a stable binary structure at a 1:1 ratio that allows it to maintain its structural integrity over water dilution [20]. Here the particle size of SFN-loaded particles was stable in SGF (pH 1.6) for 2 h and SIF (pH 6.8) for 4 h (Figure 4). The strong interaction among Miglyol 812, TPGS, and SFN could provide structural integrity against water dilution and pH change in an aqueous milieu. The notable stability of SFN-loaded particles is critical for maintaining structural integrity throughout the gastrointestinal tract during oral administration.

SFN has food effects and cancer patients are recommended to take SFN tablets without food. The components and pH of gastric fluid and intestinal fluid are different; thus, it is critical to test oral drugs in both gastric fluid and intestinal fluid. The dissolution of SFN granules was conducted by using a two-step dissolution method simulating physiological conditions. SFN granules remarkedly increased the dissolution rate compared to SFN powder in SIF (Figure 5). Coating SFN with the binary lipid mixture, the formation of SFN-loaded particles, the amorphous form, and the lipolysis of lipid components in the granules contributed to the dissolution enhancement.

Pharmacokinetic and tissue distribution studies confirmed that SFN granules enhanced oral absorption. SFN granules significantly increased blood concentration and tissue uptake compared to SFN powder (Figures 6 and 7). There are several reasons for enhanced absorption. First is the increasing dissolution by SFN granules. Secondly, the lipid and surfactant in SFN granules could enhance the permeability of SFN. Thirdly, coating the stable binary lipid mixture on the SFN surface could increase the saturated solubility and local concentration of SFN. Finally, it is known that lipid formulations increase drug lymphatic uptake [24,25]. Indeed, the tissue distribution demonstrated that SFN granules increased lymphatic uptake by over 20-fold compared to SFN powder. SFN is a key treatment for renal cell carcinoma and unresectable hepatocellular carcinoma. According to the results of biodistribution (Figure 7), SFN granules greatly increased SFN concertation in liver over 6.6-fold and in kidney over 7.8-fold. Thus, SFN granules have potential to improve the efficacy of tumor inhibition because of the increased drug concentrations in tumor tissues.

In conclusion, new lipid-based SFN granules were prepared by coating a stable binary lipid mixture of Miglyol 812 and TPGS on the SFN surface. With 10% of DL, SFN granules demonstrated remarkable stability at room temperature over three months. SFN granules produced stable SFN-loaded particles upon contact with water. Compared to SFN powder, SFN granules increased dissolution rate and oral absorption. Moreover, the preparation of lipid-based SFN granules is simple and scalable. Thus, the new lipid-based SFN granules have the potential to enhance the systemic exposure of SFN.

Author Contributions: X.D. designed the experiments and J.C.M. conducted the experiments. J.C.M. and X.D. interpreted the data, J.C.M. wrote the draft of the manuscript, and X.D. revised it. X.D. supervised the project. All authors have read and agreed to the published version of the manuscript.

Funding: Research reported in this publication was supported by the National Institute of General Medical Sciences of the National Institutes of Health under Award Number R35GM138225 to Dong, X.

Institutional Review Board Statement: The animal study protocol was approved by the Institutional Animal Care and Use Committee at the University of North Texas Health Science Center (IACUC-2020-0015) (03/27/2020).

Informed Consent Statement: Not applicable.

Data Availability Statement: Data is contained within the article.

Conflicts of Interest: The authors declare no conflict of interest.

References

1. Wilhelm, S.M.; Carter, C.; Tang, L.; Wilkie, D.; McNabola, A.; Rong, H.; Chen, C.; Zhang, X.; Vincent, P.; McHugh, M.; et al. BAY 43-9006 Exhibits Broad Spectrum Oral Antitumor Activity and Targets the RAF/MEK/ERK Pathway and Receptor Tyrosine Kinases Involved in Tumor Progression and Angiogenesis. *Cancer Res.* **2004**, *64*, 7099. [CrossRef]
2. Abdelgalil, A.A.; Alkahtani, H.M.; Al-Jenoobi, F.I. Chapter Four—Sorafenib. In *Profiles of Drug Substances, Excipients and Related Methodology*; Brittain, H.G., Ed.; Academic Press: Cambridge, MA, USA, 2019; pp. 239–266.
3. Chen, F.; Fang, Y.; Chen, X.; Deng, R.; Zhang, Y.; Shao, J. Recent advances of sorafenib nanoformulations for cancer therapy: Smart nanosystem and combination therapy. *Asian J. Pharm. Sci.* **2020**, *16*, 318–336. [CrossRef]
4. Liu, C.; Chen, Z.; Chen, Y.; Lu, J.; Li, Y.; Wang, S.; Wu, G.; Qian, F. Improving Oral Bioavailability of Sorafenib by Optimizing the "Spring" and "Parachute" Based on Molecular Interaction Mechanisms. *Mol. Pharm.* **2016**, *13*, 599–608. [CrossRef] [PubMed]
5. Ahiwale, R.J.; Chellampillai, B.; Pawar, A.P. Investigation of novel sorafenib tosylate loaded biomaterial based nano-cochleates dispersion system for treatment of hepatocellular carcinoma. *J. Dispers. Sci. Technol.* **2021**, *43*, 1568–1586. [CrossRef]
6. Pamu, S.; Pamu, P.; Darna, V.R.N.B. Self Nanoemulsifying Drug Delivery System of Sorafenib Tosylate: Development and In VivoStudies. *Pharm. Nanotechnol.* **2020**, *8*, 471–484. [CrossRef]

7. Zhang, H.; Zhang, F.-M.; Yan, S.-J. Preparation, in vitro release, and pharmacokinetics in rabbits of lyophilized injection of sorafenib solid lipid nanoparticles. *Int. J. Nanomed.* **2012**, *7*, 2901–2910. [CrossRef] [PubMed]
8. La Vine, D.B.T.; Coleman, T.A.; Davis, C.H.; Carbonell, C.E.; Davis, W.B. Frequent Dose Interruptions are Required for Patients Receiving Oral Kinase Inhibitor Therapy for Advanced Renal Cell Carcinoma. *Am. J. Clin. Oncol.* **2010**, *33*, 217–220. [CrossRef] [PubMed]
9. Zhu, Y.-J.; Zheng, B.; Wang, H.-Y.; Chen, L. New knowledge of the mechanisms of sorafenib resistance in liver cancer. *Acta Pharmacol. Sin.* **2017**, *38*, 614–622. [CrossRef] [PubMed]
10. Li, Y.; Gao, Z.-H.; Qu, X.-J. The Adverse Effects of Sorafenib in Patients with Advanced Cancers. *Basic Clin. Pharmacol. Toxicol.* **2015**, *116*, 216–221. [CrossRef]
11. Boudou-Rouquette, P.; Ropert, S.; Mir, O.; Coriat, R.; Billemont, B.; Tod, M.; Cabanes, L.; Franck, N.; Blanchet, B.; Goldwasser, F. Variability of sorafenib toxicity and exposure over time: A pharmacokinetic/pharmacodynamic analysis. *Oncologist* **2012**, *17*, 1204–1212. [CrossRef]
12. Escudier, B.; Eisen, T.; Stadler, W.M.; Szczylik, C.; Oudard, S.; Siebels, M.; Negrier, S.; Chevreau, C.; Solska, E.; Desai, A.A.; et al. Sorafenib in Advanced Clear-Cell Renal-Cell Carcinoma. *N. Engl. J. Med.* **2007**, *356*, 125–134. [CrossRef]
13. Llovet, J.M.; Ricci, S.; Mazzaferro, V.; Hilgard, P.; Gane, E.; Blanc, J.-F.; de Oliveira, A.C.; Santoro, A.; Raoul, J.-L.; Forner, A.; et al. Sorafenib in Advanced Hepatocellular Carcinoma. *N. Engl. J. Med.* **2008**, *359*, 378–390. [CrossRef]
14. Bruix, J.; Takayama, T.; Mazzaferro, V.; Chau, G.-Y.; Yang, J.; Kudo, M.; Cai, J.; Poon, R.T.; Han, K.-H.; Tak, W.Y.; et al. Adjuvant sorafenib for hepatocellular carcinoma after resection or ablation (STORM): A phase 3, randomised, double-blind, placebo-controlled trial. *Lancet Oncol.* **2015**, *16*, 1344–1354. [CrossRef]
15. Khan, M.A.; Raza, A.; Ovais, M.; Sohail, M.F.; Ali, S. Current state and prospects of nano-delivery systems for sorafenib. *Int. J. Polym. Mater. Polym. Biomater.* **2018**, *67*, 1105–1115. [CrossRef]
16. Park, S.Y.; Kang, Z.; Thapa, P.; Jin, Y.S.; Park, J.W.; Lim, H.J.; Lee, J.Y.; Lee, S.-W.; Seo, M.-H.; Kim, M.-S.; et al. Development of sorafenib loaded nanoparticles to improve oral bioavailability using a quality by design approach. *Int. J. Pharm.* **2019**, *566*, 229–238. [CrossRef] [PubMed]
17. Phan, H.T.; Haes, A.J. What Does Nanoparticle Stability Mean? *J. Phys. Chem. C Nanomater Interfaces* **2019**, *123*, 16495–16507. [CrossRef] [PubMed]
18. Wang, J.; Zhang, J.; Nguyen, N.T.D.; Chen, Y.A.; Hsieh, J.T.; Dong, X. Quantitative measurements of IR780 in formulations and tissues. *J. Pharm. Biomed. Anal.* **2021**, *194*, 113780. [CrossRef] [PubMed]
19. Guo, S.; Pham, K.; Li, D.; Penzak, S.R.; Dong, X. Novel in situ self-assembly nanoparticles for formulating a poorly water-soluble drug in oral solid granules, improving stability, palatability, and bioavailability. *Int. J. Nanomed.* **2016**, *11*, 1451–1460. [CrossRef]
20. Le, S.; Chang, C.M.; Nguyen, T.; Liu, Y.; Chen, Y.A.; Hernandez, E.; Kapur, P.; Hsieh, J.-T.; Johnston, K.; Dong, X. Anticancer Efficacy of Oral Docetaxel Nanoformulation for Metronomic Chemotherapy in Metastatic Lung Cancer. *J. Biomed. Nanotechnol.* **2020**, *16*, 583–593. [CrossRef]
21. Pham, K.; Li, D.; Guo, S.; Penzak, S.; Dong, X. Development and in vivo evaluation of child-friendly lopinavir/ritonavir pediatric granules utilizing novel in situ self-assembly nanoparticles. *J. Control. Release Off. J. Control. Release Soc.* **2016**, *226*, 88–97. [CrossRef]
22. Bobin-Dubigeon, C.; Heurgue-Berlot, A.; Bouche, O.; Amiand, M.B.; Le Guellec, C.; Bard, J.M. A new rapid and sensitive LC-MS assay for the determination of sorafenib in plasma: Application to a patient undergoing hemodialysis. *Ther. Drug Monit.* **2011**, *33*, 705–710. [CrossRef] [PubMed]
23. Shah, B.; Dong, X. Design and evaluation of two-step biorelevant dissolution methods for docetaxel oral formulations. *AAPS PharmSciTech* **2022**, *23*, 113. [CrossRef] [PubMed]
24. Ali Khan, A.; Mudassir, J.; Mohtar, N.; Darwis, Y. Advanced drug delivery to the lymphatic system: Lipid-based nanoformulations. *Int. J. Nanomed.* **2013**, *8*, 2733–2744. [CrossRef]
25. Kim, H.; Kim, Y.; Lee, J. Liposomal formulations for enhanced lymphatic drug delivery. *Asian J. Pharm. Sci.* **2013**, *8*, 96–103. [CrossRef]

Disclaimer/Publisher's Note: The statements, opinions and data contained in all publications are solely those of the individual author(s) and contributor(s) and not of MDPI and/or the editor(s). MDPI and/or the editor(s) disclaim responsibility for any injury to people or property resulting from any ideas, methods, instructions or products referred to in the content.

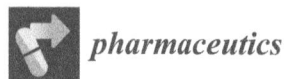

Article

Enhancing Pharmacokinetics and Pharmacodynamics of Rosuvastatin Calcium through the Development and Optimization of Fast-Dissolving Films

Ibrahim Ashraf [1], Pierre A. Hanna [1], Shadeed Gad [1], Fathy I. Abd-Allah [2] and Khalid M. El-Say [3,*]

1 Department of Pharmaceutics, Faculty of Pharmacy, Suez Canal University, Ismailia 41522, Egypt; dribrahim172@gmail.com (I.A.); pierre_hanna@pharm.suez.edu.eg (P.A.H.); shaded_abdelrahman@pharm.suez.edu.eg (S.G.)
2 Department of Pharmaceutics and Industrial Pharmacy, Faculty of Pharmacy, Al-Azhar University, Cairo 11651, Egypt; fathyfet@yahoo.com
3 Department of Pharmaceutics, Faculty of Pharmacy, King Abdulaziz University, Jeddah 21589, Saudi Arabia
* Correspondence: kelsay1@kau.edu.sa

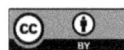

Abstract: Rosuvastatin (RSV) is a widely used cholesterol-lowering medication, but its limited bioavailability due to its susceptibility to stomach pH and extensive first-pass metabolism poses a significant challenge. A fast-dissolving film (FDF) formulation of RSV was developed, characterized, and compared to the conventional marketed tablet to address this issue. The formulation process involved optimizing the thickness, disintegration time, and folding durability. All formulations were assessed for in vitro disintegration, thickness, folding endurance, in vitro dissolution, weight, and content uniformity. The study's results revealed that the optimized RSV-FDF displayed a significantly faster time to maximum plasma concentration (t_{max}) of 2 h, compared to 4 h for the marketed tablet. The maximum plasma concentration (C_{max}) for the RSV-FDF (1.540 µg/mL ± 0.044) was notably higher than that of the marketed tablet (0.940 µg/mL ± 0.017). Additionally, the pharmacodynamic assessment in male Wistar rats demonstrated that the optimized RSV-FDF exhibited an improved lipid profile, including reduced levels of low-density lipoproteins (LDLs), elevated high-density lipoproteins (HDLs), decreased triglycerides (TGs), and lower very-low-density lipoproteins (VLDLs) compared to the conventional tablet. These findings underscore the potential of RSV-FDFs as a promising alternative to enhance the bioavailability and therapeutic efficacy of rosuvastatin in treating dyslipidemia. The faster onset of action and improved lipid-lowering effects make RSV-FDFs an attractive option for patients requiring efficient cholesterol management.

Keywords: fast-dissolving film; rosuvastatin; pharmacokinetics; hyperlipidemia; design of experiment approach

1. Introduction

Hyperlipidemia is defined as elevated levels of triglycerides and/or any of the following lipoproteins: very-low-density lipoproteins (VLDLs), low-density lipoproteins (LDLs), or high-density lipoproteins (HDLs). Hyperlipidemia expression is replaced by dyslipidemia as increasing HDL levels is a good sign [1]. Dyslipidemia is classified into familial (primary) dyslipidemia, which is caused by genetic disorders, and acquired (secondary) dyslipidemia, caused by the progression or signs of some diseases like diabetes, kidney disorder, and hypothyroidism [2,3]. Also, hyperlipidemia can increase the risk of developing some medical conditions like bladder cancer and coronary artery diseases [4]. Some cases report that dyslipidemia appears in overweight pediatrics. As a risk factor for management, triglycerides, total cholesterol, very-low-density lipoproteins (VLDLs), low-density lipoproteins (LDLs), and high-density lipoproteins (HDLs) are periodically analyzed for patients to prevent atherosclerosis [3]. The first treatment for controlling dyslipidemia is lifestyle management, e.g., decreasing fat and high-cholesterol diet intake. Several drug categories are used to manage the level of serum lipid. The first group is bile acid binders such as cholestyramine, colesovelam, and colestipol. The second group is fibrates, e.g., fenofibrate and gemfibrozil, which stimulate the cells' fatty acid uptake, convert it to acyl-CoA derivatives, and then catabolize it via oxidative pathways [5]. The third lipid-lowering group is cholesterol absorption inhibitors, e.g., ezetimibe, which significantly decreases the absorbed quantity of cholesterol. The fourth group is considered a supplement rather than a drug, which is omega-3 fatty acids that act by inhibiting VLDL synthesis. The fifth and most common group used for managing dyslipidemia is the 3-hydroxy-3-methyl-glutaryl-coenzyme A (HMG-COA) reductase inhibitors (statin). This group prevents the transformation of HMG-COA into mevalonate. The statin group contains simvastatin, pravastatin, atorvastatin, lovastatin, pitavastatin, and rosuvastatin. This medicine group is classified according to the biopharmaceutics classification system (BCS) as a class II drug characterized by low solubility and high permeability. Thus, it causes low bioavailability in this group. In addition, it shows poor acid stability and is highly affected by the first-pass effect. Thus, rosuvastatin exhibits a low bioavailability of about 20% [3].

Rosuvastatin calcium (RSV) is a synthetic lipid-lowering agent, chemically known as (3R,5S,6E)-7-[4-(4-fluorophenyl)-6-isopropyl-2-[methyl(methylsulfonyl)amino]pyrimidin-5-yl])-3,5-dihydroxyhept-6-enoic acid hemicalcium salt [6]. Rosuvastatin, among other statins, is called a "super-statin," causing a greater reduction in LDL than other statins of the same strength [7–9]. Several recent approaches have been published to improve rosuvastatin's bioavailability using different mechanisms. Elsayed and his coworkers prepared forming nanoparticles in situ with the aid of Tween 80 and cetyl alcohol and filled in delayed-release capsules that improved the dissolution rate and bioavailability [10]. In addition, reducing the particle size of rosuvastatin using a wet milling technique by adding PVP 10% as a stabilizer enhanced its dissolution behavior to release 72% after 1 h [7]. Furthermore, the development of pullulan-based tablets containing flexible chitosomes of rosuvastatin calcium improved relative bioavailability by 30% to 36% compared to marketed drugs and pure rosuvastatin tablets [3]. Also, using caffeine and Soluplus® to develop hydrotropic and micellar solubilization is another approach to directly compress rosuvastatin with improved bioavailability [11]. In addition, incorporating RSV into carboxylate cross-linked cyclodextrins improved its bioavailability [12]. Recently, González and his coworkers improved the bioavailability of RSV via its conversion to an amorphous form with a specific excipient to accelerate its dissolution onset by more than 90% in 10 min [13]. Also, RSV was incorporated with glimepiride in 3D-printed polypills formulated in a curcuma oil-based self-nanoemulsifying drug delivery system to treat patients with dyslipidemia and metabolic syndrome [14]. In addition, trials to formulate RSV as orodispersable films were performed with sophisticated and multi-stage procedures. The films produced by this work were evaluated for pharmacokinetic parameters, not for anti-dyslipidemic activity, as declared by our study [15].

Among other routes of administration, the oral route proved to yield optimum patient acceptability, as it is non-invasive and self-administered. There are many dosage forms administered orally. Some are wholly ingested; others can be chewed, dissolved in a specific solvent before taking, or adhered to the tongue or buccal cavity. Taking the dose via ingestion forced the active pharmaceutical ingredients into some challenges, like facing a low pH medium in the stomach, as many active pharmaceutical ingredients are unstable in acidic media. Also, some drugs are affected by first-pass metabolism prior to absorption. The relatively low bioavailability of some drugs after oral ingestion creates many challenges for developers to find a way to protect the drugs labile to these situations, like formulating them in delayed-release dosage forms.

Fast-dissolving films are considered a new oral dosage form that offers immediate action with a reasonable degree of protection from stomach acidity and the first-pass effect, as the dissolution and absorption phases are carried out in the oral cavity. It is a waterless dosage form and provides the action with a fast beginning. Fast-dissolving films, among other dosage forms, are highly accepted by pediatric and elderly patients due to their ease of use. Recently, many researchers published new polymer-based fast-dissolving films, e.g., fluoxetine [16], metoclopramide [17], lamotrigine [18], ondansetron hydrochloride [19], olanzapine [20], and tenoxicam [21]. Fast-dissolving films can be prepared using various techniques, such as solvent casting, characterized by combining the polymer solution with the plasticizer and drug solution, mixing, degassing, pouring into a suitable dish, and heating to evaporate the solvent [21]. Other methods include hot melt extrusion, semisolid casting, solid dispersion extrusion, and rolling [22]. A new approach was recently applied for preparing fast-dissolving dosage forms using a spinning agent that freely dissolves the drug of interest and is mixed with the polymeric solution [23].

Therefore, this work aimed to develop rosuvastatin calcium as a fast-dissolving film to be rapidly dissolved and absorbed in the buccal cavity. This approach helped to avoid the first-pass effect, protect the drug from degradation by stomach acidity, and subsequently improve the bioavailability of RSV.

2. Materials and Methods

2.1. Materials

Polyethylene glycol 400 (PEG 400) and rosuvastatin calcium were gifted from Egyptian International Pharmaceutical Industries Co. (10th of Ramadan, Egypt). Future Pharmaceutical Industries (Badr City, Egypt) provided hydroxypropyl methylcellulose (HPMC), viscosity 4000 cp, as a gift. Acetonitrile, ortho-phosphoric acid, methanol, and potassium dihydrogen phosphate were purchased from Merck (Darmstadt, Germany). Mannitol, Sorbitol, and Poloxamer 407 (P407, MW 40000) were obtained as a gift from Medical Union Pharmaceuticals (Ismailia, Egypt).

2.2. Methods

2.2.1. Experimental Design

Firstly, many trials were carried out using a single-variable test to define the effective influential variables and their range to reach an optimum film with the required attributes. The formulation process was optimized using a 2^{2+star} central composite design, which studies two variables at three levels using ten runs. Table 1 lists the number of variables included in the design and their characteristics. Table 2 describes the central composite design's layout. The effect of two factors, HPMC% (X_1) and PEG 400% (X_2), on the quality of the film was studied. A set of two center points per block and replicated center points were utilized to construct mathematical models and response surfaces using Statgraphics Centurion 18 software, Statgraphics Technologies, Inc. (Warrenton, VA, USA). After preparing and evaluating the prepared formulations, the data were statistically analyzed using one-way analysis of variance (ANOVA) to determine the significance of each variable for the p-value and F-ratio for each variable. The goal of the optimization was to minimize the disintegration time (Y_1) and the thickness (Y_2) and maximize the folding endurance (Y_3) of the film.

Table 1. Level of variables incorporated into the central composite design and their attributes.

Independent Variables	Levels		
	Low	Medium	High
X_1 = film-forming polymer (HPMC) %	1	2	3
X_2 = plasticizer (PEG 400) %	1	1.5	2
Dependent Variables	Constraints		
	Low	High	Goal
Y_1 = disintegration time (s)	26	62	Minimize
Y_2 = thickness (mm)	0.11	0.31	Minimize
Y_3 = folding endurance	155	456	Maximize

Table 2. Layout of the experimental matrix of RSV-FDFs, with the independent and dependent variables proposed as suggested by the central composite design.

Run Code	Independent Variables		Dependent Variables		
	HPMC % (X_1)	PEG 400 (X_2)	Disintegration Time (Y_1), s	Thickness (Y_2), mm	Folding Endurance (Y_3)
F1	0.59	1.5	26	0.11	189
F2	3.0	2.0	55	0.28	420
F3	3.0	1.0	49	0.27	320
F4	2.0	1.5	36	0.22	350
F5	2.0	1.5	37	0.23	354
F6	3.41	1.5	62	0.31	444
F7	1.0	1.0	29	0.14	229
F8	2.0	2.21	38	0.24	456
F9	1.0	2.0	30	0.15	269
F10	2.0	0.79	34	0.20	155

2.2.2. Preparation of RSV-FDFs

The films were prepared using the solvent-casting technique described before [22,24,25]. First, the required amount of HPMC (X_1) was dispersed in 10 mL of water containing the sweetener and flavoring agent using a mechanical shaker (IKA, Staufen, Germany) for 6 h until completely dissolved. Conversely, RSV was dissolved in 5 mL of methanol solution in water (50% v/v). Then, both solutions were transferred into a beaker centered on a magnetic stirrer (IKA, Germany) and stirred for 30 min after adding the plasticizer (X_2) and filling the volume to 25 mL. Then, the mixture was transferred to an ultrasonic bath for 15 min to degas, poured into a suitable glass dish, preserved in a refrigerator for 12 h to complete the swelling of the polymer, and then placed in an oven for 2 h at 40 °C for drying. The dried films were cut into strips, each of which contained 10 mg RSV.

2.2.3. Characterization of RSV-FDFs

Physical Appearance

The physical appearance of the prepared RSV-FDFs was inspected for transparency, air bubbles, and color uniformity [21].

Content Uniformity, Average Weight, and Thickness

The average weight of three units was determined using a semi-micro analytical balance (Sartorius, Göttingen, Germany). Then, the thickness of these films was determined using a vernier caliber in three different places for each film. The average and the standard deviation were calculated and recorded [26].

Three units were selected at random from each formulation and dissolved in 100 mL of 20 mM phosphate buffer of pH 6.8. The obtained solution was measured spectrophotometrically at 242 nm using a UV instrument (UV1900, Shimadzu, Kyoto, Japan) [27].

Folding Endurance, Tensile Strength, and Elongation Percentage

The tensile strength, elongation percentage, and folding endurance were used to examine the film's flexibility and durability. The folding endurance was determined by folding the film at an angle of 180° at one point until the film was deformed [28–30].

Using a laboratory-made instrument fabricated with two clamps, one of which was stabilized and fixed and the other freely moveable. A set of 10 gram weights was attached successively to the moveable part until the cracking or breaking of the film was examined. The tensile strength is the force applied to break the film by the Newton unit (N) over the cross-sectional area in square centimeters (cm^2), as depicted in Equation (1).

The elongation percentage is determined by dividing the increment in length by the original length and then multiplying by 100, as described in Equation (2) [21,31].

$$\text{Tensile strength} = \frac{\text{Force applied (N)}}{\text{Cross sectional area (cm}^2\text{)}} \quad (1)$$

$$\text{Elongation percentage} = \frac{\text{Increment in length}}{\text{Original lenght}} \times 100 \quad (2)$$

Surface pH

The film pH was determined by placing the film in a suitable dish and wetting it with distilled water, then measuring the pH by immersing the electrode of the calibrated pH meter into the surface of the wetted film (Schott lab 850, Mainz, Germany) [32].

In Vitro Disintegration

The prepared films were tested for their in vitro disintegration by two methods. The first was adding a film strip to the disintegration tester (Copley Scientific Limited, Nottingham, UK) containing 900 mL of deionized Milli Q water (Millipore, Molsheim, France) at 37 °C. Then, the time for complete film disintegration was determined in triplicate [20]. The second was using the Petri dish method by adding a film strip to a Petri dish containing 3 mL of simulated salivary fluid (SSF) of pH 6.8 and applying gentle stirring to mimic the oral cavity condition; the time to disintegration was calculated with a stopwatch [33].

In Vitro Dissolution

The dissolution of RSV from the prepared films was determined by placing 3 units each of 10 mg from all formulas into a rotating basket (Apparatus I) rotated at 50 rpm in a 100 mL simulated salivary solution of pH 6.8. The dissolution tester (Logan, UT, USA) was maintained at 37 °C, and 5 mL samples were withdrawn after 2 min and suitably diluted before analysis to determine the RSV content using a UV spectrophotometer (Schimadzu, Japan) at 242 nm.

2.2.4. In Vivo Pharmacokinetics Evaluation on Male Wistar Rats

Study Design

A one-period, open-label, single-dose, randomized, parallel design was implemented in the study. Two groups of male Wistar rats (6 rats per group) were administered a single dose of 20 mg/kg of the optimized RSV–FDF (test). At the same time, the marketed Crestor® tablets (reference) (AstraZeneca, Cairo, Egypt) were administered in the same dose orally with water. The study was carried out at the International Center for Bioavailability, Pharmaceutical, and Clinical Research (ICBR, Cairo, Egypt). The Institutional Review Board/Independent Ethics Committee (IRB/IEC) at the ICBR formally reviewed the proposed study's objective, design, conduct, and analysis. It approved the study protocol on 25 June 2022 with Ethical Approval Code RESH-0026.

Animal Handling and Blood Sampling

The animals were maintained in a controlled temperature with half-day morning and half-day night with access to food and water. At the time of administration, both formulations (RSV-FDF and oral tablets) were dissolved in 1% carboxymethyl cellulose. The corrected dose for each rat was administered orally using a gastric tube. Then, blood samples were collected in the following intervals: 0.5, 1, 2, 4, 6, 8, 12, 24, 36, 48, and 72 h. After each withdrawal interval, the samples were centrifugated for 10 min at 6000 RPM using a calibrated centrifuge (Eppendorf, Hamburg, Germany) and then frozen at −80 °C (Thermo, Sindelfingen, Germany). After the experiment, the samples were analyzed by the protein precipitation method. After thawing the samples and preparing the calibration curve from 25–3000 ng/mL, the samples, calibration, and quality control samples

(QCs) were precipitated using acetonitrile (1:1) and then the samples were vortexed for 20 min at 5000 RPM. The resulting supernatant was transferred to high-performance liquid chromatography (HPLC) vial inserts.

Chromatographic Conditions

A volume of 50 µL was injected into the chromatographic system conditioned by a gradient elution of 0.1% phosphoric acid and acetonitrile with a Waters C18 stationary-phase Xbridge 250 × 4.6 mm with a 5 µm particle size. The R^2 of the calibration line could not be less than 0.99, and the QC samples recovery needed to lie between 85 and 115%. The lower limit of quantitation was 25 ng/mL, and three quality control levels were determined in the following concentrations: 100, 1000, and 2000 ng/mL for QCL, QCM, and QCH, respectively. Then, the linearity equation was applied to determine the sample concentration after injecting the samples into a high-performance liquid chromatography apparatus (Waters, Milford, MA, USA) equipped with a PDA detector (Waters, Milford, MA, USA) maintained at 242 nm using Empower 3 software.

Pharmacokinetics Data Analysis

With the aid of the pharmacokinetics add-in PKsolver 2.0 software, the following parameters were measured and utilized to estimate the extravascular non-compartmental pharmacokinetics model: the time point of maximum drug concentration (T_{max}), the highest concentration of RSV (C_{max}), and the AUC, which is the area under the plasma concentration-time curve for each of the following: AUC_{0-t}: from the 0–time point to the last measurable concentration using the trapezoidal method and $AUC_{0-\infty}$: the area under the concentration-time curve from the 0–time point to infinity. This was calculated via summation of the ratio of the last concentration in the plasma over the elimination rate constant with $AUC_{0-\infty}$, the area under the moment curve from zero, to the final AUMC, as well as the mean residence time (MRT). This was calculated by plotting the AUMC over the AUC and the total body clearance (Cl), which is calculated by plotting the dose per AUC. Also, the T half elimination ($T_{1/2}$) was determined, which is calculated by dividing 0.693 by the K_{el}, the elimination rate constant (K_{el}). The apparent volume of distribution after non-intravenous administration at the terminal phase (Vd) was achieved by multiplying the total body clearance by the MRT. The relative bioavailability for the RSV-FDF versus the commercial tablets was calculated by dividing the AUC of the RSV-FDF by the AUC of the market tablets ×100.

2.2.5. In Vivo Anti-Dyslipidemic Activity

The anti-dyslipidemic activity of the optimized RSV-FDF was compared with the marketed Crestor® tablets. Male Wistar rats were used after injection with Poloxamer 407 to induce dyslipidemia 24 h before the experiment. Then, the rats were divided into three groups (3 rats per group). The optimized RSV-FDF was administered to the first group; marketed tablets were administrated to the second and third groups with no treatment as a model dyslipidemic group. Blood samples were taken at 0, 2, 6, 12, and 24 h and allowed to settle, and the serum was collected and analyzed to determine the lipid parameters (triglycerides, total cholesterol, LDLs, VLDLs, and HDLs). The in vitro diagnostic kits were used with the enzymatic colorimetric method for evaluation (Abcam Colorimetric/Fluorometric, ab65390, Waltham, Boston, USA).

2.2.6. Statistical Analysis

The data for the pharmacokinetic and anti-dyslipidemic activities were statistically analyzed using GraphPad Prism 8 (GraphPad Software, Inc., La Jolla, CA, USA) as mean ± SD. Two-way analysis of variance (ANOVA) followed by Tukey's multiple comparisons test was used to identify the significant difference between the studied groups. A p-value of less than 0.05 was statistically significant. The statistical significance between the pharmacokinetic parameters was determined using the Holm–Sidak method.

3. Results and Discussion

In the current work, optimized RSV-FDFs were developed by tailoring a polymeric matrix with the aid of hydroxypropyl methylcellulose and the plasticizing effect of glycerin. The formulation factors were investigated to determine their effects on the quality of the prepared FDFs and predict the optimum levels that produce the optimized formulation with the desired quality attributes. This optimized RSV-FDF was evaluated for its pharmacokinetic behavior and anti-dyslipidemic activity.

3.1. Formulation and Evaluation of RSV-FDFs

The evaluation of the prepared films' physicomechanical properties is provided in Table 3. The films were found to be soft, clear, thin, and colorless, with no bubbles entrapped, and there were no issues during removal from the dish or the cutting procedures. The film clarity demonstrates that the drug was already soluble in the film polymer and thus supports the results of in vitro dissolution, which demonstrated immediate release after the disintegration of the film.

Table 3. Physical characterization of the prepared RSV-FDF batches.

Run Code	Surface pH	Average Weight (g)	Tensile Strength (N/cm^2)	Percent Elongation (%)	Dissolution after 2 min (%)	RSV Content (%)
F1	6.5	0.02	1.765	10	98.61	103.69
F2	6.53	0.11	1.852	80	105.22	105.39
F3	6.6	0.10	1.843	64	105.56	103.88
F4	6.62	0.08	1.814	74	101.79	104.91
F5	6.6	0.08	1.816	72	105.69	105.16
F6	6.6	0.12	1.872	88	101.52	105.37
F7	6.58	0.03	1.758	16	98.68	104.72
F8	6.61	0.09	1.828	76	100.33	105.33
F9	6.62	0.03	1.778	70	97.22	105.55
F10	6.58	0.07	1.807	20	102.65	104.97

Note: mean ± SD used to present the data (n = 3).

To assess the uniformity of the RSV distribution within the formula, five different places in each formula were analyzed to determine the drug content in each formula, and the results show that the drug was distributed uniformly throughout the films and within the accepted and required compendial specifications, with an RSD% of less than 10%. Also, the uniformity of weight in all films yielded an acceptable RSD%.

As the normal pH range of saliva lies between 6.2 and 7.6 [21], any acidic or basic pH distortion from normal salivary pH will cause irritation and patient noncompliance with the treatment protocol. All prepared films revealed a pH range of 6.5–6.62, ensuring no irritation to the oral cavity upon administration.

3.1.1. Tensile Strength and Elongation Percentage

Table 3 shows no variability in the tensile strength (1.765–1.872 N/cm^3) of the prepared films and no breakage of any of the films during the test, confirming the satisfactory mechanical property of the films.

Elongation percentage is typically a useful tool for describing the mechanical characteristics of film. Soft films are those that have low elongation percentages and tensile strengths. A soft and tough film has high tensile strength and high elongation, whereas a hard and brittle film has moderate tensile strength and low elongation [34]. In order to increase the elasticity and decrease the brittleness of the film, it is crucial to employ the right amount of plasticizer. According to the data in Table 3, the elongation percentage for F-1 and F-6 ranged from 10 to 88%, respectively. The HPMC percentage in the film strongly impacted this result. Also, the film's PEG 400% was the most important factor, positively increasing the elongation percentage. The increased viscosity and brittleness of the manufactured films calls for more plasticizer use [35]. The plasticizer's positive impact on elasticity can be explained by how it works to weaken the forces that hold polymer chains together, interrupt polymer chains, increase chain mobility, and improve the flexibility of the polymeric matrix, softening and extending the film matrix as previously reported [36–38].

3.1.2. In Vitro Dissolution

The release of rosuvastatin from the films was rapid and precise, and all formulations showed complete dissolution within the first two minutes, as shown in Table 3. Thus, this may indicate the enhanced water solubility of the drug via dispersion with the polymer. Along with the use of water-soluble inert fillers that were reported to be used to form a highly water-soluble dispersion with active ingredients, the same also appeared with Choi et al., who correlated the solubility improvement of poorly soluble rivaroxaban to the dispersion of the drug in the polymeric solution [39].

3.2. Optimization of RSV-FDFs

Ten experimental runs were suggested by a 2^{2+star} central composite design to demonstrate the effect of the following independent variables: polymer percentage (X_1) from 1 to 3% and plasticizer percentage (X_2) from 1 to 2% on the disintegration time (Y_1), and thickness (Y_2) and folding endurance (Y_3) of the prepared films.

3.2.1. Estimation of the Quantitative Effects

Table 4 shows the statistical analysis of variance (ANOVA) of the Y_1–Y_3 response results. The factor effects of the model, F-ratio, and associated p-values for the responses are presented. A positive sign of the estimate indicates a synergistic effect, whereas a negative sign represents an antagonistic effect of the factor on the selected response. The table shows that X_1 and X_2 significantly synergistically affected all Y_1–Y_3 responses with p-values of less than 0.05.

Table 4. Statistical analysis of variance (ANOVA) of the Y_1–Y_3 response results.

Factors	Disintegration Time (Y_1), s			Thickness (Y_2), mm			Folding Endurance (Y_3)		
	Estimate	F-Ratio	p-Value	Estimate	F-Ratio	p-Value	Estimate	F-Ratio	p-Value
X_1	23.98	739.58	0.0001 *	0.14	443.28	0.0001 *	150.66	15.17	0.0176 *
X_2	3.16	12.88	0.0230 *	0.02	8.82	0.0412 *	141.42	13.36	0.0217 *
X_1X_1	7.88	45.59	0.0025 *	−0.02	4.21	0.1094	−36.25	0.50	0.5178
X_1X_2	2.50	4.02	0.1155	0.00	0.00	1.0000	30.00	0.30	0.6126
X_2X_2	−0.13	0.01	0.9198	−0.01	0.77	0.4288	−47.25	0.85	0.4081
R^2		99.51			99.13			88.17	
Adj. R^2		98.89			98.04			73.37	
SEE		1.25			0.009			54.71	
MAE		0.68			0.005			28.98	

Note: * Significant effect of factors on individual responses (p-value less than 0.05). Abbreviations: X_1, film-forming polymer (HPMC) %; X_2, plasticizer (PEG 400) %; X_1X_2, the concept describing how the factors interact; X_1X_1, and X_2X_2 are the quadratic terms between the factors; R^2, R-squared; Adj-R^2, adjusted R-squared; SEE, standard error of estimate; and MAE, mean absolute error.

The contour plots (Figure 1) demonstrate how several independent variables affected the responses of Y_1–Y_3. The response surface plots (Figure 2) made comparing each factor's impact at a specific location in the design space easier. Plotting the response involved varying just one element over its range while keeping the other variables constant. The plot was plotted by Statgraphics® 18 Centurion Software (Warrenton, VA, USA). These figures supplied information relating to the major contribution and influence of the factors on the responses. Figures 1 and 2 declare that the effect of the polymer and plasticizer had a major effect on the prepared films.

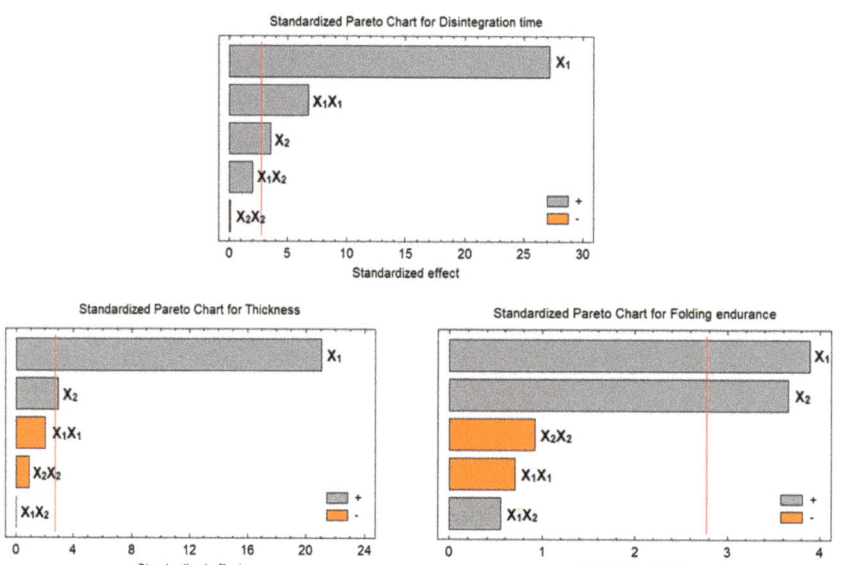

Figure 1. Pareto charts showing the effects of different variables on the responses of Y_1–Y_3. All the factors exceed the red line has a significant effect on the studied response.

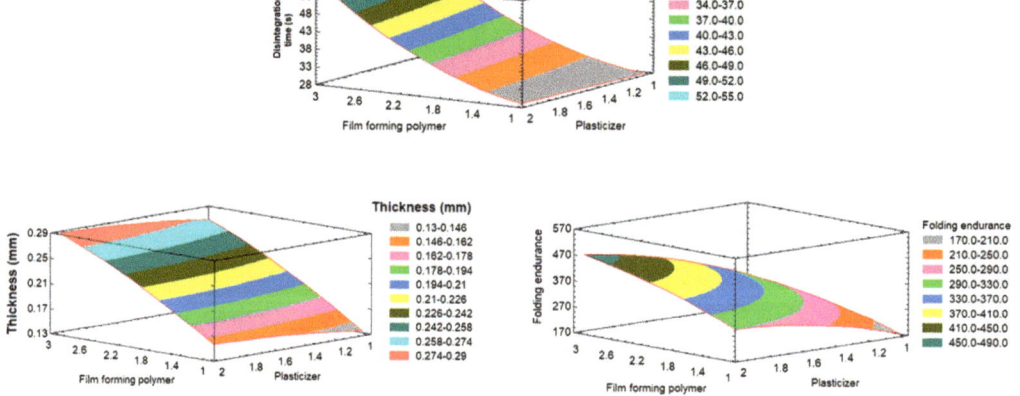

Figure 2. Effect of different variables (Y_1–Y_3) on the responses represented in the response surface plots.

Effect on the In Vitro Disintegration (Y_1):

Regarding Y_1, all formulas yielded a response of < 60 s except for F6, which disintegrated after 62 s; this may have been because of its higher content of HPMC, as reported by Rédai et al. [16]. The generated polynomial equation for Y_1 is presented in Equation (3).

$$\text{In vitro disintegration time } (Y_1) = 30.46 - 7.51\, X_1 - 1.09\, X_2 + 3.94\, X_1^2 + 2.5\, X_1 X_2 - 0.25\, X_2^2 \tag{3}$$

The dependent variable responded positively when the concentration of the independent variables X_1 and X_2 increased, as seen in Figures 1 and 2.

The fast disintegration of the films at a low HPMC content (1%) could be explained by the fact that when polymeric content increased, the viscosity of the film increased, resulting in prolonged disintegration time [18,40].

The concentration of plasticizer (X_2) had an impact on the fast-dissolving films' in vitro disintegration as well, and there was a clear correlation as the plasticizer concentration increased. This behavior could be attributed to the increase in viscosity [21].

Effect on the Film Thickness

The average thickness of the films ranged from 0.11 to 0.31 mm. The film thickness, determined by a Vernier caliber, demonstrates the direct relationship between the percentage of polymer and the thickness of the film. When the polymer percentage increased, the thickness increased. The lowest polymer % in F1 had a thickness of 0.11 mm, and the highest polymer percentage in F6 had a thickness of 0.31 mm. These results were consistent with previously published data that related fast-dissolving film thickness to the percentage of polymer added [32,41]. The low polymeric content could explain the films' thickness at a low HPMC content (1%), causing water to easily evaporate and leading to thin film [42].

The polynomial equation generated for Y_2 is presented in Equation (4).

$$\text{Film thickness } (Y_2) = -0.008 + 0.103\, X_1 + 0.06\, X_2 - 0.009\, X_1^2 + 0.0\, X_{1\times 2} - 0.015\, X_2^2 \quad (4)$$

Effect on the Folding Endurance

The durability of each formula was found to be related to the polymer and plasticizer content. The lowest amount of plasticizer, 0.79% in F10, displayed the lowest folding endurance of 155 times before breakage, whereas F8, containing 2.21% plasticizer, was folded up to 456 times with no breakage. Usually, good film can be folded 300 times or more [19]. The polynomial equation generated for Y_3 is presented in Equation (5).

$$\text{Folding endurance } (Y_3) = -205.91 + 102.83\, X_1 + 364.92\, X_2 - 18.13\, X_1^2 + 30.0\, X_{1\times 2} - 94.49\, X_2^2 \quad (5)$$

The response of Y_3 ranged from 155 to 456 times for all formulations. Both X_1 and X_2 had significant model terms and showed positive responses due to increases in impart flexibility to the film, i.e., as the amount of polymer and plasticizer increased, the folding endurance also increased (Figures 1 and 2).

The folding endurance of the films at a low content of HPMC (1%) could be related to the other effect of polymer on the thickness as the polymer decreases, yielding thin film that is more brittle compared to moderately thick film [31,43].

The content of plasticizer (X_2) had an impact on the folding endurance of fast-dissolving films (FDF), and there was a direct correlation as plasticizer concentration increased. This behavior could be attributed to the effect of plasticizer, which is added to increase film's elasticity, as it works by adding more viscosity and elasticity to the film [43].

3.2.2. Preparation and Evaluation of Optimized Formula

According to the statistical analysis for the prepared formulations, the optimized formula achieved the lowest thickness and disintegration time and the highest folding endurance, achieved with 1.15% polymer and 2.1% plasticizer. The optimized formula yielded 0.17 mm thickness, 30 s disintegration time, and 320 times sustainability versus folding. Also, it had a surface pH of 6.6 and was completely dissolved within 2 min.

3.3. In Vivo Pharmacokinetics Evaluation

The plasma concentration-time curve acquired after dosing male Wistar rats with 20mg/kg rosuvastatin from the commercial product (M) and fast-dissolving film formula (F) is demonstrated in Figure 3. The pharmacokinetic parameters were calculated using WinNonLin® 8.2 software (Princeton, NJ, USA) and are listed in Table 5. The absorption was monitored for a period of 72 h. The differences in T_{max} were used to evaluate these data. The RSV-FDF formula showed faster release, which was revealed in the reduction of the T_{max}, and the extent of the absorbed drug improved, which appeared as a higher C_{max} for the RSV-FDF (1.540 ± 0.044 µg/mL) and as 0.940 ± 0.017 µg/mL for the marketed product. In comparison to the commercial formula, relative bioavailability improved by 32.5%.

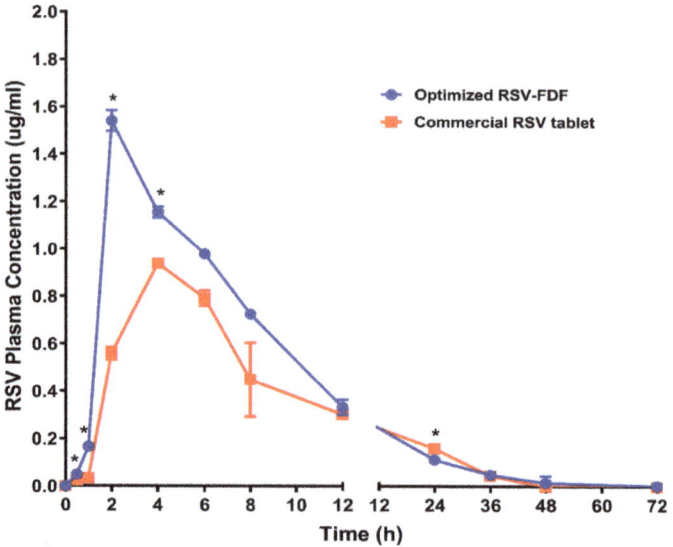

Figure 3. Rosuvastatin calcium plasma time concentration curves after administration of optimized RSV-FDFs and commercial RSV tablets. Data represent the mean value ± standard deviation (SD). * Significant at $p < 0.05$.

Table 5. Pharmacokinetic parameters of the optimized RSV-FDF versus the marketed RSV tablet after administration of 20 mg/kg in rats orally (n = 6, data expressed as average ± SD).

Parameter	Unit	Optimized RSV-FDFs		Marketed RSV Tablets	
		Average	STDEV	Average	STDEV
Lambda_z	1/h	0.072	0.020	0.084	0.004
$t_{1/2}$	h	10.172	2.716	8.231	0.417
T_{max}	h	2.000	0.000	4.000	0.000
C_{max}	µg/mL	1.540 *	0.044	0.940	0.017
AUC_{0-t}	µg/mL.h	13.680 *	0.622	10.320	0.531
AUC_{0-inf}	µg/mL.h	14.178 *	0.331	10.874	0.589
$AUMC_{0-inf}$	µg/mL.h^2	166.681	27.408	141.365	6.273
MRT_{0-inf}	h	11.731	1.656	13.005	0.188
Vz	(mg)/(µg/mL)	20.629	5.057	21.894	1.803
Cl	(mg)/(µg/mL)/h	1.411 *	0.033	1.843	0.102

Note: * denotes a significant difference between values of the optimized RSV-FDF and values of the marketed RSV tablet at $p < 0.05$.

Furthermore, the multiple *t*-test using the Holm–Sidak method revealed that C_{max}, AUC_{0-t}, AUC_{0-inf}, and the clearance (Cl) showed significant differences between the optimized RSV-FDF and the commercial oral tablet, with *p*-values of 0.000025, 0.002059, 0.001063, and 0.002239, respectively.

The improvement in T_{max} directly referred to the origin of the formula of the RSV-FDF containing the rosuvastatin in the dissolved state, so there was only 1 min for average disintegration with no dissolution time required. At the same time, the marketed product needed more time for the disintegration and dissolution stages. The improvement in the RSV-FDF is also referred to as bypassing the first pass effect and protecting rosuvastatin from degradation in acidic media.

3.4. In Vivo Pharmacodynamics Evaluation

The hypolipidemic activity of rosuvastatin was referenced to prevent the synthesis of mevalonic acid from its precursor HMG-COA by inhibiting the enzyme HMG COA reductase, which decreases the lipid profile.

To study the efficiency of the RSV-FDF on the lipid profile (triglycerides, total cholesterol, LDLs, VLDLs, and HDLs) in rats with induced hyperlipidemia, Poloxamer 407 was administered to male Wistar rats 24 h prior to the experiment by to induce hyperlipidemia; then, the rats categorized into three groups (n = 3): negative control (C), commercial product (M), and RSV-FDF (O). Then, zero time samples were collected from each group to define the baseline for each parameter and the efficacy was determined for the O group, which showed a decrease in total cholesterol of 68.1% after 6 h from the zero time point, which is a significant difference in comparison to the M group, as the total cholesterol was reduced by 58.2% and the reduction In total cholesterol persisted for 24 h. The level of triglycerides also decreased by 56.4% for the O group, whereas the M group's level of triglycerides was reduced by 37.6%. Also, for the LDLs, the O group showed better performance, as after 6 h, the level of LDLs in the O group decreased by about 60.6% compared to 50% in the marketed group. The following Figure 4 shows the graphical representation of the different parameters of the lipid profiles in the three groups.

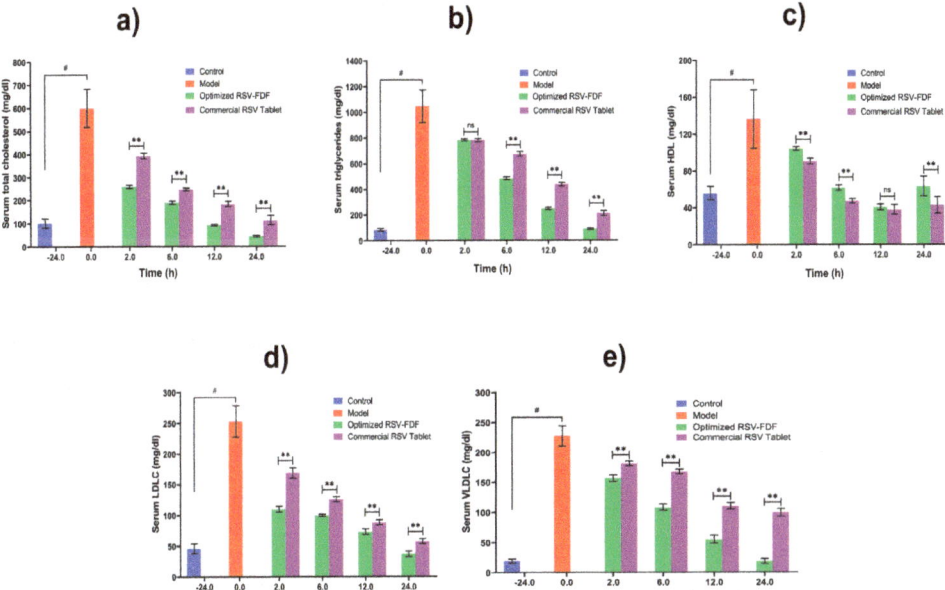

Figure 4. Lipid profiles of induced hyperlipidemic rats after single-dose administration of optimized RSV-FDFs and commercial RSV tablets. Data are presented as mean ± SD (n = 3). Note: # denotes a significant difference between normal and model at $p < 0.05$, ** denotes a significant difference between the optimized RSV-FDF and the commercial RSV tablets at $p < 0.01$, and ns denotes a non-significant difference. (**a**) the total serum cholesterol level in mg/dl, (**b**) the total serum triglyceride level mg/dl, (**c**) the serum HDL level mg/dl, (**d**) the serum LDL level mg/dl, and (**e**) the serum VLDL level mg/dl.

4. Conclusions

The prepared fast-dissolving film formula containing rosuvastatin (RSV-FDF) yielded acceptable results regarding in vitro characterization and evaluation. The pharmacokinetics supported these findings, which revealed a significant improvement in relative bioavailability of 32.5%. The pharmacodynamic experiments also showed significant improvements for RSV-FDF compared to the commercial rosuvastatin tablets of a 50% reduction in triglyceride levels and a 21% reduction in LDL values. Therefore, the RSV-FDF can be considered a promising substitute for commercial tablets, although additional studies in humans and extra stability determinations should be carried out in the future.

Author Contributions: Conceptualization, K.M.E.-S. and I.A.; methodology, I.A. and K.M.E.-S.; software, K.M.E.-S., I.A. and P.A.H.; validation, S.G., K.M.E.-S. and P.A.H.; formal analysis, S.G., P.A.H. and K.M.E.-S.; investigation, I.A., P.A.H., S.G. and F.I.A.-A.; resources, I.A. and K.M.E.-S.; data curation, P.A.H., S.G. and F.I.A.-A.; writing—original draft preparation, I.A. and K.M.E.-S.; writing—review and editing, I.A., P.A.H., S.G., F.I.A.-A. and K.M.E.-S.; visualization, I.A. and K.M.E.-S.; supervision, P.A.H., S.G. and F.I.A.-A.; project administration, K.M.E.-S.; funding acquisition, K.M.E.-S. All authors have read and agreed to the published version of the manuscript.

Funding: This research work was funded by Institutional Fund Projects under grant No. IFPIP: 233-166-1443. The authors gratefully acknowledge the technical and financial support provided by the Ministry of Education and King Abdulaziz University, DSR, Jeddah, Saudi Arabia.

Institutional Review Board Statement: The study was conducted and approved by the International Center for Bioavailability, Pharmaceutical, and Clinical Research (ICBR), Cairo, Egypt, with Ethical Approval Code RESH-0026.

Informed Consent Statement: Not applicable.

Data Availability Statement: Data are contained within the article.

Conflicts of Interest: The authors declare no conflict of interest.

References

1. Mosca, S.; Araújo, G.; Costa, V.; Correia, J.; Bandeira, A.; Martins, E.; Mansilha, H.; Tavares, M.; Coelho, M.P. Dyslipidemia Diagnosis and Treatment: Risk Stratification in Children and Adolescents. *J. Nutr. Metab.* **2022**, *2022*, 1–10. [CrossRef] [PubMed]
2. Su, X.; Peng, H.; Chen, X.; Wu, X.; Wang, B. Hyperlipidemia and hypothyroidism. *Clin. Chim. Acta* **2022**, *527*, 61–70. [CrossRef] [PubMed]
3. Ahmed, T.A.; Elimam, H.; Alrifai, A.O.; Nadhrah, H.M.; Masoudi, L.Y.; Sairafi, W.O.; M.El-Say, K. Rosuvastatin lyophilized tablets loaded with flexible chitosomes for improved drug bioavailability, anti-hyperlipidemic and anti-oxidant activity. *Int. J. Pharm.* **2020**, *558*, 119791. [CrossRef] [PubMed]
4. Shih, H.-J.; Lin, K.-H.; Wen, Y.-C.; Fan, Y.-C.; Tsai, P.-S.; Huang, C.-J. Increased risk of bladder cancer in young adult men with hyperlipidemia: A population-based cohort study. *Medicine* **2021**, *100*, e28125. [CrossRef]
5. Staels, B.; Dallongeville, J.; Auwerx, J.; Schoonjans, K.; Leitersdorf, E.; Fruchart, J.-C. Mechanism of action of fibrates on lipid and lipoprotein metabolism. *Circulation* **1998**, *98*, 2088–2093. [CrossRef] [PubMed]
6. Lennernäs, H.; Fager, G. Pharmacodynamics and Pharmacokinetics of the HMG-CoA Reductase Inhibitors. *Clin. Pharmacokinet.* **1997**, *32*, 403–425. [CrossRef] [PubMed]
7. Alshora, D.H.; Ibrahim, M.A.; Elzayat, E.; Almeanazel, O.T.; Alanazi, F. Rosuvastatin calcium nanoparticles: Improving bioavailability by formulation and stabilization codesign. *PLoS ONE* **2018**, *13*, e0200218. [CrossRef]
8. Chizner, M.A.; Duvall, W.L. Highlights of prescribing information crestor (rosuvastatin calcium). *Cardiovasc. Rev. Rep.* **2003**, *24*, 591.
9. Scott, L.J.; Curran, M.P.; Figgitt, D.P. Rosuvastatin. *Am. J. Cardiovasc. Drugs* **2004**, *4*, 117–138. [CrossRef]
10. Elsayed, I.; El-Dahmy, R.M.; Elshafeey, A.H.; El Gawad, N.A.A.; El Gazayerly, O.N. Tripling the bioavailability of rosuvastatin calcium through development and optimization of an In-Situ forming nanovesicular system. *Pharmaceutics* **2019**, *11*, 275. [CrossRef]
11. Butt, S.; Hasan, S.M.F.; Hassan, M.M.; Alkharfy, K.M.; Neau, S.H. Directly compressed rosuvastatin calcium tablets that offer hydrotropic and micellar solubilization for improved dissolution rate and extent of drug release. *Saudi Pharm. J.* **2019**, *27*, 619–628. [CrossRef] [PubMed]
12. Gabr, M.M.; Mortada, S.M.; Sallam, M.A. Carboxylate cross-linked cyclodextrin: A nanoporous scaffold for enhancement of rosuvastatin oral bioavailability. *Eur. J. Pharm. Sci.* **2018**, *111*, 1–12. [CrossRef] [PubMed]

13. González, R.; Peña, M.; Torres, N.S.; Torrado, G. Design, development, and characterization of amorphous rosuvastatin calcium tablets. *PLoS ONE* **2022**, *17*, e0265263. [CrossRef] [PubMed]
14. El-Say, K.M.; Felimban, R.; Tayeb, H.H.; Chaudhary, A.G.; Omar, A.M.; Rizg, W.Y.; Alnadwi, F.H.; I Abd-Allah, F.; Ahmed, T. Pairing 3D-Printing with Nanotechnology to Manage Metabolic Syndrome. *Int. J. Nanomed.* **2022**, *17*, 1783–1801. [CrossRef] [PubMed]
15. Zaki, R.M.; Alfadhel, M.; Seshadri, V.D.; Albagami, F.; Alrobaian, M.; Tawati, S.M.; Warsi, M.H.; Almurshedi, A.S. Fabrication and characterization of orodispersible films loaded with solid dispersion to enhance Rosuvastatin calcium bioavailability. *Saudi Pharm. J.* **2023**, *31*, 135–146. [CrossRef]
16. Rédai, E.-M.; Antonoaea, P.; Todoran, N.; Vlad, R.A.; Bîrsan, M.; Tătaru, A.; Ciurba, A. Development and evaluation of fluoxetine fast dissolving films: An alternative for noncompliance in pediatric patients. *Processes* **2021**, *9*, 778. [CrossRef]
17. Reveny, J.; Tanuwijaya, J.; Remalya, A. Formulation of Orally Dissolving Film (ODF) Metoclopramide Using Hydroxy Propyl Methyl Cellulose and Polyvinyl Alcohol with Solvent Casting Method. *Int. J. ChemTech Res.* **2017**, *10*, 316–321.
18. Hamza, M. Development and Evaluation of Orodispersible Films of Lamotrigine: Hydroxypropyl B Cyclodextrin Inclusion Complex. *Al-Azhar J. Pharm. Sci.* **2017**, *56*, 31–46. [CrossRef]
19. Koland, M.; Sandeep, V.; Charyulu, N. Fast Dissolving Sublingual Films of Ondansetron Hydrochloride: Effect of Additives on in vitro Drug Release and Mucosal Permeation. *J. Young- Pharm.* **2010**, *2*, 216–222. [CrossRef]
20. Cho, H.-W.; Baek, S.-H.; Lee, B.-J.; Jin, H.-E. Orodispersible polymer films with the poorly water-soluble drug, olanzapine: Hot-Melt pneumatic extrusion for single-process 3D printing. *Pharmaceutics* **2020**, *12*, 692. [CrossRef]
21. Abdulelah, F.M.; Abdulbaqi, M.R. Fast dissolving film nanocrystal (FDFN) preparation as a new trend for solubility enhancement of poorly soluble class ii drug tenoxicam. *AVFT–Arch. Venez. Farmacol. Ter.* **2021**, *40*, 333–339.
22. Hoffmann, E.M.; Breitenbach, A.; Breitkreutz, J.; Pharm, D. Advances in orodispersible films for drug delivery. *Expert Opin. Drug Deliv.* **2011**, *8*, 299–316. [CrossRef] [PubMed]
23. Geng, Y.; Zhou, F.; Williams, G.R. Developing and scaling up fast-dissolving electrospun formulations based on poly(vinylpyrrolidone) and ketoprofen. *J. Drug Deliv. Sci. Technol.* **2020**, *61*, 102138. [CrossRef]
24. Adrover, A.; Varani, G.; Paolicelli, P.; Petralito, S.; Di Muzio, L.; Casadei, M.A.; Tho, I. Experimental and modeling study of drug release from HPMC-based erodible oral thin films. *Pharmaceutics* **2018**, *10*, 222. [CrossRef] [PubMed]
25. Hosny, K.M.; El-Say, K.M.; Ahmed, O.A. Optimized sildenafil citrate fast orodissolvable film: A promising formula for overcoming the barriers hindering erectile dysfunction treatment. *Drug Deliv.* **2014**, *23*, 355–361. [CrossRef] [PubMed]
26. Rathod, S.; Phansekar, M.; Bhagwan, A.; Surve, G. A Review on mouth dissolving tablets. *Indian Drugs* **2013**, *50*, 5–14. [CrossRef]
27. Maher, E.M.; Ali, A.M.A.; Salem, H.F.; Abdelrahman, A.A. In vitro/in vivo evaluation of an optimized fast dissolving oral film containing olanzapine co-amorphous dispersion with selected carboxylic acids. *Drug Deliv.* **2016**, *23*, 3088–3100. [CrossRef]
28. Wasilewska, K.; Winnicka, K. How to assess orodispersible film quality? A review of applied methods and their modifications. *Acta Pharm.* **2019**, *69*, 155–176. [CrossRef]
29. Vishvakarma, P. Design and development of montelukast sodium fast dissolving films for better therapeutic efficacy. *J. Chil. Chem. Soc.* **2018**, *63*, 3988–3993. [CrossRef]
30. Kumar, A.; Verma, R.; Jain, V. Formulation Development and Evaluation of Fast Dissolving Oral Film of Dolasetron Mesylate. *Asian J. Pharm. Educ. Res.* **2019**, *8*, 38. [CrossRef]
31. Liew KBin Tan, Y.T.F.; Peh, K.K. Effect of polymer, plasticizer and filler on orally disintegrating film. *Drug. Dev. Ind. Pharm.* **2014**, *40*, 110–119. [CrossRef] [PubMed]
32. Elshafeey, A.H.; El-Dahmy, R.M. Formulation and development of oral fast-dissolving films loaded with nanosuspension to augment paroxetine bioavailability: In vitro characterization, ex vivo permeation, and pharmacokinetic evaluation in healthy human volunteers. *Pharmaceutics* **2021**, *13*, 1869. [CrossRef] [PubMed]
33. Olechno, K.; Maciejewski, B.; Głowacz, K.; Lenik, J.; Ciosek-Skibińska, P.; Basa, A.; Winnicka, K. Orodispersible Films with Rupatadine Fumarate Enclosed in Ethylcellulose Microparticles as Drug Delivery Platform with Taste-Masking Effect. *Materials* **2022**, *15*, 2126. [CrossRef] [PubMed]
34. Lin, S.-Y.; Lee, C.-J.; Lin, Y.-Y. Drug-polymer interaction affecting the mechanical properties, adhesion strength and release kinetics of piroxicam-loaded Eudragit E films plasticized with different plasticizers. *J. Control. Release* **1995**, *33*, 375–381. Available online: http://www.sciencedirect.com/science/article/pii/0168365994001098 (accessed on 23 October 2023). [CrossRef]
35. Pichayakorn, W.; Suksaeree, J.; Boonme, P.; Amnuaikit, T.; Taweepreda, W.; Ritthidej, G.C. Deproteinized natural rubber film forming polymeric solutions for nicotine transdermal delivery. *Pharm. Dev. Technol.* **2011**, *18*, 1111–1121. [CrossRef] [PubMed]
36. Rujivipat, S.; Bodmeier, R. Moisture plasticization for enteric Eudragit®L30D-55-coated pellets prior to compression into tablets. *Eur. J. Pharm. Biopharm.* **2012**, *81*, 223–229. [CrossRef]
37. Nesseem, D.I.; Eid, S.; El-Houseny, S. Development of novel transdermal self-adhesive films for tenoxicam, an anti-inflammatory drug. *Life Sci.* **2011**, *89*, 430–438. [CrossRef]
38. Bhupinder, B.; Sarita, J. Formulation and evaluation of fast dissolving sublingual films of Rizatriptan Benzoate. *Int. J. Drug. Dev. Res.* **2012**, *4*, 133–143.
39. Choi, M.-J.; Woo, M.R.; Choi, H.-G.; Jin, S.G. Effects of Polymers on the Drug Solubility and Dissolution Enhancement of Poorly Water-Soluble Rivaroxaban. *Int. J. Mol. Sci.* **2022**, *23*, 9491. [CrossRef]

40. Al-Mogherah, A.I.; Ibrahim, M.A.; Hassan, M.A. Optimization and evaluation of venlafaxine hydrochloride fast dissolving oral films. *Saudi Pharm. J.* **2020**, *28*, 1374–1382. [CrossRef]
41. Centkowska, K.; Ławrecka, E.; Sznitowska, M. Technology of orodispersible polymer films with micronized loratadine—influence of different drug loadings on film properties. *Pharmaceutics* **2020**, *12*, 250. [CrossRef] [PubMed]
42. Basu, B.; Mankad, A.; Dutta, A. Methylphenidate Fast Dissolving Films: Development, Optimization Using Simplex Centroid Design and In Vitro Characterization. *Turk. J. Pharm. Sci.* **2022**, *19*, 251–266. [CrossRef] [PubMed]
43. Bharti, K.; Mittal, P.; Mishra, B. Formulation and characterization of fast dissolving oral films containing buspirone hydrochloride nanoparticles using design of experiment. *J. Drug Deliv. Sci. Technol.* **2018**, *49*, 420–432. [CrossRef]

Disclaimer/Publisher's Note: The statements, opinions and data contained in all publications are solely those of the individual author(s) and contributor(s) and not of MDPI and/or the editor(s). MDPI and/or the editor(s) disclaim responsibility for any injury to people or property resulting from any ideas, methods, instructions or products referred to in the content.

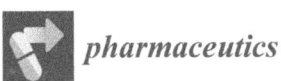

Review

Exploiting Benefits of Vaterite Metastability to Design Degradable Systems for Biomedical Applications

Yulia Svenskaya [1,*] and Tatiana Pallaeva [2,*]

1. Scientific Medical Center, Saratov State University, 410012 Saratov, Russia
2. FSRC "Crystallography and Photonics" RAS, 119333 Moscow, Russia
* Correspondence: svenskaya@info.sgu.ru (Y.S.); borodina@crys.ras.ru (T.P.)

Abstract: The widespread application of calcium carbonate is determined by its high availability in nature and simplicity of synthesis in laboratory conditions. Moreover, calcium carbonate possesses highly attractive physicochemical properties that make it suitable for a wide range of biomedical applications. This review provides a conclusive analysis of the results on using the tunable vaterite metastability in the development of biodegradable drug delivery systems and therapeutic vehicles with a controlled and sustained release of the incorporated cargo. This manuscript highlights the nuances of vaterite recrystallization to non-porous calcite, dissolution at acidic pH, biodegradation at in vivo conditions and control over these processes. This review outlines the main benefits of vaterite instability for the controlled liberation of the encapsulated molecules for the development of biodegradable natural and synthetic polymeric materials for biomedical purposes.

Keywords: calcium carbonate; $CaCO_3$ particles; vaterite; metastability; recrystallization; calcite; degradation; dissolution; pH-sensitivity; resorption; biodegradation; controlled release; ayer-by-layer assembly; calcium ions; carbon dioxide bubbles; ossification; theranostics; anticancer therapy; antimicrobial therapy; US imaging; cavitation; buffering

---

Citation: Svenskaya, Y.; Pallaeva, T. Exploiting Benefits of Vaterite Metastability to Design Degradable Systems for Biomedical Applications. *Pharmaceutics* **2023**, *15*, 2574. https://doi.org/10.3390/pharmaceutics15112574

Academic Editors: Christian Celia, Carlos Alonso-Moreno, Gábor Vasvári and Ádám Haimhoffer

Received: 18 September 2023
Revised: 3 October 2023
Accepted: 12 October 2023
Published: 2 November 2023

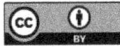

Copyright: © 2023 by the authors. Licensee MDPI, Basel, Switzerland. This article is an open access article distributed under the terms and conditions of the Creative Commons Attribution (CC BY) license (https://creativecommons.org/licenses/by/4.0/).

1. Introduction

Over the recent decades, calcium carbonate-based materials have gained a tremendous interest in a broad range of biomedical applications [1]. Being degradable, biologically compatible and low-cost, $CaCO_3$ is widely used to manufacture drug delivery systems [2–4], biosensors [5], tissue-engineering scaffolds [6,7] and imaging platforms [8,9]. The low toxicity and unique physico-chemical properties of this inert material make it suitable for various routes of administration, whether gastrointestinal, parenteral or topical [2]. Thus, for instance, previous studies have considered its intravenous [10], intramuscular [11] and subcutaneous [12] injection, as well as oral [13], nasal [14], dermal (e.g., intradermal [15] and intrafollicular [16]) and even tracheal [17] administration for the delivery of $CaCO_3$ particles. Calcium carbonate is a highly available material since it abundantly occurs in nature as a component of limestone, marble and chalk in sedimentary rocks and as a content of marine sediments [18] and spring deposits [19]. Furthermore, it can be easily synthesized in the lab choosing the most suitable protocol among a wide range of methods [18,20]. $CaCO_3$ appears in living organisms, e.g., as a component of bones, teeth, shells, coral skeletons and eggshells [21,22] and can also be produced by various bacteria [23], which has opened up the great opportunities for biomimetic synthesis of this material to make it even more safe and compatible for biomedical applications.

Calcium carbonate presents the phenomenon of polymorphism and appears either in crystalline solid forms of anhydrous (calcite, vaterite and aragonite) and hydrated (ikaite and $CaCO_3$ monohydrate) polymorphs, or in amorphous calcium carbonate (ACC) modification [24]. Cubic calcite crystals with rhombohedral lattice and needle-like aragonite crystals with orthorhombic lattice are more thermodynamically stable and, thus, represent the most widespread form of anhydrous $CaCO_3$ [25]. In contrast, mesoporous vaterite polycrystals and ACC are non-stable and can only be found in nature when their surface is stabilized with some additives [26]. In spite of, and even benefitting from such instability, these two forms are highly demanded in biomedicine. ACC comprises the seeds for crystal growth of the other $CaCO_3$ polymorphs and plays a significant role in biomineralization processes [27]. Thus, ACC clusters are effectively used to design the implant materials and coating for the implants [28,29]. Vaterite is metastable and the most soluble $CaCO_3$ polymorph [30]. This material is widely applied to create novel vehicles for drug delivery and templates for therapeutic platforms with a broad range of biomedical applications [2,4].

The crystal structure of vaterite is long being debated. Kabalah-Amitai et al. showed that this form of $CaCO_3$ contains at least two coexisting crystallographic structures forming a pseudo-single crystal [31]. In particular, they stated that vaterite represented a hexagonal lattice structure with the nanodomains of an unknown structure distributed within its matrix. Vaterite rarely occurs as single crystals (both in geologic/biominerals and when synthetically produced) and is often formed as spherulitic polycrystalline aggregates [32]. Due to this feature, vaterite particles are mostly obtained as mesoporous with a large surface area, which is usually around 20 m^2g^{-1} [33,34], but can be increased even up to 200 m^2g^{-1} by varying the reaction medium for its synthesis [35]. The porosity of this material allows for the incorporation of various substances making it especially advantageous in terms of drug, proteins and gene delivery [36]. It should also be noted that vaterite particles are used as carriers on their own or as a part of a composite (hydrogels, fibers and implanted materials), where it is incorporated in order to improve mechanical or therapeutic functions.

Owing to its instability, vaterite can be either transformed into non-porous calcite crystals via dissolution–reprecipitation [37] or even completely dissolved/resorbed, depending on the immersion medium used [16,38]. The release of the incorporated cargo is driven by such transitions. Importantly, the rate of these processes strongly depends on the surrounding conditions, such as the pH [39], temperature [37] and ionic strength [40] of the media and presence of different ions or additives [26,41,42], thus can be controlled externally. Furthermore, depending on the intended use of the vaterite carriers, the payload liberation can either by delayed by means of their surface modification [43,44] or accelerated, e.g., by means of ultrasound treatment [45]. In addition to the transition-driven drug release property, vaterite particles can serve as a source of Ca^{2+} ions. This feature is effectively exploited when creating the scaffolds for bone and tooth tissue regeneration [6,46] due to the ability of calcium ions to improve osteo- and odontoblasts' activity [47]. Moreover, such capability of vaterite to release Ca^{2+} ions is of high importance when designing hydrogels with an autogelation property as far as these cations can efficiently bind polymer chains in hydrogels providing the hydrogel formation [48,49]. In addition, this feature is extensively used to create $CaCO_3$-based hemostatic materials [18,50,51].

Being degradable at mild conditions, vaterite particles are also used as sacrificial templates for the fabrication of other functional materials and biosensors [52]. For instance, layer-by-layer adsorption of biocompatible polyelectrolytes onto these particles together with further dissolution of vaterite cores allows one to fabricate bio-friendly hollow polymer capsules [53]. Vaterite-based templating is also utilized to design porous alginate hydrogels with a well-controlled architecture aiming at fabrication either of drug delivery systems or three-dimensional cell scaffolds [49]. Dissolution of the template in such systems can be achieved by complexation with ethylenediaminetetraacetic acid (**EDTA**) at a neutral pH [54] or by reducing the pH [55] due to the feature of vaterite to decompose rapidly under acidic conditions [38].

Another important outcome of vaterite instability is associated with the generation of carbon dioxide bubbles during dissolution in acidic media. This property determines the potential of $CaCO_3$-based carriers' application in ultrasound imaging and therapy [18]. Besides, the dissolution of vaterite in an acidic environment can increase the local pH due to its regenerative buffering capacity [56]. This effect was shown promising for the use in anticancer therapy, as it enables modulation of the extracellular pH in tumors inducing the cellular metabolic reprogramming [57].

The numerous advantages that we listed above explain the high interest of researchers in calcium carbonate-based materials. To date, a great number of comprehensive reviews have been published that summarize the synthesis techniques and protocols, discuss the main applications of $CaCO_3$ and offer different perspectives on this object [2,3,18,42,58–61]. Nevertheless, none of them emphasized vaterite separately and suggested that attention should be paid to the possibility of using the metastability of this material to advantage. In view of this fact, our review highlights the main benefits of vaterite instability potentiating its employment in the design of degradable systems for biomedical purposes.

2. Incorporation of Various Substances into the Vaterite Matrix

There are two main approaches for the entrapment of functional substances into the calcium carbonate particles, namely: sorption [53] and co-precipitation [62] (Figure 1). The first one is based on the inclusion of drug molecules as a result of their physical sorption in the pores of preformed $CaCO_3$ matrices. In the co-precipitation method, the formation of carbonates occurs in the presence of an active compound resulting in vaterite crystallization with simultaneous inclusion of the active molecules. Both techniques allow the co-immobilization of several bioactive compounds within one particle [2].

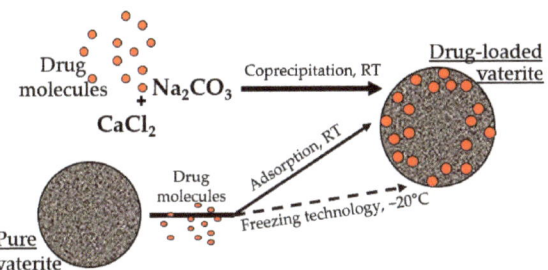

Figure 1. Incorporation of the drug molecules within the vaterite particles by adsorption and co-precipitation methods at room temperature (RT), and via freezing induced loading at −20 °C.

It was demonstrated previously that the loading efficiency by the co-precipitation is higher than by the sorption, especially for high molecular weight molecules of a hydrophilic nature [63,64]. It is probable that during the formation of the particles in the presence of the drug molecules, the encapsulated substance is distributed throughout the entire volume of the carbonate matrix, and during physical sorption, it occurs mainly on its surface [65]. Taking into account the stability of the calcium carbonate in non-polar solvents, the surface sorption of the biologically active substances allows the loading of hydrophobic compounds, which is restricted for the co-precipitation approach [66–68]. Moreover, the entrapment efficacy of the vaterite particles could be enhanced by several methods, including a freezing technology, where successive cycles of freezing and thawing resulted in the substance embedment in the particles' pores by the growing pressure of the forming solvent crystals [69–72]. Various additives during particle synthesis were also utilized to intensify the loading capacity of the carbonate matrices, such as proteins [73–76], polysaccharides [77–81], glycosaminoglycans [82], glycoproteins [63,83], etc. [84–86].

To date, almost all known classes of substances have been successfully loaded into calcium carbonate particles, including but not limited to herbal extracts [65,87], genetic materials [88,89], vaccines [90,91], enzymes and other proteins and peptides [92–96], anti-cancer drugs [58,97], including photosensitizers [38,98] and therapeutic radionuclides [99], antimicrobial compounds [43,100–102] and others [103,104].

3. Vaterite Recrystallization to Calcite: Mechanism and Associated Release of the Loaded Drugs and Calcium Ions

The instability of vaterite manifests itself in contact with water. Being quite stable in the dry state, it dissolves/recrystallizes upon incubation in aqueous solutions [30,105]. In particular, under non-acidic conditions, vaterite easily and irreversibly transforms into calcite form [106]. This transformation takes place through the dissolution of vaterite followed by the nucleation and growth of the calcite crystals (solution-mediated transformation). Such a recrystallization process is gradual and starts at the surface of vaterite particles. Specifically, the external layer of the particles starts to solvate and ionize, the constituent ions (Ca^{2+} and CO_3^{2-}) diffuse away from the surface and then seeds the formation of calcite monocrystals [105]. In such a manner, porous spherical particles reassemble into smooth cubic ones, which are generally larger in size (Figure 2A).

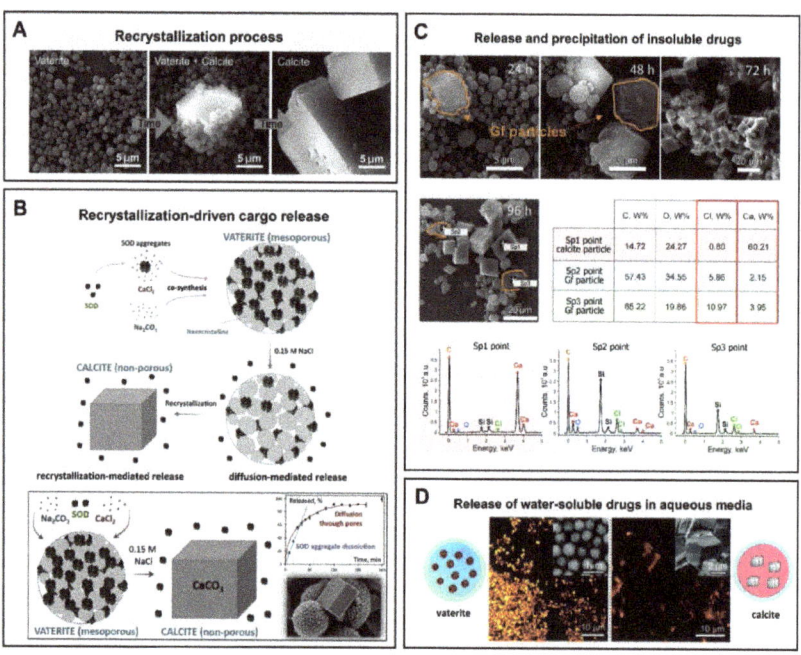

Figure 2. (**A**) Schematic representation of the vaterite–calcite recrystallization process. Reproduced with permission from [101]. (**B**) Schematics for the process of drug liberation from vaterite carriers, which is mediated by the vaterite–calcite recrystallization. Reproduced from Open Access Article [107]. (**C**) Release of water-insoluble drugs from vaterite carriers in aqueous media resulting in the formation of insoluble crystals (particles) by payload molecules. SEM images and results of EDX analysis illustrating the degradation process of the carriers loaded with griseofulvin (Gf) antifungal drug in deionized water. The precipitated Gf particles are contoured with orange. Reproduced with permission from [43]. (**D**) Release of water-soluble drugs from vaterite carriers in aqueous media. Schematics of the release process and corresponding two-photon fluorescence microscopy and SEM (insets) images of the carriers loaded with rhodamine 6G before and after their incubation in water. Adapted with permission from [33].

The rate of the recrystallization process depends on the temperature and ionic strength of the immersion medium [37], as well as on the supersaturation level [108]. Namely, the vaterite–calcite transformation speeds up when these parameters increase. Specifically, at a higher temperature and ionic strength, the ion exchange between the particle surface and the incubation solution is accelerated, which leads to the faster transition to calcite.

Relatively high supersaturation ratios (1.5–1.9) also speeds up this transformation as it is controlled by the vaterite dissolution in this case, whereas at lower supersaturation ratios (1.2–1.5), the rate of dissolution of vaterite is similar with that of the crystallization of calcite [108].

The major practical benefits of the transformation process appears when the vaterite carriers are applied for drug encapsulation and delivery as it opens up the possibility of a degradation-driven release of the payload. It is well-demonstrated that liberation of the loaded molecules from the porous $CaCO_3$ particles results from drug desorption and carrier recrystallization [33,38,107] (Figure 2B). Thus, the release profile represents an interplay of these two processes and strongly depends on the immersion medium [109]. In particular, when the solvent is not payload-specific, the desorption process is obviously slow. In contrast, intensification of this process occurs if a suitable solvent penetrates into the vaterite matrix dissolving the drug, which then diffuses faster in the medium [109]. In addition, vaterite carriers liberate the loaded molecules during their degradation while forming calcite crystals. The released drug can either diffuse into the solvent [43] (Figure 2D) or precipitate out (if its solubility is limited in this media) [43,110] (Figure 2C).

In such a manner, the recrystallization-driven release mechanism allows for control of the payload delivery time by changing the properties of the environment [109]. However, the release rate also depends on the molecular properties of the cargo (e.g., its molecular weight and ζ-potential) [33], carriers' size [38], and method of its loading into vaterite carriers (as this determines the filling density of the particles) [95]. Obviously, the lower the molecular weight of the payload, the smaller the size of the vaterite carriers and the more superficial the drug distribution across the carrier, the faster release occurs.

The virtue of vaterite–calcite recrystallization is successfully employed for intracellular drug delivery. Thus, for instance, Parakhonskiy et al. have demonstrated the possibility of delivering drugs into living cells by means of vaterite carriers exploiting the delayed burst-release mechanism [33]. Furthering this line of research, this team has studied the intercellular behavior of vaterite particles in the cellular cytoplasm [111] (Figure 3). In particular, they have monitored the process of vaterite recrystallization within the cell in real-time by means of confocal Raman and laser scanning microscopies. The formation of the stable calcite phase from the clusters of vaterite particles was registered after 72 h of their incubation with cells, confirming an ion-exchange mechanism of vaterite–calcite transformation inside the cell. Importantly, multiple cytotoxicity studies have revealed that vaterite particles demonstrated no significant influence on the viability or metabolic activity of different cell lines [33,112–114]. That defines the possibility of their application in cellular drug delivery [115–117].

Regarding the intracellular delivery, it is important to note that the immersion media might stabilize the particle surface affecting the crystal phase transition [114]. In particular, it was repeatedly demonstrated that the incubation of vaterite particles in cell culture medium leads to the adsorption of protein molecules from the medium onto their surface [118]. The protein corona formed on the surface of vaterite carriers as a result of such adsorption decelerates the process of their transformation into calcite and hence slows down the rate of the payload release [43,114,119]. This effect commonly occurs in biological fluids when the foreign materials are introduced into the body [120,121]. The beneficial impact of protein corona formation is especially evident in targeted drug delivery. For example, it has been shown that such a prevention of rapid release positively contributed to the drug localization within the cell upon uptake of vaterite carriers [114]. In terms of photodynamic therapy (**PDT**), such an effect enabled the controlled consequential cell destroying by the laser in a point-wise manner [116].

The payload can also affect the process of vaterite–calcite transformation. Thus, the incorporation of proteins into the vaterite matrix might stabilize it, slowing down the transformation to calcite [122]. Namely, the delivery of an antiproliferative lectin (the *Dioclea violacea* lectin, **DVL**) into cancer cells utilizing the recrystallization-driven mechanism resulted in a more pronounced therapeutic effect due to such stabilization, which provided a more constant release over time. The local increase in lectin concentration and a constant exposure of the cells to the lectin was supposed to be responsible for the superior effect observed upon the usage of DVL-loaded vaterite carriers in comparison with DVL solution.

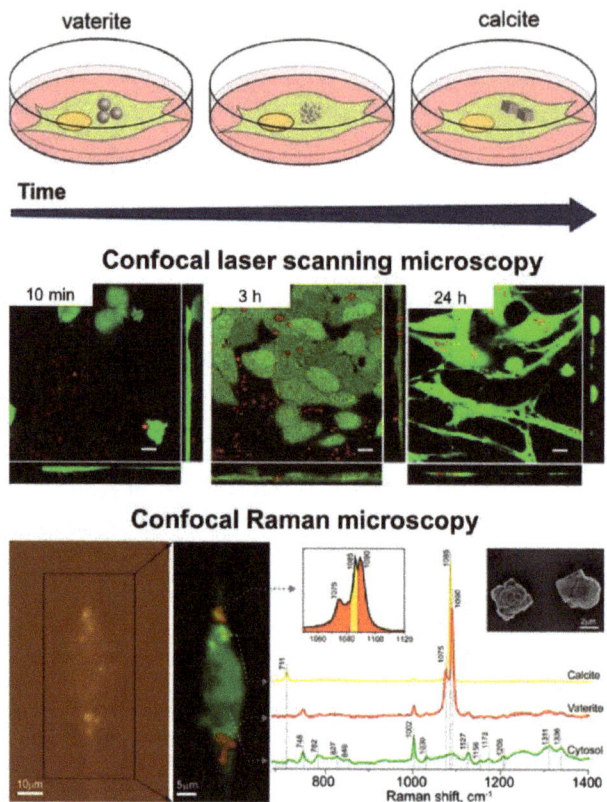

Figure 3. Intracellular recrystallization of vaterite carriers. Schematics of the vaterite–calcite transformation (**the upper row**), CLSM images of HeLa cells after their incubation with the carriers for 10 min, 3 and 24 h (**the middle row**) and the results of Raman analysis of a single cell after 72 h incubation with the carriers (**the bottom row**). Adapted with permission from [111].

It is worth noting that in addition to the transition-driven drug release property, vaterite particles can serve as a source of Ca^{2+} ions while transforming to calcite. This feature has been recently exploited to accelerate the ossification both in vitro [123] and in vivo [6]. In particular, the immobilization and intracellular delivery of alkaline phosphatase (**ALP**) by means of vaterite carriers resulted in improvement of the ossification process in osteoblastic cells as the released ALP and Ca^{2+} ions represent essential components for extracellular matrix formation (Figure 4) [123]. The osteoinductive effect was demonstrated also in vivo when vaterite-coated polycaprolactone (**PCL**) scaffolds were loaded with ALP and implanted into a femoral defect in rats [6]. A significant increase in the osteoblast's synthetic activity and intensification of bone tissue formation was observed due to the effective release of the enzyme and Ca^{2+} ions. This resulted in a complete restoration of the external defect cleft in the rat's femoral bone.

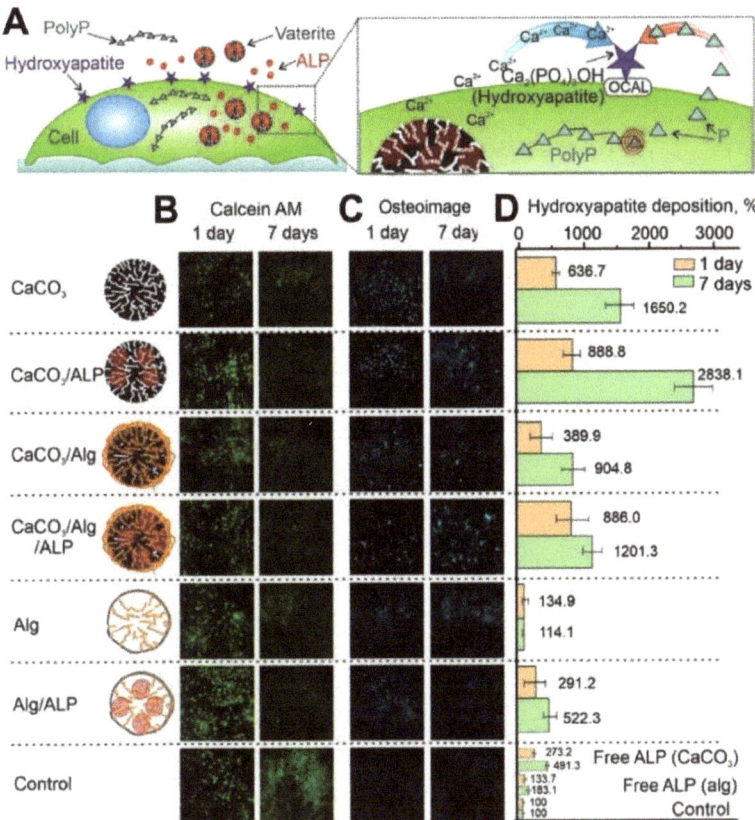

Figure 4. Exploiting of Ca^{2+} release, which occurs during the vaterite–calcite recrystallization, for improvement of the ossification process in vitro. (**A**) Schematic representation of the cellular treatment using vaterite carriers loaded with alkaline phosphatase (ALP). (**B**) Live cells stained by calcein AM (green), (**C**) fixed cells stained by the Osteoimage mineralization assay (Cyan) and (**D**) hydroxyapatite deposition measured at different times using the Osteoimage mineralization assay on MC3T3-E1 cells. Reproduced with permission from [123].

Although vaterite recrystallization to calcite is generally observed in in vitro systems, the calcite formation can also occur during the degradation process at in vivo conditions [7,16]. In particular, at a high local concentration and dense arrangement vaterite particles can aggregate and recrystallize forming cubic-like crystals as the outflow of Ca^{2+} and CO_3^{2-} ions from the carrier surface is not fast enough in this case. Thus, the above-described recrystallization-driven release property might remain actual for vaterite carriers when delivering drugs in vivo as well. For instance, Saveleva et al. demonstrated the liberation of tannic acid from the vaterite-coated PCL fibers in vivo, which took place through the vaterite–calcite recrystallization, lasted for 21 days when the scaffolds were subcutaneously implanted in rats (Figure 5) [7]. In our previous work, dealing with drug administration through the skin appendages (in particular, via hair follicles), in vivo monitoring reveals the active dissolution/recrystallization of vaterite carriers, resulting in their total resorption within 12 days [16]. The proposed particulate system served as an intrafollicular depot for a model drug storage and prolonged in situ release over this period.

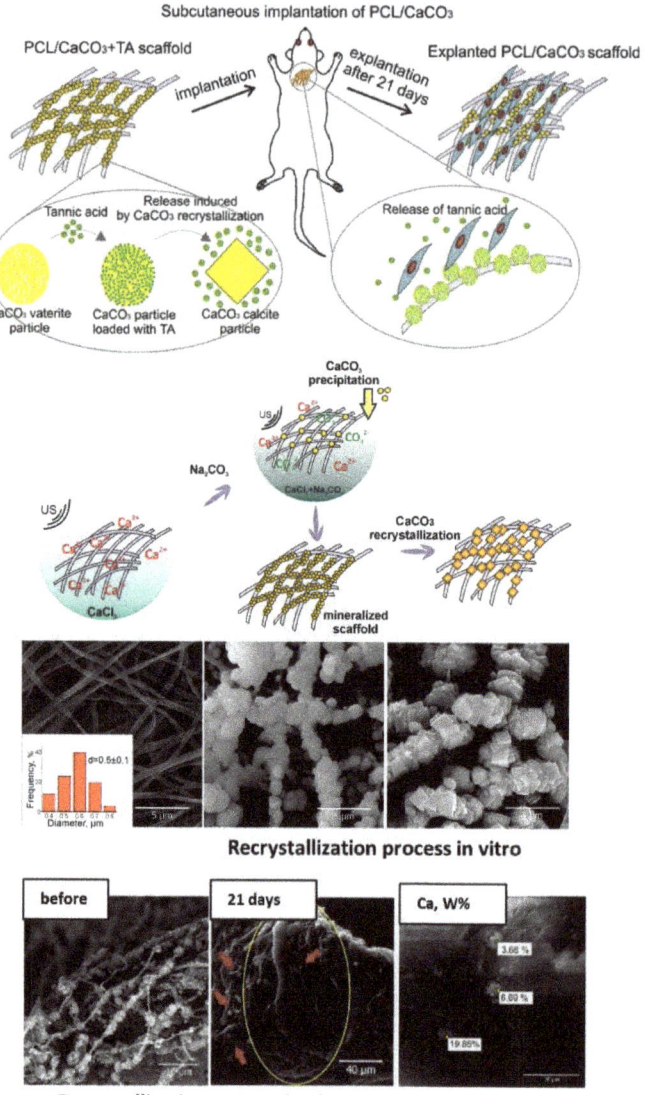

Figure 5. Recrystallization-driven drug release from the vaterite carriers in vivo. Schematic representation of tannic acid (TA) release from the vaterite-coated polycaprolactone (PCL) fibers subcutaneously implanted in rats (**the upper row**). Schematics and SEM images illustrating the process of the vaterite-coating formation and its transformation to calcite in an aqueous medium in vitro (**the middle row**). SEM images and results of EDX analysis illustrating the vaterite–calcite transformation of the fiber coating in vivo (**the lower row**). Reproduced with permission from [7].

It should also be mentioned that even though the main applications of the vaterite–calcite transition are related to the release of the loaded substance, such a transition can still be used, conversely, to incorporate different substances into $CaCO_3$ particles [124,125]. In this case, the drug molecules are captured by calcite crystals formed during the incubation of vaterite particles in aqueous solution. This procedure can be applied when it is necessary to obtain the drug-containing calcite particles.

4. Vaterite Dissolution at Acidic pH: Mechanism, pH-Dependent Release of the Loaded Drugs, Calcium Ions and Carbon Dioxide Bubbles

Besides being transferable to calcite in neutral solutions, vaterite can also decompose rapidly with a decreasing pH (Figure 6A) [126]. For a quarter of a century, this property has been actively used to form hollow polyelectrolyte capsules [127,128]. Vaterite-templated consecutive adsorption of polyelectrolytes followed by the core decomposition is applied for the formation of polyelectrolyte micro- and nanocapsules of various shapes [53,129–131] aiming to deliver a great variety of payloads, from the fluorescent molecules to proteins [64], enzymes [132], different drugs [133] and genetic material [134].

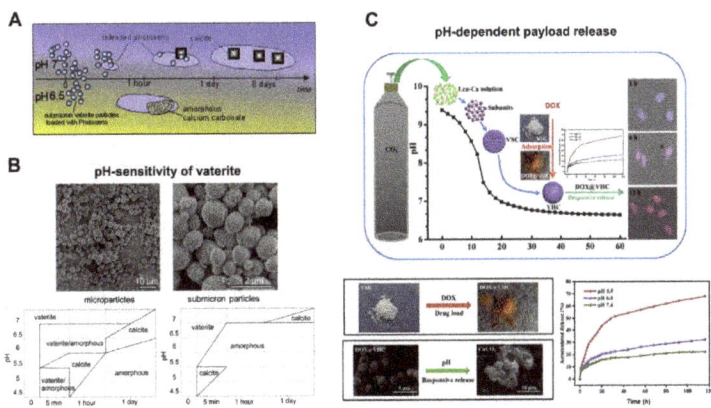

Figure 6. pH-dependent dissolution of vaterite carriers triggering the payload release. (**A**) Schematic representation of the decomposition-mediated drug release process from the vaterite carriers depending on the pH of the medium. Reproduced with permission from [38]. (**B**) SEM images of micro- and submicron vaterite carriers loaded with a photosensitizer before their incubation in various media and the phase-schemes illustrating the process of their transformation in acetate buffers (pH 4.5–6.5) and in water (pH 7.0) during 24 h. Reproduced with permission from [38]. (**C**) Schematics and SEM images illustrating the dissolution of vaterite-based carriers (VHC) and kinetics of the pH-dependent release of the loaded doxorubicin (DOX) drug. Reproduced with permission from [97].

Apart from that, vaterite particles themselves are used as the carriers releasing the loaded substances upon their decomposition in acidic media [44,61]. The dissolution of the carriers starts at their surface, where disintegration of the crystal lattice and hydration of constituent ions takes place [37]. Then, the dissolved matter is transported away from the particle surface into the bulk solution and the cargo molecules are liberated simultaneously. The dissolution-mediated release property granted the successful application of vaterite carriers in drug delivery and sensing [61]. Importantly, the dynamics of such release was demonstrated to be sensitive to the environmental pH [38].

In particular, in the work [38], the drug liberation process was studied by incubating photosensitizer-loaded vaterite carriers of two different sizes at room temperature in acetate buffers with a pH ranging from 4.5 to 6.5 and in deionized water with pH 7 for 6 days. It was found that vaterite particles dissolved rapidly with acidity increasing, as the $CaCO_3$ solubility increases with pH lowering [135], and the amorphous phase appeared either before the recrystallization to calcite or as a final state (the phase-scheme is shown in Figure 6B). The time to complete vanishing of vaterite carriers decreased strongly with reducing the pH, so the photosensitizer liberation was increasingly dependent on the carrier dissolution process. A decrease of the particle size influenced the duration of their degradation in acidic buffers, where the complete dissolution of microparticles (3.6 ± 0.5 µm) was accomplished within 24 h of incubation at pH 6.5, while submicron particles (0.65 ± 0.03 µm) were completely dissolved within 1 h at the same pH. The fastest vaterite dissolution was observed at a low pH of 5 to 4.5, where the carriers of both sizes decomposed within the first 5 min causing an immediate burst release of the loaded photosensitizer. Meanwhile, at a neutral pH = 7, the photosensitizer release from vaterite submicron carriers lasted for several days and occurred during the transition to calcite.

Such a pH-dependent release of a payload from vaterite-based carriers was demonstrated multiple times by other authors. Thus, Feng et al. have shown that pH lowering leads to the greater amount of the liberated drug doxorubicin (**DOX**) from vaterite microparticles (~1.4 μm) [97]. Specifically, at pH 7.4 only 22% of the loaded DOX was released within 168 h, while at pH 6.5 liberation of 32% of the drug amount occurred for this period. When the pH level was set at 5.5, more than 40% of the payload released during 24 h and 68% liberated within 168 h. The authors proved that DOX release was induced by the carriers' decomposition in an acidic environment, since transformation of the hollow vaterite structure to an amorphous form was observed (Figure 6C).

Yang et al. have demonstrated the possibility to trigger the release of the sanguinarine (**SAN**) anticancer drug from the vaterite carriers [136]. Comparison of the release behavior at pH 7 and pH 4 clearly demonstrated more sustained kinetics at the neutral conditions, where ~15% of the loaded drug appeared within 3.5 h and was followed by a slow release of 36% in the next 147 h. Meanwhile, at pH 4.0, these carriers exhibited a fast release of 72% in the first 3.5 h and the sustained release of up to 99% of the loaded SAN amount in the following 147 h. Moreover, vaterite exhibited a better pH-responsiveness than calcite illustrating the lower stability of the vaterite versus calcite crystalline phase. As mentioned above, this feature is an important advantage of vaterite which accounts for its wide application in biomedicine.

The same features were demonstrated for the hydrophobic drugs fluorouracil (**5-Fu**) and sodium levothyroxine (**L-Thy**) encapsulated into cyclodextrin (**CD**)-containing vaterite carriers [137]. Release studies demonstrated a more intense payload liberation upon the carrier incubation in acidic media (at pH 4.8 for 5-Fu and pH 1.2 for L-Thy) in comparison with a neutral solution (pH 7.4). The authors did not observe complete dissolution of the containers at such a low pH. This was most likely due to the stabilizing effect of the introduced CD. The pH buffering properties of $CaCO_3$ could also be the reason for such observations. The dissolution of vaterite might increase the pH of the immersion medium affecting the further degradation of the carriers [56]. This feature should always be kept in mind when setting the mass of vaterite powder incubated and the volume of the immersion medium used, so that this effect can be leveled out.

Chesneau et al. have also demonstrated the pH-dependent release of the hydrophobic drug from CD-containing vaterite particles [67]. However, their carriers liberated the whole amount of the loaded tocopherol acetate (vitamin E) within 2 h while decomposing in acidic media at pH 5. This illustrates the importance of considering the leaching feature of vaterite. At pH 7.4 (0.15 M NaCl), the carriers remained stable and no hydrophobic cargo release was observed for this period.

In terms of biomedical application, the pH-sensitivity of vaterite is of high importance in the targeted delivery of anticancer agents, since the microenvironment in tumors is generally more acidic than in normal tissues and in blood (pH 6.5–6.8 versus 7.4, respectively) [58,138] (Figure 7A). Similar to the other pH-responsive inorganic materials, vaterite can provide the pH-triggered release in the tumor site [139].

For example, by virtue of their pH sensitivity, Parakhonskiy et al. have demonstrated the possibility of using submicron vaterite particles (~500 μm) loaded with porphyrazine anticancer drug as an in vivo theranostic system (Figure 7B) [98]. A high sensitivity of the porphyrazine release to an even slightly acidic pH (6.8) represented a rationale behind the choice of these carriers in their study. Namely, the release of slightly more than 50% of the loaded drug within 3 h was shown there due to the partial carrier dissolution at pH 6.8. Injection of the carriers into the tail vein of tumor-bearing mice resulted in their passive accumulation in the tumor followed by an hours-scale release of the drug, which permeated then to the entire interstitium of the solid tumor. That enabled the intravital imaging and PDT of xenograft tumors.

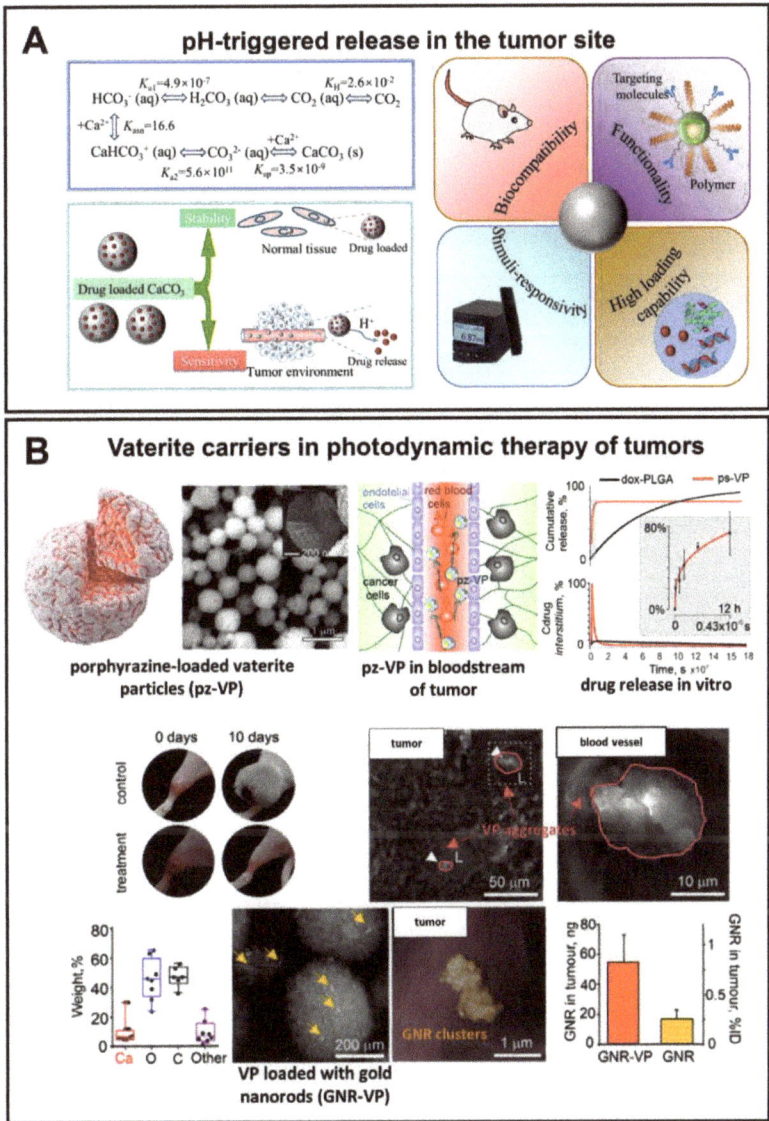

Figure 7. Exploiting pH-sensitivity of vaterite carriers for drug delivery to tumors. (**A**) Schematic presentation of vaterite application in tumor targeting. Reproduced from Open Access Article [18]. (**B**) An example of successful application of the vaterite particles loaded with a porphyrazine (pz) drug and gold nanorods (GNR) in photodynamic therapy of tumors. Adapted with permission from [98].

We should note that in the above-mentioned work, the rapid drug release from the vaterite particles was required to provide the high drug concentration in the vessel for creating a gradient from the intracapillary space to the interstitium. However, the need for a more precise control over the payload release encourages researchers to optimize the structure of vaterite-based carriers, including by modifying their surface, for providing better tumor selectivity and prevention of drug liberation in the bloodstream. For instance, Choukrani et al. have synthetized the vaterite nanoparticles loaded with bovine serum albumin (**BSA**) and demonstrated that modification of their surface with carboxyl group-containing polymers using a layer-by-layer (**LbL**) assembly technique could provide their stabilization in neutral aqueous solutions (Tris pH 7.5) postponing the recrystallization from 5 h to 2 months [140]. The investigation of the BSA release kinetics in conditions mimicking the blood flow (flow rate of 0.2 mL min^{-1}) demonstrated almost twice reduction of the BSA release from the polymer-coated carriers compared to the pristine particles at pH 6.5 and 7.4 (Figure 8A). The authors suggested that it would ensure the prevention of a burst payload release in the bloodstream; meanwhile, the entry of such carriers into the tumor could trigger drug liberation.

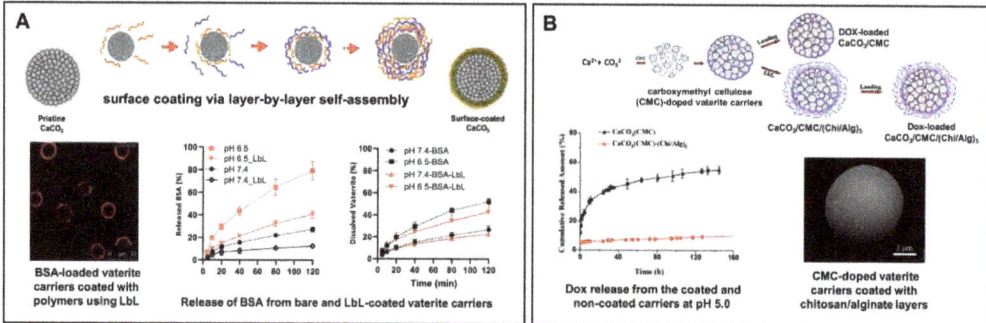

Figure 8. Prevention of the burst release from vaterite carriers via their surface modification. (**A**) Effect of the layer-by-layer (LbL) coating formation on the BSA release from the vaterite carriers: schematics of the polyelectrolyte layers deposition, CLSM image of the LbL-coated carriers and BSA release kinetics from the bare and coated carriers at different pH (6.5 and 7.4). Adapted with permission from [44,127,140]. (**B**) Effect of carboxymethyl cellulose (CMC) incorporation and further coating of the vaterite matrices with chitosan/alginate (Chi/Alg) multilayers on the payload release: schematics, SEM-image and kinetics of DOX liberation from the CMC-doped carriers, both coated and non-coated with Chi/Alg, at pH 5.0. Adapted with permission from [78].

Peng et al. have demonstrated the effect of carboxymethyl cellulose (**CMC**) incorporation into the vaterite matrix on the release of the encapsulated DOX (Figure 8B) [78]. Negatively charged CMC possesses hydrophobic properties at acidic conditions as a result of protonation of the carboxyl groups with subsequent inhibition of the vaterite particles dissolution leading to the slowing down of the DOX release rate at pH 5 (0.1 M sodium citrate–HCl buffer). Further modification of the CMC-containing carriers with chitosan and alginate multilayers via the LbL self-assembly technique allowed the authors to drastically decrease the rate of DOX liberation, when 10% of the loaded drug released at pH 5 during 150 h.

In addition to control over the payload release, surface modification of the vaterite-based carriers with various polymers, antibodies, peptides and aptamers can simultaneously facilitate the drug targeting [18]. Thus, Dong Z. et al. have designed pH-responsive calcium carbonate carriers loaded with a Mn^{2+}-chelated chlorin e6 photosensitizer and DOX drug, the surface of which was functionalized with polyethylene glycol (**PEG**) [141]. The carriers demonstrated relatively good stability under physiological pH 7.4 (less than 20% of the loaded drug amount was liberated during 12 h for both therapeutic compounds), but high sensitivity to pH as they were displaying rapid degradation and payload release at acidic conditions (Figure 9). PEGelation provided a sufficient blood circulation time for the carriers injected in tumor-bearing mice in vivo (the first and the second phases of the circulation half-lives were ~1 h and ~14 h, respectively). The designed carriers exhibited a pH-dependent enhancement of the T1-weighted magnetic resonance (**MR**) contrast due to Mn^{2+}-chelated photosensitizer liberation at an acidic pH both in vitro and in vivo. This feature allowed the authors to study the efficacy of tumor-targeted delivery for the loaded drugs by means of intravenously injected carriers utilizing MR and fluorescence imaging modalities. As a result, the gradual accumulation of the carriers in the tumor was shown which enabled the effective realization of combined PDT and chemotherapy, which granted the synergistic anti-tumor effect.

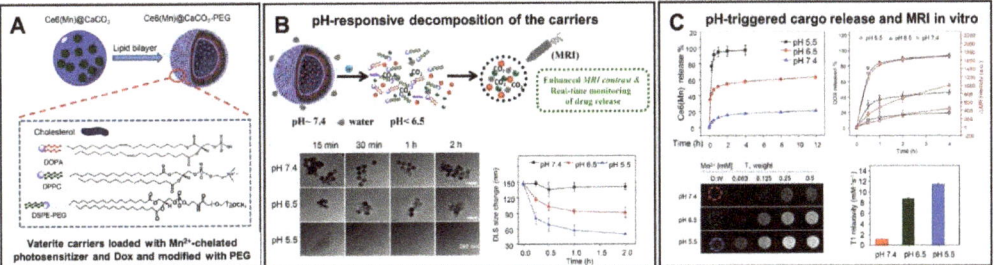

Figure 9. Enhancement of the vaterite carriers targeting to tumors via their surface modification. (**A**) Schematics representing the structure of vaterite carriers loaded with Mn^{2+}-chelated chlorin e6 photosensitizer (Ce6(Mn)) and modified with PEG. (**B**) Schematic illustration of the pH-responsive decomposition of the carriers (incubation in PBS at pH 5.5, 6.5 and 7.4). (**C**) pH-triggered MR enhancement and MR-imaging monitored photosensitizer release in vitro. Adapted with permission from [141].

$CaCO_3$ particles are effectively integrated with the other encapsulation systems to generate the advanced pH-responsive vaterite-derived platforms. Some interesting examples have been recently reviewed by Tan and co-authors [44]. This review highlighted different polymer-doped vaterite containers, as well as introduced various hybrid systems obtained when integrating $CaCO_3$ with emulsions, hydrogels and liposomes. Besides, $CaCO_3$ mineralization of the micellar core allows the formation of pH-responsive vehicles, which were demonstrated to be especially valuable in terms of the intracellular delivery of anticancer drugs [142], including the co-delivery of various therapeutic agents [143,144]. Concerning the acidic pH of cellular endosomes (pH 5.5–6.5) and lysosomes (pH 4.5–5.5), such mineralized polypeptide nanoparticles enable the pH-triggered intracellular release of the payload, while protecting it from the leakage at the physiological pH, which extend the circulation half-life and, thus, enhance the drug accumulation in tumors (Figure 10). We will discuss further the other possibilities of controlling the process of decomposition for vaterite-based carriers.

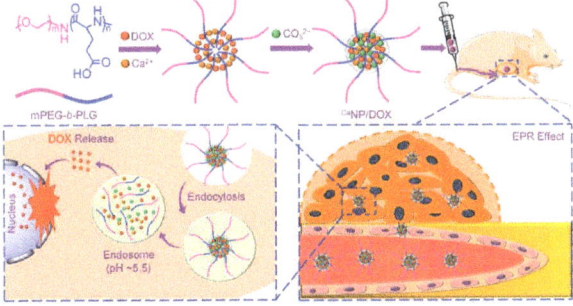

Figure 10. Schematic illustration for fabrication of the DOX-loaded calcium carbonate-crosslinked polypeptide carriers (CaNP/DOX), their circulation in vivo, intratumoral accumulation and pH-triggered intracellular DOX release. Reproduced from Open Access Article [142].

The pH sensitivity of vaterite is also successfully utilized for the development of different antibacterial coatings. This possibility arises due to local acidification (pH 5.0–5.5) of the environment by bacteria during their growth and metabolic processes [145]. Antibacterial film, which was based on vaterite microspheres loaded with a sanguinarine (**SAN**) drug, has demonstrated a strong bactericidal activity against *Staphylococcus aureus* [146]. Lowering the pH from 7.0 to 5.0 upon the film incubation in PBS resulted in the liberation of 46% instead of 21% of the loaded SAN during 67 h. Importantly, when growing the bacteria on the surface of this film, its gradual decomposition was observed. Namely, the coating became transparent with the growth of bacteria as the result of vaterite dissolution. At the same time, a large zone of inhibition was formed indicating the release of SAN from the carriers. The authors suggested that these processes were induced by the acidic environment of bacteria.

Ferreira A. et al. have designed pH-sensitive vaterite–nanosilver hybrids, which demonstrated good activity against *Escherichia coli*, methicillin-resistant *Staphylococcus aureus* and *Pseudomonas aeruginosa* [147]. However, the pristine silver-loaded particles were characterized by initial burst release even in non-acidic buffers (at pH 7.4 and pH 9.0) liberating ~50% of the incorporated AgNPs within a few hours (Figure 11). The incorporation of poly(4-styrenesulfonic acid) sodium salt (**PSS**) during the formation of the hybrids allowed the prevention of premature AgNPs release at non-acidic pH. Namely, the PSS-containing carriers did not recrystallize during 50 h at pH 7.4 and pH 9.0, so no AgNP release was observed during this period. In contrast, at pH 5.0 an immediate burst release occurred resulting in the liberation of over 90% of loaded AgNPs from the hybrids.

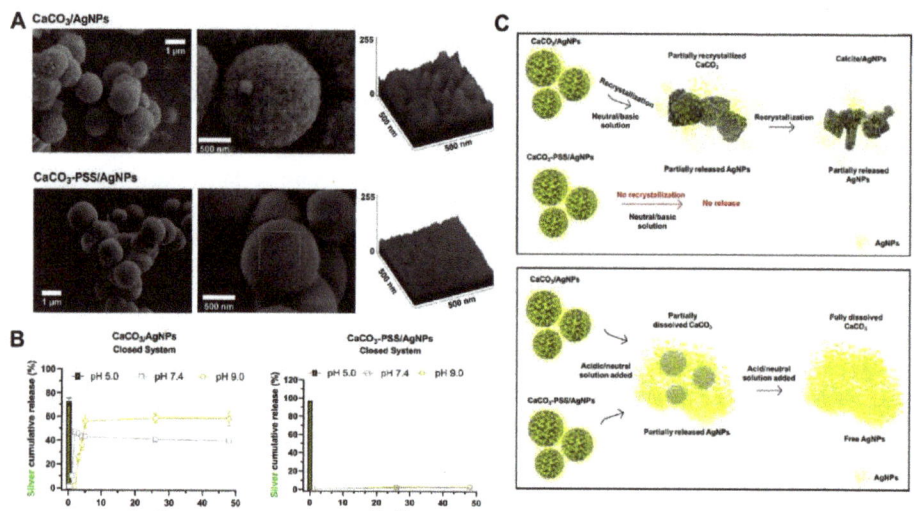

Figure 11. Vaterite–nanosilver hybrids with antibacterial properties and pH-triggered release. (**A**) SEM images and surface roughness plots of the pristine (CaCO$_3$/AgNPs) and PSS-modified (CaCO$_3$-PSS/AgNPs) vaterite–nanosilver hybrids. (**B**) Cumulative release of silver ions from the hybrids in PBS at pH 5.0, 7.4 and 9.0. (**C**) Schematic illustration of the AgNPs release driven by the recrystallization and dissolution of the hybrids. Adapted from Open Access Article [147].

Similar to the vaterite–calcite recrystallization process, the decomposition of vaterite carriers at an acidic pH not only induces the payload liberation, but also ensures the release of Ca^{2+} ions. This feature, for example, is often applied to trigger alginate gelation [55,123,148] (Figure 12A). The released Ca^{2+} ions could also participate in hemostasis, catalyzing different coagulation-related reactions that promote the blood coagulation process [18,149,150] (Figure 12B).

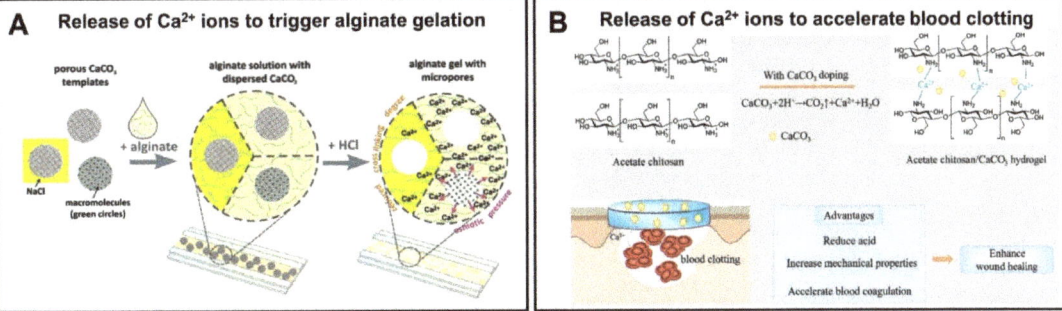

Figure 12. Exploiting of Ca^{2+} release, which occurs during the dissolution of vaterite particles, for triggering the alginate gelation (**A**) and accelerating the blood clotting (**B**). (**A**) reproduced with permission from [55], (**B**) from [149].

Moreover, during the decomposition in acidic media, vaterite generates carbon dioxide (CO_2) bubbles that open up the potential of its application in ultrasound (**US**) imaging [151,152], as well as in US cavitation and sonodynamic therapy [45,153]. For instance, Min K.H. with co-authors have shown the possibility to exploit such gas generation in US imaging of tumors [152]. Their DOX-loaded vaterite-based carriers exhibited strong echogenic signals at a tumoral acid pH in vivo in mice through the production of CO_2 bubbles (Figure 13). Importantly, in normal (non-tumoral) tissues the carriers did not provide any US contrast as no bubble generation occurred there. Furthermore, the DOX release, which was induced by the carriers' dissolution in the tumor, granted the antitumor therapeutic effect in that study. The proposed concept is very promising as it opens new perspectives for the development of novel theranostic platforms combining ultrasound imaging and therapy for various cancers. Thus, for instance, in further elaboration of this idea, the authors have designed the photosensitizer-loaded vaterite carriers with a potential for US imaging-guided photodynamic destruction of cancer cells [151].

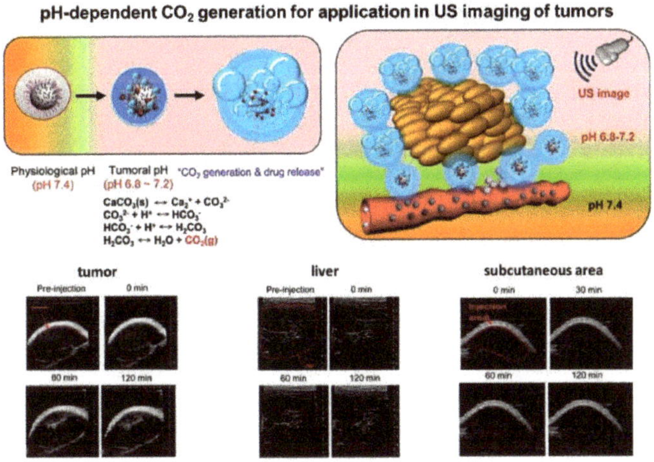

Figure 13. Exploiting of CO_2 bubbles' generation, which occurs during the dissolution of vaterite particles, for US imaging of tumors. Schematic illustration of the pH-dependent CO_2 generation and the images showing the US contrast in tumor, liver and subcutaneous area after the injection of DOX-loaded vaterite carriers in vivo to the corresponding site. Reproduced with permission from [152].

In the work [45], photosensitizer-loaded vaterite carriers were tested for their ability to destruct tumors under the US treatment (0.89 MHz) followed by the light irradiation US of certain intensity producing the acoustic cavitation, which effects, such as the formation of microjets and shock waves [154], can cause cytotoxic effects in tumor cells [155]. Varying the US power density (0.05–1.00 W/cm^2) and the pH of the immersion medium (7.0 and 5.0), the controlled cavitation-mediated release of aluminum phthalocyanine from the carriers was shown. At pH 7.0, the bubbles' formation was weakly intense until the power density of sonication reached 1 W/cm^2. Then, intensification of the bubbling process occurred, also accelerating the vaterite–calcite recrystallization and subsequent liberation of the photosensitizer. At the same time, at pH 5.0, the carrier dissolution accompanied by the payload release and CO_2 bubbles generation was observed even without the US treatment, while the sonication with the power densities above 0.2 W/cm^2 drastically intensified these processes. Given the acidity of the tumor microenvironment, the carriers will be dissolved upon the accumulation inside and thus produce CO_2 bubbles, which generation could be enhanced by the US exposure. In vivo investigation in tumor-bearing rats approved this suggestion, revealing the damaging effect of sonication after the intratumoral injection of the carriers. Further irradiation with a light at the wavelength corresponding to the photosensitizer absorption maximum allowed the enhancement of the therapeutic effect.

Following this approach, Feng Q. et al. introduced the vaterite-based carriers capable of decomposing in a tumor under the combined action of an acidic pH and US irradiation as a result of the simultaneous release of the loaded drug and CO_2 bubbles' generation (Figure 14) [153]. That led to cavitation-mediated irreversible necrosis of tumor cells and destruction of its blood vessels. To achieve the anticancer synergism, the carriers were loaded with a sonosensitizer; thus, they could provide the reactive oxygen species generation leading to apoptotic destruction of the cancer cells. Moreover, the echogenic property of CO_2 provides the US imaging guidance for therapeutic inertial cavitation and sonodynamic therapy simultaneously.

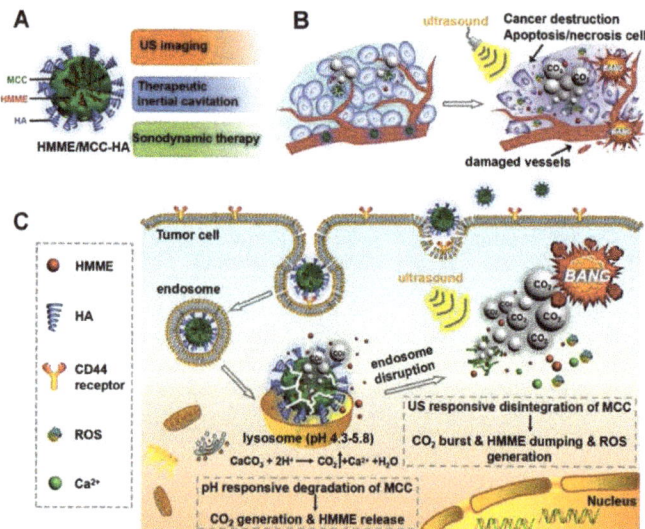

Figure 14. Schematic of the pH/ultrasound dual-responsive CO_2 generation for US imaging-guided therapeutic inertial cavitation and sonodynamic therapy. (**A**) Formation of the hematoporphyrin monomethyl ether (HMME)-loaded vaterite carriers coated with hyaluronic acid (HA). (**B**,**C**) Mechanism of the tumor destruction utilizing the carriers and US treatment. Reproduced with permission from [153].

To date, a great number of different pH-responsive CaCO$_3$-based delivery systems and composites have been designed for anticancer, antibacterial and other drug encapsulation. Recent advances in this field have been discussed in a number of well-organized and comprehensive reviews [3,18,58,59,61,156]. Such microenvironment-activated systems are mainly applied in chemotherapy, photothermal therapy or PDT, wound healing, blood clotting, tissue engineering, as well as in ultrasound, fluorescence and MRI imaging [18]. Both relatively simple vaterite-based systems and composite multicomponent platforms, which are highly demanded in multimodal theranostics, find their application in biomedicine.

5. Biodegradation of Vaterite Carriers

Vaterite-based drug carriers exhibit high biocompatibility and good biodegradability participating in the normal metabolism of the living body by dissolving into nontoxic ions. There are two possible routes for the calcium-based materials degradation: the dissolution by body fluids, and phagocytosis and absorption by cells (mainly macrophage) [157]. The first route includes a split of the carbonate materials into particles, molecules or ions due to the acidic environment of the body fluids containing a number of acidic metabolites such as citrate, lactate and acid hydrolysis enzyme. The second route can be divided into intracellular and extracellular degradation, where the particles can be split into ions after phagocytosis by macrophages under the effect of cytoplasmic and lysosomal enzymes, and then the degradation products, such as Ca^{2+} and CO$_3^{2-}$, can be transferred to outside the cell. Additionally, the environment of macrophages enriched with acid hydrolases (including lysosomal enzyme and acid phosphatase enzymes) promotes a secretion of H$^+$ and induces the pH decrease.

Fu K. et al. demonstrated the biodegradation of the composite comprising a calcium carbonate scaffold enveloped by a thin layer of hydroxyapatite [158]. Despite the slow biodegradability of hydroxyapatite, the complete resorption and remodeling of the implanted calcium carbonate-based composite takes 18–24 months, which was revealed by in vivo clinical observations. Moreover, the promotion of conductive osteogenesis was assessed in vitro by the successful attachment and proliferation of human mesenchymal stem cells on the composite and in vivo using an immunodeficient mouse model.

The metabolites of vaterite degradation can participate in the formation of new bone, thus completing the transformation of inorganic materials in organisms. Stengelin E. et al. successfully applied the conversion of vaterite to bone-like hydroxycarbonate apatite (**HCA**) under physiological conditions in the development of bone scaffolds based on biodegradable vaterite/PEG-composite microgels [159]. FT-IR spectroscopy indicated the transformation of vaterite in the polymer matrix to HCA, and co-encapsulation of vaterite with the osteoblast cells (MG-63 GFP) characterized by a similar cell viability and high cell compatibility compared to a microgel containing only cells without vaterite. The application of calcium carbonate implants in rabbit bone defects revealed their rapid degradation even before osteoconduction was completed [160]. The results indicated abundant woven bone in the cortical shell of the surgical site, indicative of spontaneous healing without an osteoconductive implant. To prolong the osteoconductivity, Fujioka-Kobayashi M. et al. used CaCO$_3$ core coated with carbonate apatite [161]. The biodegradation of CaCO$_3$ is caused by dissolution or cell mediation depending on the mineral phase [162], while calcium phosphate biomaterials resorption is associated with the combination of physical, chemical and biological processes [163]. The combination of CaCO$_3$ and carbonate apatite allowed the authors to balance new bone formation and material resorption leading to suitable bone replacement, where the higher contents of CaCO$_3$ resulted in a shortened resorption rate with the subsequent promotion of Ca^{2+} release and carbonate apatite and, in turn, demonstrated a perfect osteoconductive potential (Figure 15). Another work described the hybrid system composed of the vaterite particles formed in the presence of inorganic polyphosphate (**polyP**), which restrain vaterite–calcite recrystallization [164]. The hybrid particles degraded within 5 days of the incubation in the cell culture medium with 65% of suppression of calcite formation in the first 3 days. The rapid degradation of CaCO$_3$/polyP particles was confirmed by a Ca^{2+} release investigation portraying 68% of the total Ca^{2+} in the reaction mixture compared to almost no Ca^{2+} content for the calcite sample.

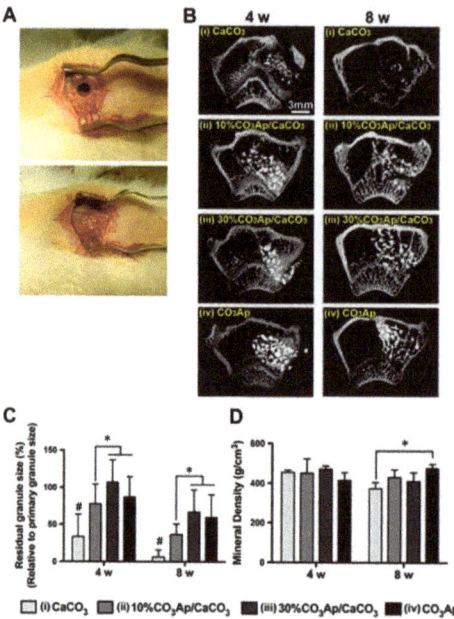

Figure 15. In vivo degradation of the $CaCO_3$-based implanting material for improvement of ossification in bone tissue engineering. (**A**) Implantation of the fabricated granules in cylindrical bone defects of the rabbit femur. (**B**) Horizontal μCT views of the rabbit femur defect with $CaCO_3$, 10% $CO_3Ap/CaCO_3$, 30% $CO_3Ap/CaCO_3$ and CO_3Ap granules at 4 and 8 weeks. (**C**) The residual granules area (%) quantified by μCT at 4 and 8 weeks. (**D**) Mineral density the bone defect area at 4 and 8 weeks. An asterisk (*) denotes significant differences between groups, $p < 0.05$; a hash (#) denotes significantly lower than all other modalities, $p < 0.05$. Reproduced with permission from [161].

Unger R. et al. [165] declared the in vivo biodegradation of an injectable bone substitute composed of PEG-acetal-dimethacrylate and vaterite nanoparticles mediated by mononuclear cells of the macrophage lineage via a pro-inflammatory process. During degradation of the material, M1 macrophages involved in this process may express lytic enzymes such as the members of the group of reactive oxygen species and other relevant mediators [166].

The mechanism of the in vitro resorption of natural $CaCO_3$ by avian osteoclasts was investigated by Guillemin et al. demonstrating that carbonic anhydrases produced by osteoclasts play a crucial role in generating protons for the acidification of the calcium carbonate [167]. The calcium carbonate from *Tridacna* shell is a biomaterial that can undergo dissolution through the mechanism of osteoclastic resorption. The degradation of the carbonate-based materials induced by bacterial activity was demonstrated in [168]. In aerobic systems, the decomposition of $CaCO_3$ is attributed to a metabolic byproduct through the bacterial-induced decomposition of skeletal-binding organic matter.

The pH-dependent biodegradation of vaterite nanoparticles was discussed in the case of the drug delivery to tumors, where the authors concluded that the blood flow rate plays a crucial role in this process [98]. Different perfusion rates influence the pH of tumor venous blood from neutral to acidic values resulting in the partial or complete degradation of the vaterite. Moreover, it is shown that the main pathway of the $CaCO_3$ particles internalization is micropinocytosis with their subsequent resorption in lysosomes, which are characterized by an acidic pH (4.0–5.5) [169] and good stability in the extracellular space for longer times (Figure 16).

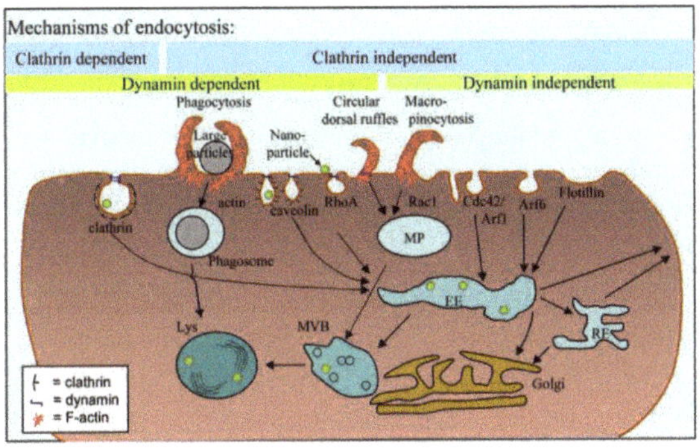

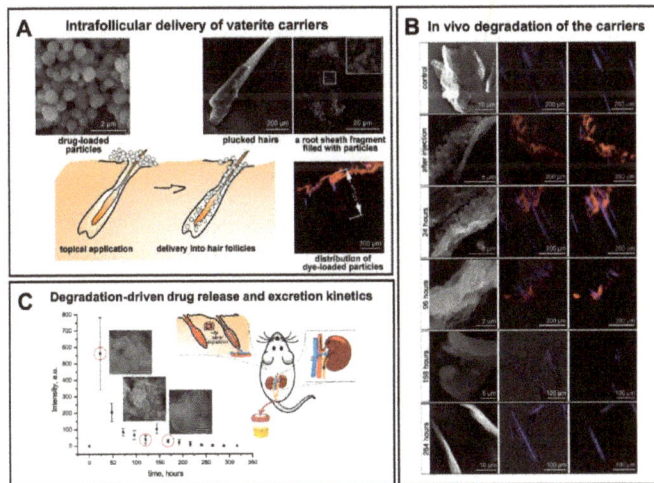

Figure 16. The scheme of the micro- and nanoparticle internalization by endocytic mechanism and intracellular transport. Reproduced with permission from [169].

In vivo degradation of the vaterite carriers was demonstrated in the rat skin, both after their delivery to the dermis using fractional laser microablation (**FLMA**) [15] and after non-invasive intrafollicular administration of the carriers [16]. In the first case, the carrier degradation was enhanced by the inflammatory reaction occurred in skin as a result of the FLMA-microchannels' formation. Meanwhile, in the second case, the hair cycle stimulated processes, which activated the secretion within the hair follicle forming the release medium for the particles and delivering drugs. That led to a gradual degradation of the vaterite particles inside the hair follicles, which ended up with their total resorption within 12 days (Figure 17). The biodegradation of the vaterite particles was followed by the in situ release of the payload ensuring its distribution in the hair follicle tissue and subsequent systemic uptake.

Figure 17. In vivo degradation of vaterite carriers in hair follicles. (**A**) SEM, CLSM images and schematics illustrating the intrafollicular delivery of the carriers. Reproduced with permission from [170]. (**B**) SEM (**the left column**) and CLSM (**the middle and right columns**) images illustrating the process of the carriers' degradation inside the hair follicles of rats in vivo. (**C**) Excretion kinetics of the fluorescent dye intrafollicularly delivered by means of degradable vaterite carries. (**B**) and (**C**) reproduced with permission from [16].

As a practical implementation of intrafollicular drug transportation following the vaterite degradation, such carriers were applied for influenza vaccine delivery proposing the new strategy for transcutaneous immunization [90], as well as for the photosensitizer targeting enabling the improvement of psoralen–ultraviolet A therapy of dermatoses [171,172]. Besides, the vaterite particles were applied for the intrafollicular delivery of antifungal drugs [43,101,113,173]. In particular, the immobilization of a griseofulvin drug (**Gf**) into such biodegradable carriers enabled its dermal bioavailability enhancement [43,113]. The degradation-driven liberation of the loaded Gf from the carriers was evaluated in water, saline and cell culture medium [43]. The influence of the release medium has a dramatic effect on the degradation rate of the vaterite matrix driven mainly by its transition to calcite. The acceleration of the $CaCO_3$ recrystallization process was demonstrated in saline caused by its higher ionic strength, speeding up ion exchange between the $CaCO_3$ surface and the incubation solution. Oppositely, the incomplete degradation of carbonate carrier in cell culture medium was attributed to the adsorption of protein molecules from this medium on the carrier surface. The modification of the particle surface with polyelectrolyte shell (poly-L-arginine, dextran sulfate and heparin) via the LbL approach extended the recrystallization duration for Gf-loaded carriers twice in water (144 h vs. 72 h) and 2.5 times in saline (120 h vs. 48 h). The sustained effect of the stabilizing shell was also verified in vivo, when delivering these carriers into the hair follicles of rats (Figure 18). According to the drug excretion profiles, the use of such a formulation provided detectable Gf concentrations in urine for over a week (168–192 h). Importantly, no obvious adverse effects were observed upon the multi-dose dermal toxicity assessment of the Gf-loaded vaterite carriers in rabbits, while a high antifungal efficiency was demonstrated when studying their therapeutic potential in a guinea pig model of trichophytosis [113]. This methodology was extended to deliver the antifungal drug naftifine hydrochloride into the deep layers of the skin through the hair follicles [101]. Scanning electron microscopy (SEM) investigation revealed the vaterite bulk resorption within 72 h inside the follicles of mice followed by its gradual degradation within 120 h with the simultaneous release of the payload drug into the surrounding tissues. To accelerate the vaterite carrier degradation in skin, the authors in Ref. [174] proposed an application of sonophoretic post-treatment (1 MHz, 1 W/cm^2, 9 min) after the particles' delivery into hair follicles. The results of optical coherence tomography monitoring of the skin and SEM investigation of the plucked hairs revealed the twice-reduction of the degradation period of the carriers.

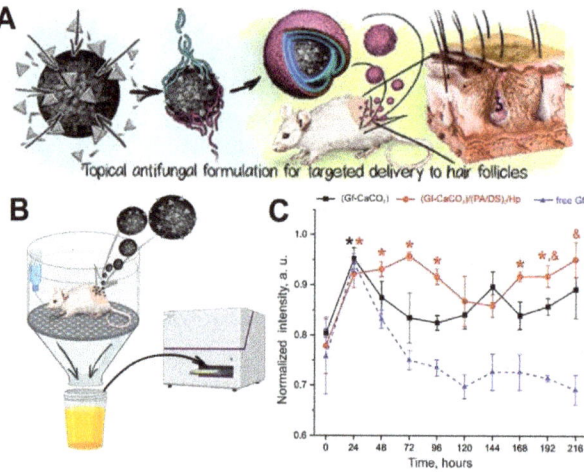

Figure 18. Prolongation of in vivo degradation of the vaterite carriers and sustainment of the payload release via formation of the stabilizing coating on the carriers' surface. (**A**) Schematics illustrating the

formation of vaterite carriers loaded with a griseofulvin (Gf) drug and coated with poly-L-arginine (PA), dextran sulfate (DS) and heparin (HP) polyelectrolytes. (**B**) Schematics of the Gf urinary excretion rate investigation. (**C**) Urinary excretion profiles of Gf after its administration by means of (Gf-CaCO$_3$) and (Gf-CaCO$_3$)/(PA/DS)$_2$/HP carriers or after pure Gf application in rats in vivo. An asterisk (*) indicates significant differences in the Gf peak intensity at a particular time point after drug delivery as compared to the control urine value (zero time point) within the same group ($p < 0.05$). An ampersand (&) shows a significant difference in the Gf peak intensities between the group of (Gf-CaCO$_3$)/(PA/DS)$_2$/HP carriers and the pure Gf group ($p < 0.05$) on the last day of the experiment. Reproduced with permission from [43].

6. Control over the Dissolution/Recrystallization/Degradation Process of Vaterite

Various applications of vaterite require its stabilization to prevent degradation/recrystallization in aqueous environments, including implantable drug delivery systems, tissue engineering platforms, food/cosmetic additives and storage materials, which are designed for prolonged action [175]. As mentioned above, the regulation of the CaCO$_3$ stability could be driven by the addition of macromolecules of a different nature during the particle synthesis or by the CaCO$_3$ surface modification by the polymer film. The polymer network suppresses the ions diffusion from the carbonate crystal surface, which resulted in the stabilization of vaterite nanocrystals.

The different additives were applied to control the degradation/recrystallization of the vaterite particles. So, the amino acids and polypeptides were found to have a pronounced effect on the stabilization of the vaterite polymorphs. The presence of polar C=O groups in the structure of amino acids has a crucial influence on the electrostatic interactions of Ca^{2+} ions with the negatively charged oxygen atoms within the C=O bonds, which along with the diffused CO$_3^{2-}$ ions toward the fixed Ca^{2+} may initiate the critical nuclei of vaterite formation [176]. Thus, the supersaturated solutions of lysine, glycine, alanine, polyglycine, polymethionine, polylysine and polyaspartate were demonstrated to control the vaterite recrystallization [176,177]. In [26], the authors demonstrated the stabilizing effect of negatively charged ovalbumin over positively charged lysozyme to prevent the metastable vaterite from transformation via dissolution-recrystallization processes. The results confirmed that only the net of negatively charged proteins enhance its stability as a result of the strong binding between carboxylate groups of ovalbumin and the calcium ions on the CaCO$_3$ surface (Figure 19).

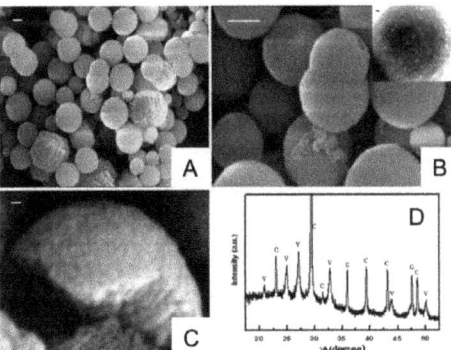

Figure 19. Stabilization of metastable vaterite in CaCO$_3$ biomineralization through the addition of ovalbumin protein. (**A–C**) Calcium carbonate particles formed in the presence of 0.2 gL^{-1} ovalbumin. (**D**) XRD spectrum of the CaCO$_3$-ovalbumin precipitates, where "C" indicates calcite peaks (JCPDS: 05-0586), "V"—vaterite ones (JCPDS: 33-0268). Scale bars correspond to 1 μm (**A**,**B**) and 100 nm (**C**,**D**). Reproduced with permission from [26].

Similar results were shown for the particles co-precipitated with BSA, where the formation of stable vaterite was attributed to the interaction of BSA functional groups (namely, C=O, HO-, N-H, C-N) with the carbonate surface [178]. In another study, the proteins extracted from gastroliths of the crayfish *C. quadricarinatus* induced the stabilization of amorphous calcium carbonate (**ACC**) in vitro mediated by the phosphorylated residues of phosphoproteins [179]. The major proteinaceous fraction of the organic matrix with a heavily phosphorylated doublet band at 70–75 kDa was also incorporated into the mineral phase during the precipitation. The single amino acids, phosphoserine or phosphothreonine, have a similar stabilizing effect proving that phosphoamino acid moieties are the key factors in the control of ACC formation and stabilization.

Among polysaccharides, the incorporation of dextran and its derivatives into the vaterite particles by co-precipitation revealed the possibility of their selective stabilization depending on the polymer charge [175]. The co-synthesis of vaterite with the nonionic dextran resulted in the decreasing of the nanocrystallite size with partial blocking of the crystal pores. The inclusion of negatively charged carboxymethyl-dextran significantly retarded the vaterite–calcite recrystallization under a basic pH, whilst positively charged diethylaminoethyl–dextran did not affect this process (Figure 20).

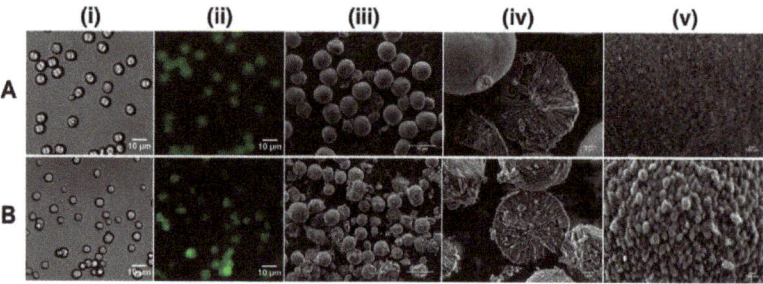

Figure 20. CLSM and SEM images of carboxymethyl–dextran–FITC/vaterite hybrids (**A**) and diethylaminoethyl–dextran–FITC/vaterite hybrids (**B**). Scale bar is 10 μm for (**i**), (**ii**) and (**iii**), 1 μm for (**iv**), and 100 nm for (**v**). Reproduced with permission from [175].

Similar observations were demonstrated in the co-synthesis of calcium carbonate with the anionic functional biopolymer carboxymethylinulin, which resulted in enhanced stability of the vaterite phase [180]. Elsewhere, the degradation of vaterite was suppressed by co-precipitation with mucin, as glycoprotein possesses functional groups of different charge [83]. The filling of porous vaterite crystals with a gel-like matrix of mucin reduced ion mobility near the crystal surface in aqueous solution and hampered the recrystallization rate of vaterite to calcite. An increase of mucin content in the obtained hybrid particles reduced the release rate of the encapsulated cationic drug DOX via stabilization of the porous vaterite crystals against recrystallization to non-porous calcite (Figure 21).

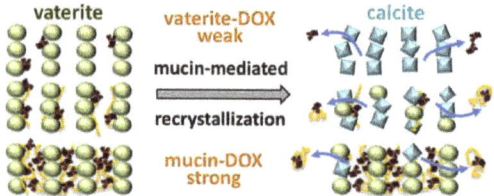

Figure 21. Scheme illustrating the process of vaterite stabilization by mucin incorporation. Reproduced with permission from [83].

The carbonate controlled-addition method was applied to synthesize poly(acrylic acid) (**PAA**)–calcium carbonate composite particles, which were extremely stable in the aqueous medium [181]. The stabilization of ACC was achieved by the complexation of Ca^{2+} ions with PAA and dependent on the polymer molar mass and duration of the complexation process. The shorter complexation time together with the usage of medium molar mass PAA induced the stabilization of ACC due to a more random coordination of Ca^{2+} ions with PAA. In other work, the stability of polycrystalline vaterite was achieved due to the specific interaction between poly(vinyl alcohol) and $CaCO_3$ through hydrogen-bonding, probably to the carbonate ions, allowing a high density of polymer chains right near the interface by increasing the number of segments that are intimately attached to the solid [182]. The incorporation of poly (vinylsulfonic acid) through co-synthesis with calcium carbonate controls growth of the vaterite polymorph and its stability over degradation owing to sequestering calcium ions followed by slowing down the nucleation rate and preventing surface calcification or aggregation into microparticles [183]. The obtained vaterite maintained a crystal structure for about 5 months of storage in aqueous medium. An interesting approach was proposed to obtain vaterite particles with long-term stability via the addition of $Ca(OH)_2$ to branched polyethylenimine (**PEI**)–CO_2 adduct solutions [184]. The hydrolysis of the alkylammonium carbamate zwitterions in PEI-CO_2 adducts led to the release of bicarbonate ions to feed the in situ vaterite crystal nucleation and growth, thus serving as both the CO_2 source and template for vaterite $CaCO_3$ nucleation and growth. The synthesized particles retained the vaterite phase for at least 8 months of storage.

The vaterite crystalline dissolution and recrystallization could be inhibited by the inclusion of the polycarboxylate-type superplasticizer (**PCS**) during its synthesis [185]. The crystal growth process of vaterite microspheres was assisted by the PCS molecules, which rearranged on the surfaces of the vaterite particles and modulated the formation of lenticular aggregates through the hydrogen bonding effect. The carboxylate groups of the polymer interacted with Ca^{2+} ions blocking the transformation of vaterite to calcite. The authors of [186] presented the stabilized vaterite by the poly(amidoamine) dendrimers with external carboxylate groups. The control over dissolution was achieved for more than 1 week at storage in water. The increase of the -COONa groups concentration and the generation number of the dendrimer resulted in the reduction of the vaterite size.

An interesting research study introduced the application of B. subtilis bacterial cells as the templates to the formation of biogenic ACC or vaterite, where the carbonic anhydrase secreted by the bacteria plays an important role in the mineralization of $CaCO_3$ [187]. The results indicated the growth of the vaterite phase only in the presence of carbohydrate (crude extracellular protein contains some polysaccharide), whilst both polysaccharides and proteins secreted by bacterial metabolism maintained the stability of vaterite (Figure 22). Other biotic experiments explained the long-term stabilization of vaterite due to binding between the vaterite surface and organic by-products of bacterial activity (extracellular polymeric substances, which include polysaccharides, proteins, glycoproteins, nucleic acids, phospholipids and humic acids) [188].

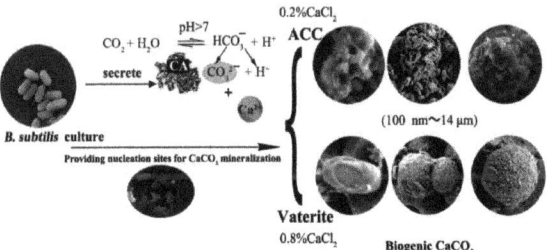

Figure 22. Schematics of possible mechanisms of $CaCO_3$ biomineralization. Reproduced with permission from [187].

7. Conclusions

The development of degradable systems for biomedical applications eliminates the need to retrieve or dispose of them once their function has been fulfilled. Nowadays, the amount of different materials available for this purpose is immense. Having the lack of the toxicity, expensive production and sophisticated degradability, calcium carbonate in its vaterite polymorph is highly attractive to the design of such systems. The metastability of vaterite manifests in its recrystallization into non-porous calcite crystals via dissolution–reprecipitation or even complete dissolution, depending on the surrounding medium. Because the environment of the living body in different organs and tissues varies in pH, ionic strength, as well as in the presence of molecules, degradation of the vaterite-based carriers is realized differently providing the sustained release of the incorporated cargo driven by such transitions. This manuscript discussed the benefits of vaterite instability including dissolution at an acidic pH, biodegradation at in vivo conditions, transformation to non-porous calcite and the main approaches to control over these processes. The additional profits of $CaCO_3$-based systems include the regulation of the payload liberation by means of their surface modification or accelerated by means of external treatment, e.g., ultrasonication, microwave irradiation etc. Vaterites being a versatile platform can be utilized both in its native form and as part of complex hybrid systems. Additional functionalization with different photo- [38,114,151] and sonosensitive drugs [153], as well as with metallic nanoparticles (silver, gold, magnetite, etc.) [9,69,189–193], enables the creation of multimodal theranostic platforms capable of different biomedical applications. The degradation of $CaCO_3$ at mild conditions determines its widespread use for the formation of the polyelectrolyte hollow capsules and core/shell containers by layer-by-layer assembly technique. Besides the transition-driven drug release property, the vaterite particles can serve as a source of Ca^{2+} ions, which are found to be effective in the scaffolds for bone and tooth tissue regeneration due to the ability of calcium ions to improve osteo- and odontoblasts' activity. An interesting research trend is associated with creation of vaterite-based active colloids (also called micro/nano-motors or swimmers), which exhibit propulsion by transforming energy from their environment into enhanced diffusive motion [194–197]. The formation of any anisotropy on the particles' surface (e.g., by its partial coverage with silica layer) enables the generation of self-propulsion upon the vaterite decomposition in acidic media [196]. The ability of vaterite to locally increase the pH medium during its dissolution deserves particular attention. This feature provides the in vivo pH modulation of solid tumors with the selective localization of vaterite particles with distinct sizes (20, 100 and 300 nm) in the extracellular region of tumors, followed by buffering of their environment which resulted in the prevention or reduction of tumor growth [56]. The size-dependence behavior of alkalinization of the acidic pH of human fibrosarcoma (HT1080) cells demonstrated the most pronounced ΔpH and longest effect for the 100 nm particles, while larger (300 nm) and smaller (20 nm) ones were less efficient due to limited diffusion and transient retention in the tumor environment, respectively. The effectiveness of nano-$CaCO_3$ was confirmed against RFP-expressing breast cancer cells (MDA-MB-231) without an impact on the growth and behavior of the surrounding fibroblasts [57]. Co-incubation of MDA-MB-231 with fibroblasts with subsequent vaterite treatment indicated the selective inhibition of the MDA-MB-231 cells growth with severe suppression of their cellular migration (which increases by co-incubation with fibroblasts) without affecting the stromal cells. The authors highlighted that this approach could serve as a treatment paradigm for long-term tumor static therapy. Based on the discussed facts, vaterites are not only perfect carriers for various bioactive molecules, but also are of paramount importance in their initial state for the biomedical applications.

The discussed benefits of vaterite's instability justify its favorable use in the design of multipurpose degradable systems for biomedical purposes. Taking into account the diversity of techniques enabling the synthesis of vaterite carriers in scalable [198] and even automated [199,200] ways, one can consider these systems as especially beneficial for potentially resolving a key bottleneck in industrial applications.

Author Contributions: Conceptualization, Y.S.; writing—original draft preparation, Y.S. and T.P.; writing—review and editing, Y.S. and T.P. All authors have read and agreed to the published version of the manuscript.

Funding: The study of Y.S. related to vaterite recrystallization to calcite, vaterite dissolution at acidic pH and degradation of vaterite carriers in skin (including intrafollicular delivery) was supported by the Russia Science Foundation (Project No. 22-73-10194). The study of T.P. related to the drug incorporation into the vaterite matrix, biodegradation of vaterite carriers and control over their degradation was supported by the Russian Ministry of Education and Science within the State assignment FSRC «Crystallography and Photonics» RAS.

Data Availability Statement: The data presented in this study are available in this paper.

Conflicts of Interest: The authors declare no conflict of interest.

Abbreviations

ACC	amorphous calcium carbonate
BSA	bovine serum albumin
CD	cyclodextrin
CLSM	confocal laser scanning microscopy
CMC	carboxymethyl cellulose
DOX	doxorubicin
EDX	energy-dispersive X-ray spectroscopy
Gf	griseofulvin
LbL	layer-by-layer
MR	magnetic resonance
PCL	polycaprolactone
PDT	photodynamic therapy
PEG	polyethylene glycol
SEM	scanning electron microscopy
US	ultrasound

References

1. Liendo, F.; Arduino, M.; Deorsola, F.A.; Bensaid, S. Factors Controlling and Influencing Polymorphism, Morphology and Size of Calcium Carbonate Synthesized through the Carbonation Route: A Review. *Powder Technol.* **2022**, *398*, 117050. [CrossRef]
2. Trushina, D.B.; Borodina, T.N.; Belyakov, S.; Antipina, M.N. Calcium Carbonate Vaterite Particles for Drug Delivery: Advances and Challenges. *Mater. Today Adv.* **2022**, *14*, 100214. [CrossRef]
3. Ferreira, A.M.; Vikulina, A.S.; Volodkin, D. CaCO$_3$ Crystals as Versatile Carriers for Controlled Delivery of Antimicrobials. *J. Control. Release* **2020**, *328*, 470–489. [CrossRef] [PubMed]
4. Huang, Y.; Cao, L.; Parakhonskiy, B.V.; Skirtach, A.G. Hard, Soft, and Hard-and-Soft Drug Delivery Carriers Based on CaCO$_3$ and Alginate Biomaterials: Synthesis, Properties, Pharmaceutical Applications. *Pharmaceutics* **2022**, *14*, 909. [CrossRef] [PubMed]
5. Boyjoo, Y.; Pareek, V.K.; Liu, J. Synthesis of Micro and Nano-Sized Calcium Carbonate Particles and Their Applications. *J. Mater. Chem. A* **2014**, *2*, 14270–14288. [CrossRef]
6. Saveleva, M.S.; Ivanov, A.N.; Chibrikova, J.A.; Abalymov, A.A.; Surmeneva, M.A.; Surmenev, R.A.; Parakhonskiy, B.V.; Lomova, M.V.; Skirtach, A.G.; Norkin, I.A. Osteogenic Capability of Vaterite-Coated Nonwoven Polycaprolactone Scaffolds for In Vivo Bone Tissue Regeneration. *Macromol. Biosci.* **2021**, *21*, 2100266. [CrossRef]
7. Saveleva, M.S.; Ivanov, A.N.; Kurtukova, M.O.; Atkin, V.S.; Ivanova, A.G.; Lyubun, G.P.; Martyukova, A.V.; Cherevko, E.I.; Sargsyan, A.K.; Fedonnikov, A.S.; et al. Hybrid PCL/CaCO$_3$ Scaffolds with Capabilities of Carrying Biologically Active Molecules: Synthesis, Loading and in Vivo Applications. *Mater. Sci. Eng. C* **2018**, *85*, 57–67. [CrossRef]
8. Zhao, P.; Tian, Y.; You, J.; Hu, X.; Liu, Y. Recent Advances of Calcium Carbonate Nanoparticles for Biomedical Applications. *Bioengineering* **2022**, *9*, 691. [CrossRef]
9. Noskov, R.E.; Machnev, A.; Shishkin, I.I.; Novoselova, M.V.; Gayer, A.V.; Ezhov, A.A.; Shirshin, E.A.; German, S.V.; Rukhlenko, I.D.; Fleming, S.; et al. Golden Vaterite as a Mesoscopic Metamaterial for Biophotonic Applications. *Adv. Mater.* **2021**, *33*, 2008484. [CrossRef]
10. Timin, A.S.; Postovalova, A.S.; Karpov, T.E.; Antuganov, D.; Bukreeva, A.S.; Akhmetova, D.R.; Rogova, A.S.; Muslimov, A.R.; Rodimova, S.A.; Kuznetsova, D.S.; et al. Calcium Carbonate Carriers for Combined Chemo- and Radionuclide Therapy of Metastatic Lung Cancer. *J. Control. Release* **2022**, *344*, 1–11. [CrossRef]
11. Jia, J.; Liu, Q.; Yang, T.; Wang, L.; Ma, G. Facile Fabrication of Varisized Calcium Carbonate Microspheres as Vaccine Adjuvants. *J. Mater. Chem. B* **2017**, *5*, 1611–1623. [CrossRef]

12. Ueno, Y.; Futagawa, H.; Takagi, Y.; Ueno, A.; Mizushima, Y. Drug-Incorporating Calcium Carbonate Nanoparticles for a New Delivery System. *J. Control. Release* **2005**, *103*, 93–98. [CrossRef] [PubMed]
13. Zhang, Y.; Zhu, W.; Lin, Q.; Han, J.; Jiang, L.; Zhang, L. Hydroxypropyl-β-Cyclodextrin Functionalized Calcium Carbonate Microparticles as a Potential Carrier for Enhancing Oral Delivery of Water-Insoluble Drugs. *Int. J. Nanomed.* **2015**, *10*, 3291–3302. [CrossRef] [PubMed]
14. Ishikawa, F.; Murano, M.; Hiraishi, M.; Yamaguchi, T.; Tamai, I.; Tsuji, A. Insoluble Powder Formulation as an Effective Nasal Drug Delivery System. *Pharm. Res.* **2002**, *19*, 1097–1104. [CrossRef] [PubMed]
15. Genina, E.A.; Svenskaya, Y.I.; Yanina, I.Y.; Dolotov, L.E.; Navolokin, N.A.; Bashkatov, A.N.; Terentyuk, G.S.; Bucharskaya, A.B.; Maslyakova, G.N.; Gorin, D.A.; et al. In Vivo Optical Monitoring of Transcutaneous Delivery of Calcium Carbonate Microcontainers. *Biomed. Opt. Express* **2016**, *7*, 2082. [CrossRef]
16. Svenskaya, Y.I.; Genina, E.A.; Parakhonskiy, B.V.; Lengert, E.V.; Talnikova, E.E.; Terentyuk, G.S.; Utz, S.R.; Gorin, D.A.; Tuchin, V.V.; Sukhorukov, G.B. A Simple Non-Invasive Approach toward Efficient Transdermal Drug Delivery Based on Biodegradable Particulate System. *ACS Appl. Mater. Interfaces* **2019**, *11*, 17270–17282. [CrossRef] [PubMed]
17. Gusliakova, O.; Atochina-Vasserman, E.N.; Sindeeva, O.; Sindeev, S.; Pinyaev, S.; Pyataev, N.; Revin, V.; Sukhorukov, G.B.; Gorin, D.; Gow, A.J. Use of Submicron Vaterite Particles Serves as an Effective Delivery Vehicle to the Respiratory Portion of the Lung. *Front. Pharmacol.* **2018**, *9*, 559. [CrossRef]
18. Niu, Y.-Q.; Liu, J.-H.; Aymonier, C.; Fermani, S.; Kralj, D.; Falini, G.; Zhou, C.-H. Calcium Carbonate: Controlled Synthesis, Surface Functionalization, and Nanostructured Materials. *Chem. Soc. Rev.* **2022**, *51*, 7883–7943. [CrossRef]
19. Jones, B. Review of Calcium Carbonate Polymorph Precipitation in Spring Systems. *Sediment. Geol.* **2017**, *353*, 64–75. [CrossRef]
20. Konopacka-Łyskawa, D. Synthesis Methods and Favorable Conditions for Spherical Vaterite Precipitation: A Review. *Crystals* **2019**, *9*, 223. [CrossRef]
21. Dorozhkin, S.V.; Epple, M. Biological and Medical Significance of Calcium Phosphates. *Angew. Chem. Int. Ed.* **2002**, *41*, 3130–3146. [CrossRef]
22. Hunton, P. Research on Eggshell Structure and Quality: An Historical Overview. *Rev. Bras. Ciência Avícola* **2005**, *7*, 67–71. [CrossRef]
23. Seifan, M.; Berenjian, A. Microbially Induced Calcium Carbonate Precipitation: A Widespread Phenomenon in the Biological World. *Appl. Microbiol. Biotechnol.* **2019**, *103*, 4693–4708. [CrossRef] [PubMed]
24. Fiori, C.; Vandini, M.; Prati, S.; Chiavari, G. Vaterite in the Mortars of a Mosaic in the Saint Peter Basilica, Vatican (Rome). *J. Cult. Herit.* **2009**, *10*, 248–257. [CrossRef]
25. Wolf, G.; Günther, C. Thermophysical Investigations of the Polymorphous Phases of Calcium Carbonate. *J. Therm. Anal. Calorim.* **2001**, *65*, 687–698. [CrossRef]
26. Wang, X.; Kong, R.; Pan, X.; Xu, H.; Xia, D.; Shan, H.; Lu, J.R. Role of Ovalbumin in the Stabilization of Metastable Vaterite in Calcium Carbonate Biomineralization. *J. Phys. Chem. B* **2009**, *113*, 8975–8982. [CrossRef]
27. Weiner, S.; Levi-Kalisman, Y.; Raz, S.; Addadi, L. Biologically Formed Amorphous Calcium Carbonate. *Connect. Tissue Res.* **2003**, *44*, 214–218. [CrossRef]
28. Jia, S.; Guo, Y.; Zai, W.; Su, Y.; Yuan, S.; Yu, X.; Xu, Y.; Li, G. Preparation and Characterization of a Composite Coating Composed of Polycaprolactone (PCL) and Amorphous Calcium Carbonate (ACC) Particles for Enhancing Corrosion Resistance of Magnesium Implants. *Prog. Org. Coat.* **2019**, *136*, 105225. [CrossRef]
29. Wang, X.; Ackermann, M.; Wang, S.; Tolba, E.; Neufurth, M.; Feng, Q.; Schröder, H.C.; Müller, W.E.G. Amorphous Polyphosphate/Amorphous Calcium Carbonate Implant Material with Enhanced Bone Healing Efficacy in a Critical-Size Defect in Rats. *Biomed. Mater.* **2016**, *11*, 035005. [CrossRef]
30. Ogino, T.; Suzuki, T.; Sawada, K. The Formation and Transformation Mechanism of Calcium Carbonate in Water. *Geochim. Cosmochim. Acta* **1987**, *51*, 2757–2767. [CrossRef]
31. Kabalah-Amitai, L.; Mayzel, B.; Kauffmann, Y.; Fitch, A.N.; Bloch, L.; Gilbert, P.U.P.A.; Pokroy, B. Vaterite Crystals Contain Two Interspersed Crystal Structures. *Science* **2013**, *340*, 454–457. [CrossRef]
32. Schenk, A.S.; Albarracin, E.J.; Kim, Y.-Y.; Ihli, J.; Meldrum, F.C. Confinement Stabilises Single Crystal Vaterite Rods. *Chem. Commun.* **2014**, *50*, 4729–4732. [CrossRef]
33. Parakhonskiy, B.V.; Foss, C.; Carletti, E.; Fedel, M.; Haase, A.; Motta, A.; Migliaresi, C.; Antolini, R. Tailored Intracellular Delivery via a Crystal Phase Transition in 400 Nm Vaterite Particles. *Biomater. Sci.* **2013**, *1*, 1273. [CrossRef] [PubMed]
34. Beuvier, T.; Calvignac, B.; Delcroix, G.J.-R.; Tran, M.K.; Kodjikian, S.; Delorme, N.; Bardeau, J.-F.; Gibaud, A.; Boury, F. Synthesis of Hollow Vaterite CaCO$_3$ Microspheres in Supercritical Carbon Dioxide Medium. *J. Mater. Chem.* **2011**, *21*, 9757. [CrossRef]
35. Wang, A.; Yang, Y.; Zhang, X.; Liu, X.; Cui, W.; Li, J. Gelatin-Assisted Synthesis of Vaterite Nanoparticles with Higher Surface Area and Porosity as Anticancer Drug Containers In Vitro. *Chempluschem* **2016**, *81*, 194–201. [CrossRef] [PubMed]
36. Vikulina, A.; Voronin, D.; Fakhrullin, R.; Vinokurov, V.; Volodkin, D. Naturally Derived Nano- and Micro-Drug Delivery Vehicles: Halloysite, Vaterite and Nanocellulose. *New J. Chem.* **2020**, *44*, 5638–5665. [CrossRef]
37. Kralj, D.; Brečević, L.; Kontrec, J. Vaterite Growth and Dissolution in Aqueous Solution III. Kinetics of Transformation. *J. Cryst. Growth* **1997**, *177*, 248–257. [CrossRef]
38. Svenskaya, Y.; Parakhonskiy, B.; Haase, A.; Atkin, V.; Lukyanets, E.; Gorin, D.; Antolini, R. Anticancer Drug Delivery System Based on Calcium Carbonate Particles Loaded with a Photosensitizer. *Biophys. Chem.* **2013**, *182*, 11–15. [CrossRef] [PubMed]

39. Sheng Han, Y.; Hadiko, G.; Fuji, M.; Takahashi, M. Crystallization and Transformation of Vaterite at Controlled pH. *J. Cryst. Growth* **2006**, *289*, 269–274. [CrossRef]
40. Parakhonskiy, B.; Tessarolo, F.; Haase, A.; Antolini, R. Dependence of Sub-Micron Vaterite Container Release Properties on pH and Ionic Strength of the Surrounding Solution. *Adv. Sci. Technol.* **2012**, *86*, 81–85.
41. Katsifaras, A.; Spanos, N. Effect of Inorganic Phosphate Ions on the Spontaneous Precipitation of Vaterite and on the Transformation of Vaterite to Calcite. *J. Cryst. Growth* **1999**, *204*, 183–190. [CrossRef]
42. Al Omari, M.M.H.; Rashid, I.S.; Qinna, N.A.; Jaber, A.M.; Badwan, A.A. Calcium Carbonate. In *Profiles of Drug Substances, Excipients and Related Methodology*; Elsevier: Amsterdam, The Netherlands, 2016; pp. 31–132.
43. Saveleva, M.S.; Lengert, E.V.; Verkhovskii, R.A.; Abalymov, A.A.; Pavlov, A.M.; Ermakov, A.V.; Prikhozhdenko, E.S.; Shtykov, S.N.; Svenskaya, Y.I. CaCO$_3$-Based Carriers with Prolonged Release Properties for Antifungal Drug Delivery to Hair Follicles. *Biomater. Sci.* **2022**, *10*, 3323–3345. [CrossRef] [PubMed]
44. Tan, C.; Dima, C.; Huang, M.; Assadpour, E.; Wang, J.; Sun, B.; Kharazmi, M.S.; Jafari, S.M. Advanced CaCO$_3$-Derived Delivery Systems for Bioactive Compounds. *Adv. Colloid Interface Sci.* **2022**, *309*, 102791. [CrossRef] [PubMed]
45. Svenskaya, Y.I.; Navolokin, N.A.; Bucharskaya, A.B.; Terentyuk, G.S.; Kuz'mina, A.O.; Burashnikova, M.M.; Maslyakova, G.N.; Lukyanets, E.A.; Gorin, D.A. Calcium Carbonate Microparticles Containing a Photosensitizer Photosens: Preparation, Ultrasound Stimulated Dye Release, and In Vivo Application. *Nanotechnol. Russ.* **2014**, *9*, 398–409. [CrossRef]
46. Dizaj, S.M.; Barzegar-Jalali, M.; Hossein Zarrintan, M.; Adibkia, K.; Lotfipour, F. Calcium Carbonate Nanoparticles; Potential in Bone and Tooth Disorders. *Pharm. Sci.* **2015**, *20*, 175–182.
47. An, S. The Emerging Role of Extracellular Ca^{2+} in Osteo/Odontogenic Differentiation and the Involvement of Intracellular Ca^{2+} Signaling: From Osteoblastic Cells to Dental Pulp Cells and Odontoblasts. *J. Cell. Physiol.* **2019**, *234*, 2169–2193. [CrossRef]
48. Abalymov, A.; Lengert, E.; Van der Meeren, L.; Saveleva, M.; Ivanova, A.; Douglas, T.E.L.; Skirtach, A.G.; Volodkin, D.; Parakhonskiy, B. The Influence of Ca/Mg Ratio on Autogelation of Hydrogel Biomaterials with Bioceramic Compounds. *Biomater. Adv.* **2022**, *133*, 112632. [CrossRef]
49. Sergeeva, A.; Vikulina, A.S.; Volodkin, D. Porous Alginate Scaffolds Assembled Using Vaterite CaCO$_3$ Crystals. *Micromachines* **2019**, *10*, 357. [CrossRef]
50. Yu, Q.; Su, B.; Zhao, W.; Zhao, C. Janus Self-Propelled Chitosan-Based Hydrogel Spheres for Rapid Bleeding Control. *Adv. Sci.* **2023**, *10*, 2205989. [CrossRef]
51. Li, Q.; Hu, E.; Yu, K.; Xie, R.; Lu, F.; Lu, B.; Bao, R.; Zhao, T.; Dai, F.; Lan, G. Self-Propelling Janus Particles for Hemostasis in Perforating and Irregular Wounds with Massive Hemorrhage. *Adv. Funct. Mater.* **2020**, *30*, 2004153. [CrossRef]
52. Volodkin, D. CaCO$_3$ Templated Micro-Beads and -Capsules for Bioapplications. *Adv. Colloid Interface Sci.* **2014**, *207*, 306–324. [CrossRef] [PubMed]
53. Volodkin, D.V.; Petrov, A.I.; Prevot, M.; Sukhorukov, G.B. Matrix Polyelectrolyte Microcapsules: New System for Macromolecule Encapsulation. *Langmuir* **2004**, *20*, 3398–3406. [CrossRef] [PubMed]
54. Volodkin, D.V.; Larionova, N.I.; Sukhorukov, G.B. Protein Encapsulation via Porous CaCO$_3$ Microparticles Templating. *Biomacromolecules* **2004**, *5*, 1962–1972. [CrossRef] [PubMed]
55. Sergeeva, A.; Feoktistova, N.; Prokopovic, V.; Gorin, D.; Volodkin, D. Design of Porous Alginate Hydrogels by Sacrificial CaCO$_3$ Templates: Pore Formation Mechanism. *Adv. Mater. Interfaces* **2015**, *2*, 1500386. [CrossRef]
56. Som, A.; Raliya, R.; Tian, L.; Akers, W.; Ippolito, J.E.; Singamaneni, S.; Biswas, P.; Achilefu, S. Monodispersed Calcium Carbonate Nanoparticles Modulate Local pH and Inhibit Tumor Growth in Vivo. *Nanoscale* **2016**, *8*, 12639–12647. [CrossRef]
57. Lam, S.F.; Bishop, K.W.; Mintz, R.; Fang, L.; Achilefu, S. Calcium Carbonate Nanoparticles Stimulate Cancer Cell Reprogramming to Suppress Tumor Growth and Invasion in an Organ-on-a-Chip System. *Sci. Rep.* **2021**, *11*, 9246. [CrossRef]
58. Maleki Dizaj, S.; Barzegar-Jalali, M.; Zarrintan, M.H.; Adibkia, K.; Lotfipour, F. Calcium Carbonate Nanoparticles as Cancer Drug Delivery System. *Expert Opin. Drug Deliv.* **2015**, *12*, 1649–1660. [CrossRef]
59. Maleki Dizaj, S.; Sharifi, S.; Ahmadian, E.; Eftekhari, A.; Adibkia, K.; Lotfipour, F. An Update on Calcium Carbonate Nanoparticles as Cancer Drug/Gene Delivery System. *Expert Opin. Drug Deliv.* **2019**, *16*, 331–345. [CrossRef]
60. Zafar, B.; Campbell, J.; Cooke, J.; Skirtach, A.G.; Volodkin, D. Modification of Surfaces with Vaterite CaCO$_3$ Particles. *Micromachines* **2022**, *13*, 473. [CrossRef]
61. Fu, J.; Leo, C.P.; Show, P.L. Recent Advances in the Synthesis and Applications of pH-Responsive CaCO$_3$. *Biochem. Eng. J.* **2022**, *187*, 108446. [CrossRef]
62. Petrov, A.I.; Volodkin, D.V.; Sukhorukov, G.B. Protein-Calcium Carbonate Coprecipitation: A Tool for Protein Encapsulation. *Biotechnol. Prog.* **2008**, *21*, 918–925. [CrossRef] [PubMed]
63. Balabushevich, N.; Sholina, E.; Mikhalchik, E.; Filatova, L.; Vikulina, A.; Volodkin, D. Self-Assembled Mucin-Containing Microcarriers via Hard Templating on CaCO$_3$ Crystals. *Micromachines* **2018**, *9*, 307. [CrossRef]
64. Sukhorukov, G.B.; Volodkin, D.V.; Günther, A.M.; Petrov, A.I.; Shenoy, D.B.; Möhwald, H. Porous Calcium Carbonate Microparticles as Templates for Encapsulation of Bioactive Compounds. *J. Mater. Chem.* **2004**, *14*, 2073–2081. [CrossRef]
65. Borodina, T.N.; Rumsh, L.D.; Kunizhev, S.M.; Sukhorukov, G.B.; Vorozhtsov, G.N.; Feldman, B.M.; Rusanova, A.V.; Vasil'eva, T.V.; Strukova, S.M.; Markvicheva, E.A. Entrapment of Herbal Extracts into Biodegradable Microcapsules. *Biochem. Suppl. Ser. B Biomed. Chem.* **2008**, *2*, 176–182. [CrossRef]

66. Elbaz, N.M.; Owen, A.; Rannard, S.; McDonald, T.O. Controlled Synthesis of Calcium Carbonate Nanoparticles and Stimuli-Responsive Multi-Layered Nanocapsules for Oral Drug Delivery. *Int. J. Pharm.* **2020**, *574*, 118866. [CrossRef]
67. Chesneau, C.; Sow, A.O.; Hamachi, F.; Michely, L.; Hamadi, S.; Pires, R.; Pawlak, A.; Belbekhouche, S. Cyclodextrin-Calcium Carbonate Micro- to Nano-Particles: Targeting Vaterite Form and Hydrophobic Drug Loading/Release. *Pharmaceutics* **2023**, *15*, 653. [CrossRef]
68. Dunuweera, S.P.; Rajapakse, R.M.G. Encapsulation of Anticancer Drug Cisplatin in Vaterite Polymorph of Calcium Carbonate Nanoparticles for Targeted Delivery and Slow Release. *Biomed. Phys. Eng. Express* **2017**, *4*, 015017. [CrossRef]
69. German, S.V.; Novoselova, M.V.; Bratashov, D.N.; Demina, P.A.; Atkin, V.S.; Voronin, D.V.; Khlebtsov, B.N.; Parakhonskiy, B.V.; Sukhorukov, G.B.; Gorin, D.A. High-Efficiency Freezing-Induced Loading of Inorganic Nanoparticles and Proteins into Micron- and Submicron-Sized Porous Particles. *Sci. Rep.* **2018**, *8*, 17763. [CrossRef]
70. Demina, P.A.; Voronin, D.V.; Lengert, E.V.; Abramova, A.M.; Atkin, V.S.; Nabatov, B.V.; Semenov, A.P.; Shchukin, D.G.; Bukreeva, T.V. Freezing-Induced Loading of TiO$_2$ into Porous Vaterite Microparticles: Preparation of CaCO$_3$/TiO$_2$ Composites as Templates to Assemble UV-Responsive Microcapsules for Wastewater Treatment. *ACS Omega* **2020**, *5*, 4115–4124. [CrossRef] [PubMed]
71. Novoselova, M.V.; Voronin, D.V.; Abakumova, T.O.; Demina, P.A.; Petrov, A.V.; Petrov, V.V.; Zatsepin, T.S.; Sukhorukov, G.B.; Gorin, D.A. Focused Ultrasound-Mediated Fluorescence of Composite Microcapsules Loaded with Magnetite Nanoparticles: In Vitro and In Vivo Study. *Colloids Surf. B Biointerfaces* **2019**, *181*, 680–687. [CrossRef]
72. Mikheev, A.V.; Pallaeva, T.N.; Burmistrov, I.A.; Artemov, V.V.; Khmelenin, D.N.; Fedorov, F.S.; Nasibulin, A.G.; Trushina, D.B. Hybrid Core–Shell Microparticles Based on Vaterite Polymorphs Assembled via Freezing-Induced Loading. *Cryst. Growth Des.* **2023**, *23*, 96–103. [CrossRef]
73. Qiu, N.; Yin, H.; Ji, B.; Klauke, N.; Glidle, A.; Zhang, Y.; Song, H.; Cai, L.; Ma, L.; Wang, G.; et al. Calcium Carbonate Microspheres as Carriers for the Anticancer Drug Camptothecin. *Mater. Sci. Eng. C* **2012**, *32*, 2634–2640. [CrossRef]
74. Song, J.; Wang, R.; Liu, Z.; Zhang, H. Preparation and Characterization of Calcium Carbonate Microspheres and Their Potential Application as Drug Carriers. *Mol. Med. Rep.* **2018**, *17*, 8403–8408. [CrossRef]
75. Li, L.; Yang, Y.; Lv, Y.; Yin, P.; Lei, T. Porous Calcite CaCO$_3$ Microspheres: Preparation, Characterization and Release Behavior as Doxorubicin Carrier. *Colloids Surf. B Biointerfaces* **2020**, *186*, 110720. [CrossRef]
76. Xue, J.; Li, X.; Li, Q.; Lyu, J.; Wang, W.; Zhuang, L.; Xu, Y. Magnetic Drug-Loaded Osteoinductive Fe$_3$O$_4$/CaCO$_3$ Hybrid Microspheres System: Efficient for Sustained Release of Antibiotics. *J. Phys. D Appl. Phys.* **2020**, *53*, 245401. [CrossRef]
77. Sudareva, N.; Suvorova, O.; Saprykina, N.; Smirnova, N.; Bel'tyukov, P.; Petunov, S.; Radilov, A.; Vilesov, A. Two-Level Delivery Systems Based on CaCO$_3$ Cores for Oral Administration of Therapeutic Peptides. *J. Microencapsul.* **2018**, *35*, 619–634. [CrossRef]
78. Peng, C.; Zhao, Q.; Gao, C. Sustained Delivery of Doxorubicin by Porous CaCO$_3$ and Chitosan/Alginate Multilayers-Coated CaCO$_3$ Microparticles. *Colloids Surf. A Physicochem. Eng. Asp.* **2010**, *353*, 132–139. [CrossRef]
79. Wu, J.-L.; Wang, C.-Q.; Zhuo, R.-X.; Cheng, S.-X. Multi-Drug Delivery System Based on Alginate/Calcium Carbonate Hybrid Nanoparticles for Combination Chemotherapy. *Colloids Surf. B Biointerfaces* **2014**, *123*, 498–505. [CrossRef]
80. Bosio, V.E.; Cacicedo, M.L.; Calvignac, B.; León, I.; Beuvier, T.; Boury, F.; Castro, G.R. Synthesis and Characterization of CaCO$_3$–Biopolymer Hybrid Nanoporous Microparticles for Controlled Release of Doxorubicin. *Colloids Surf. B Biointerfaces* **2014**, *123*, 158–169. [CrossRef]
81. Ying, X.; Shan, C.; Jiang, K.; Chen, Z.; Du, Y. Intracellular PH-Sensitive Delivery CaCO$_3$ Nanoparticles Templated by Hydrophobic Modified Starch Micelles. *RSC Adv.* **2014**, *4*, 10841–10844. [CrossRef]
82. Shi, P.; Luo, S.; Voit, B.; Appelhans, D.; Zan, X. A Facile and Efficient Strategy to Encapsulate the Model Basic Protein Lysozyme into Porous CaCO$_3$. *J. Mater. Chem. B* **2018**, *6*, 4205–4215. [CrossRef] [PubMed]
83. Balabushevich, N.G.; Kovalenko, E.A.; Le-Deygen, I.M.; Filatova, L.Y.; Volodkin, D.; Vikulina, A.S. Hybrid CaCO$_3$-Mucin Crystals: Effective Approach for Loading and Controlled Release of Cationic Drugs. *Mater. Des.* **2019**, *182*, 108020. [CrossRef]
84. Osada, N.; Otsuka, C.; Nishikawa, Y.; Kasuga, T. Protein Adsorption Behaviors on Siloxane-Containing Vaterite Particles. *Mater. Lett.* **2020**, *264*, 127280. [CrossRef]
85. Singh, P.; Sen, K. Drug Delivery of Sulphanilamide Using Modified Porous Calcium Carbonate. *Colloid Polym. Sci.* **2018**, *296*, 1711–1718. [CrossRef]
86. Vergaro, V.; Papadia, P.; Leporatti, S.; De Pascali, S.A.; Fanizzi, F.P.; Ciccarella, G. Synthesis of Biocompatible Polymeric Nano-Capsules Based on Calcium Carbonate: A Potential Cisplatin Delivery System. *J. Inorg. Biochem.* **2015**, *153*, 284–292. [CrossRef]
87. Chitprasert, P.; Dumrongchai, T.; Rodklongtan, A. Effect of In Vitro Dynamic Gastrointestinal Digestion on Antioxidant Activity and Bioaccessibility of Vitexin Nanoencapsulated in Vaterite Calcium Carbonate. *LWT* **2023**, *173*, 114366. [CrossRef]
88. Borodina, T.; Markvicheva, E.; Kunizhev, S.; Möhwald, H.; Sukhorukov, G.B.; Kreft, O. Controlled Release of DNA from Self-Degrading Microcapsules. *Macromol. Rapid Commun.* **2007**, *28*, 1894–1899. [CrossRef]
89. Cheng, B.; Cai, W.; Yu, J. DNA-Mediated Morphosynthesis of Calcium Carbonate Particles. *J. Colloid Interface Sci.* **2010**, *352*, 43–49. [CrossRef]
90. Svenskaya, Y.I.; Lengert, E.V.; Tarakanchikova, Y.V.; Muslimov, A.R.; Saveleva, M.S.; Genina, E.A.; Radchenko, I.L.; Stepanova, L.A.; Vasin, A.V.; Sukhorukov, G.B.; et al. Non-Invasive Transcutaneous Influenza Immunization Using Vaccine-Loaded Vaterite Particles. *J. Mater. Chem. B* **2023**, *11*, 3860–3870. [CrossRef]
91. Wang, S.; Ni, D.; Yue, H.; Luo, N.; Xi, X.; Wang, Y.; Shi, M.; Wei, W.; Ma, G. Exploration of Antigen Induced CaCO$_3$ Nanoparticles for Therapeutic Vaccine. *Small* **2018**, *14*, 1704272. [CrossRef]

92. Borodina, T.N.; Rumsh, L.D.; Kunizhev, S.M.; Sukhorukov, G.B.; Vorozhtsov, G.N.; Feldman, B.M.; Markvicheva, E.A. Polyelectrolyte Microcapsules as the Systems for Delivery of Biologically Active Substances. *Biochem. Suppl. Ser. B Biomed. Chem.* **2008**, *2*, 88–93. [CrossRef]
93. Lee, C.H.; Lee, H.S.; Lee, J.W.; Kim, J.; Lee, J.H.; Jin, E.S.; Hwang, E.T. Evaluating Enzyme Stabilizations in Calcium Carbonate: Comparing In Situ and Crosslinking Mediated Immobilization. *Int. J. Biol. Macromol.* **2021**, *175*, 341–350. [CrossRef] [PubMed]
94. Tewes, F.; Gobbo, O.L.; Ehrhardt, C.; Healy, A.M. Amorphous Calcium Carbonate Based-Microparticles for Peptide Pulmonary Delivery. *ACS Appl. Mater. Interfaces* **2016**, *8*, 1164–1175. [CrossRef] [PubMed]
95. Feoktistova, N.A.; Vikulina, A.S.; Balabushevich, N.G.; Skirtach, A.G.; Volodkin, D. Bioactivity of Catalase Loaded into Vaterite $CaCO_3$ Crystals via Adsorption and Co-Synthesis. *Mater. Des.* **2020**, *185*, 108223. [CrossRef]
96. Yanina, I.Y.; Svenskaya, Y.I.; Prikhozhdenko, E.S.; Bratashov, D.N.; Lomova, M.V.; Gorin, D.A.; Sukhorukov, G.B.; Tuchin, V.V. Optical Monitoring of Adipose Tissue Destruction under Encapsulated Lipase Action. *J. Biophotonics* **2018**, *11*, e201800058. [CrossRef]
97. Feng, Z.; Yang, T.; Dong, S.; Wu, T.; Jin, W.; Wu, Z.; Wang, B.; Liang, T.; Cao, L.; Yu, L. Industrially Synthesized Biosafe Vaterite Hollow $CaCO_3$ for Controllable Delivery of Anticancer Drugs. *Mater. Today Chem.* **2022**, *24*, 100917. [CrossRef]
98. Parakhonskiy, B.V.; Shilyagina, N.Y.; Gusliakova, O.I.; Volovetskiy, A.B.; Kostyuk, A.B.; Balalaeva, I.V.; Klapshina, L.G.; Lermontova, S.A.; Tolmachev, V.; Orlova, A.; et al. A Method of Drug Delivery to Tumors Based on Rapidly Biodegradable Drug-Loaded Containers. *Appl. Mater. Today* **2021**, *25*, 101199. [CrossRef]
99. Zyuzin, M.V.; Antuganov, D.; Tarakanchikova, Y.V.; Karpov, T.E.; Mashel, T.V.; Gerasimova, E.N.; Peltek, O.O.; Alexandre, N.; Bruyere, S.; Kondratenko, Y.A.; et al. Radiolabeling Strategies of Micron- and Submicron-Sized Core–Shell Carriers for In Vivo Studies. *ACS Appl. Mater. Interfaces* **2020**, *12*, 31137–31147. [CrossRef]
100. Begum, G.; Reddy, T.N.; Kumar, K.P.; Dhevendar, K.; Singh, S.; Amarnath, M.; Misra, S.; Rangari, V.K.; Rana, R.K. In Situ Strategy to Encapsulate Antibiotics in a Bioinspired $CaCO_3$ Structure Enabling pH-Sensitive Drug Release Apt for Therapeutic and Imaging Applications. *ACS Appl. Mater. Interfaces* **2016**, *8*, 22056–22063. [CrossRef]
101. Gusliakova, O.; Verkhovskii, R.; Abalymov, A.; Lengert, E.; Kozlova, A.; Atkin, V.; Nechaeva, O.; Morrison, A.; Tuchin, V.; Svenskaya, Y. Transdermal Platform for the Delivery of the Antifungal Drug Naftifine Hydrochloride Based on Porous Vaterite Particles. *Mater. Sci. Eng. C* **2021**, *119*, 111428. [CrossRef]
102. Verkhovskii, R.A.; Lengert, E.V.; Saveleva, M.S.; Kozlova, A.A.; Tuchin, V.V.; Svenskaya, Y.I. Cellular Uptake Study of Antimycotic-Loaded Carriers Using Imaging Flow Cytometry and Confocal Laser Scanning Microscopy. *Opt. Spectrosc.* **2020**, *128*, 799–808. [CrossRef]
103. Borodina, T.N.; Trushina, D.B.; Marchenko, I.V.; Bukreeva, T.V. Calcium Carbonate-Based Mucoadhesive Microcontainers for Intranasal Delivery of Drugs Bypassing the Blood–Brain Barrier. *Bionanoscience* **2016**, *6*, 261–268. [CrossRef]
104. Borodina, T.; Marchenko, I.; Trushina, D.; Volkova, Y.; Shirinian, V.; Zavarzin, I.; Kondrakhin, E.; Kovalev, G.; Kovalchuk, M.; Bukreeva, T. A Novel Formulation of Zolpidem for Direct Nose-to-Brain Delivery: Synthesis, Encapsulation and Intranasal Administration to Mice. *J. Pharm. Pharmacol.* **2018**, *70*, 1164–1173. [CrossRef] [PubMed]
105. Kralj, D.; Brečević, L.; Nielsen, A.E. Vaterite Growth and Dissolution in Aqueous Solution II. Kinetics of Dissolution. *J. Cryst. Growth* **1994**, *143*, 269–276. [CrossRef]
106. Kralj, D.; Brečević, L.; Nielsen, A.E. Vaterite Growth and Dissolution in Aqueous Solution I. Kinetics of Crystal Growth. *J. Cryst. Growth* **1990**, *104*, 793–800. [CrossRef]
107. Binevski, P.V.; Balabushevich, N.G.; Uvarova, V.I.; Vikulina, A.S.; Volodkin, D. Bio-Friendly Encapsulation of Superoxide Dismutase into Vaterite $CaCO_3$ Crystals. Enzyme Activity, Release Mechanism, and Perspectives for Ophthalmology. *Colloids Surf. B Biointerfaces* **2019**, *181*, 437–449. [CrossRef]
108. Spanos, N.; Koutsoukos, P.G. The Transformation of Vaterite to Calcite: Effect of the Conditions of the Solutions in Contact with the Mineral Phase. *J. Cryst. Growth* **1998**, *191*, 783–790. [CrossRef]
109. Parakhonskiy, B.V.; Haase, A.; Antolini, R. Sub-Micrometer Vaterite Containers: Synthesis, Substance Loading, and Release. *Angew. Chem.* **2012**, *124*, 1221–1223. [CrossRef]
110. Saveleva, M.S.; Lengert, E.V.; Abramova, A.M.; Shtykov, S.N.; Svenskaya, Y.I. Spectroscopic Study of the Release Kinetics of Water-Insoluble Drug Griseofulvin from Vaterite Containers in Aqueous Medium. *Opt. Spectrosc.* **2021**, *129*, 813–820. [CrossRef]
111. Abalymov, A.A.; Verkhovskii, R.A.; Novoselova, M.V.; Parakhonskiy, B.V.; Gorin, D.A.; Yashchenok, A.M.; Sukhorukov, G.B. Live-Cell Imaging by Confocal Raman and Fluorescence Microscopy Recognizes the Crystal Structure of Calcium Carbonate Particles in HeLa Cells. *Biotechnol. J.* **2018**, *13*, 1800071. [CrossRef]
112. Schröder, R.; Besch, L.; Pohlit, H.; Panthöfer, M.; Roth, W.; Frey, H.; Tremel, W.; Unger, R.E. Particles of Vaterite, a Metastable $CaCO_3$ Polymorph, Exhibit High Biocompatibility for Human Osteoblasts and Endothelial Cells and May Serve as a Biomaterial for Rapid Bone Regeneration. *J. Tissue Eng. Regen. Med.* **2018**, *12*, 1754–1768. [CrossRef] [PubMed]
113. Verkhovskii, R.A.; Kozlova, A.A.; Lengert, E.V.; Saveleva, M.S.; Makarkin, M.A.; Mylnikov, A.M.; Navolokin, N.A.; Bucharskaya, A.B.; Terentyuk, G.S.; Bosak, I.A.; et al. Cytotoxicity, Dermal Toxicity, and In Vivo Antifungal Effect of Griseofulvin-Loaded Vaterite Carriers Administered via Sonophoresis. *ACS Infect. Dis.* **2023**, *9*, 1137–1149. [CrossRef] [PubMed]
114. Svenskaya, Y.I.; Pavlov, A.M.; Gorin, D.A.; Gould, D.J.; Parakhonskiy, B.V.; Sukhorukov, G.B. Photodynamic Therapy Platform Based on Localized Delivery of Photosensitizer by Vaterite Submicron Particles. *Colloids Surf. B Biointerfaces* **2016**, *146*, 171–179. [CrossRef]

115. Souza, E.F.; Ambrósio, J.A.R.; Pinto, B.C.S.; Beltrame, M.; Sakane, K.K.; Pinto, J.G.; Ferreira-Strixino, J.; Gonçalves, E.P.; Simioni, A.R. Vaterite Submicron Particles Designed for Photodynamic Therapy in Cells. *Photodiagnosis Photodyn. Ther.* **2020**, *31*, 101913. [CrossRef] [PubMed]
116. Svenskaya, Y.; Gorin, D.; Parakhonskiy, B.; Sukhorukov, G. Point-Wise Laser Effect on NIH/3T3 Cells Impregnated with Photosensitizer-Loaded Porous Calcium Carbonate Microparticles. In Proceedings of the 2015 IEEE 15th International Conference on Nanotechnology (IEEE-NANO), Rome, Italy, 27–30 July 2015; IEEE: New York City, NY, USA, 2015; pp. 1513–1516.
117. Tarakanchikova, Y.; Muslimov, A.; Sergeev, I.; Lepik, K.; Yolshin, N.; Goncharenko, A.; Vasilyev, K.; Eliseev, I.; Bukatin, A.; Sergeev, V.; et al. A Highly Efficient and Safe Gene Delivery Platform Based on Polyelectrolyte Core–Shell Nanoparticles for Hard-to-Transfect Clinically Relevant Cell Types. *J. Mater. Chem. B* **2020**, *8*, 9576–9588. [CrossRef]
118. Lauth, V.; Maas, M.; Rezwan, K. An Evaluation of Colloidal and Crystalline Properties of $CaCO_3$ Nanoparticles for Biological Applications. *Mater. Sci. Eng. C* **2017**, *78*, 305–314. [CrossRef]
119. Gusliakova, O.I.; Lengert, E.V.; Atkin, V.S.; Tuchin, V.V.; Svenskaya, Y.I. Spectral Monitoring of Naftifine Immobilization into Submicron Vaterite Particles. *Opt. Spectrosc.* **2019**, *126*, 539–544. [CrossRef]
120. Barbero, F.; Russo, L.; Vitali, M.; Piella, J.; Salvo, I.; Borrajo, M.L.; Busquets-Fité, M.; Grandori, R.; Bastús, N.G.; Casals, E.; et al. Formation of the Protein Corona: The Interface between Nanoparticles and the Immune System. *Semin. Immunol.* **2017**, *34*, 52–60. [CrossRef]
121. Caracciolo, G. The Protein Corona Effect for Targeted Drug Delivery. *Bioinspired Biomim. Nanobiomater.* **2013**, *2*, 54–57. [CrossRef]
122. Osterne, V.J.S.; Verduijn, J.; Lossio, C.F.; Parakhonskiy, B.; Oliveira, M.V.; Pinto-Junior, V.R.; Nascimento, K.S.; Skirtach, A.G.; Van Damme, E.J.M.; Cavada, B.S. Antiproliferative Activity of Dioclea Violacea Lectin in $CaCO_3$ Particles on Cancer Cells after Controlled Release. *J. Mater. Sci.* **2022**, *57*, 8854–8868. [CrossRef]
123. Abalymov, A.; Van Poelvoorde, L.; Atkin, V.; Skirtach, A.G.; Konrad, M.; Parakhonskiy, B. Alkaline Phosphatase Delivery System Based on Calcium Carbonate Carriers for Acceleration of Ossification. *ACS Appl. Bio Mater.* **2020**, *3*, 2986–2996. [CrossRef]
124. Fujiwara, M.; Shiokawa, K.; Kubota, T.; Morigaki, K. Preparation of Calcium Carbonate Microparticles Containing Organic Fluorescent Molecules from Vaterite. *Adv. Powder Technol.* **2014**, *25*, 1147–1154. [CrossRef]
125. Fujiwara, M.; Shiokawa, K.; Araki, M.; Ashitaka, N.; Morigaki, K.; Kubota, T.; Nakahara, Y. Encapsulation of Proteins into $CaCO_3$ by Phase Transition from Vaterite to Calcite. *Cryst. Growth Des.* **2010**, *10*, 4030–4037. [CrossRef]
126. Volodkin, D.V.; Schmidt, S.; Fernandes, P.; Larionova, N.I.; Sukhorukov, G.B.; Duschl, C.; Möhwald, H.; von Klitzing, R. One-Step Formulation of Protein Microparticles with Tailored Properties: Hard Templating at Soft Conditions. *Adv. Funct. Mater.* **2012**, *22*, 1914–1922. [CrossRef]
127. Donath, E.; Sukhorukov, G.B.; Caruso, F.; Davis, S.A.; Möhwald, H. Novel Hollow Polymer Shells by Colloid-Templated Assembly of Polyelectrolytes. *Angew. Chem. Int. Ed.* **1998**, *37*, 2201–2205. [CrossRef]
128. Zhao, S.; Caruso, F.; Dähne, L.; Decher, G.; De Geest, B.G.; Fan, J.; Feliu, N.; Gogotsi, Y.; Hammond, P.T.; Hersam, M.C.; et al. The Future of Layer-by-Layer Assembly: A Tribute to ACS Nano Associate Editor Helmuth Möhwald. *ACS Nano* **2019**, *13*, 6151–6169. [CrossRef]
129. Möhwald, H.; Donath, E.; Sukhorukov, G. Smart Capsules. In *Multilayer Thin Films*; Wiley: Hoboken, NJ, USA, 2002; pp. 363–392.
130. Parakhonskiy, B.V.; Yashchenok, A.M.; Konrad, M.; Skirtach, A.G. Colloidal Micro- and Nano-Particles as Templates for Polyelectrolyte Multilayer Capsules. *Adv. Colloid Interface Sci.* **2014**, *207*, 253–264. [CrossRef] [PubMed]
131. Campbell, J.; Kastania, G.; Volodkin, D. Encapsulation of Low-Molecular-Weight Drugs into Polymer Multilayer Capsules Templated on Vaterite $CaCO_3$ Crystals. *Micromachines* **2020**, *11*, 717. [CrossRef] [PubMed]
132. Kazakova, L.I.; Shabarchina, L.I.; Sukhorukov, G.B. Co-Encapsulation of Enzyme and Sensitive Dye as a Tool for Fabrication of Microcapsule Based Sensor for Urea Measuring. *Phys. Chem. Chem. Phys.* **2011**, *13*, 11110. [CrossRef]
133. Li, J.; Parakhonskiy, B.V.; Skirtach, A.G. A Decade of Developing Applications Exploiting the Properties of Polyelectrolyte Multilayer Capsules. *Chem. Commun.* **2023**, *59*, 807–835. [CrossRef]
134. Tarakanchikova, Y.; Alzubi, J.; Pennucci, V.; Follo, M.; Kochergin, B.; Muslimov, A.; Skovorodkin, I.; Vainio, S.; Antipina, M.N.; Atkin, V.; et al. Biodegradable Nanocarriers Resembling Extracellular Vesicles Deliver Genetic Material with the Highest Efficiency to Various Cell Types. *Small* **2020**, *16*, 1904880. [CrossRef] [PubMed]
135. Coto, B.; Martos, C.; Peña, J.L.; Rodríguez, R.; Pastor, G. Effects in the Solubility of $CaCO_3$: Experimental Study and Model Description. *Fluid Phase Equilib.* **2012**, *324*, 1–7. [CrossRef]
136. Yang, T.; Ao, Y.; Feng, J.; Wang, C.; Zhang, J. Biomineralization Inspired Synthesis of $CaCO_3$-Based DDS for pH-Responsive Release of Anticancer Drug. *Mater. Today Commun.* **2021**, *27*, 102256. [CrossRef]
137. Lakkakula, J.R.; Kurapati, R.; Tynga, I.; Abrahamse, H.; Raichur, A.M.; Maçedo Krause, R.W. Cyclodextrin Grafted Calcium Carbonate Vaterite Particles: Efficient System for Tailored Release of Hydrophobic Anticancer or Hormone Drugs. *RSC Adv.* **2016**, *6*, 104537–104548. [CrossRef]
138. Zhang, X.; Lin, Y.; Gillies, R.J. Tumor pH and Its Measurement. *J. Nucl. Med.* **2010**, *51*, 1167–1170. [CrossRef]
139. Verkhovskii, R.A.; Ivanov, A.N.; Lengert, E.V.; Tulyakova, K.A.; Shilyagina, N.Y.; Ermakov, A.V. Current Principles, Challenges, and New Metrics in pH-Responsive Drug Delivery Systems for Systemic Cancer Therapy. *Pharmaceutics* **2023**, *15*, 1566. [CrossRef] [PubMed]

140. Choukrani, G.; Álvarez Freile, J.; Avtenyuk, N.U.; Wan, W.; Zimmermann, K.; Bremer, E.; Dähne, L. High Loading Efficiency and Controlled Release of Bioactive Immunotherapeutic Proteins Using Vaterite Nanoparticles. *Part. Part. Syst. Charact.* **2021**, *38*, 2100012. [CrossRef]
141. Dong, Z.; Feng, L.; Zhu, W.; Sun, X.; Gao, M.; Zhao, H.; Chao, Y.; Liu, Z. CaCO$_3$ Nanoparticles as an Ultra-Sensitive Tumor-pH-Responsive Nanoplatform Enabling Real-Time Drug Release Monitoring and Cancer Combination Therapy. *Biomaterials* **2016**, *110*, 60–70. [CrossRef]
142. Li, K.; Li, D.; Zhao, L.; Chang, Y.; Zhang, Y.; Cui, Y.; Zhang, Z. Calcium-Mineralized Polypeptide Nanoparticle for Intracellular Drug Delivery in Osteosarcoma Chemotherapy. *Bioact. Mater.* **2020**, *5*, 721–731. [CrossRef]
143. Cheng, Z.; Zhao, D.; Wu, M.; Zhao, W.; Zhang, W.; Cui, Y.; Zhang, P.; Zhang, Z. Intracellular Co-Delivery of Proteins and Chemotherapeutics Using Calcium Carbonate Mineralized Nanoparticles for Osteosarcoma Therapy. *Mater. Des.* **2022**, *222*, 111040. [CrossRef]
144. Lee, H.J.; Kim, D.E.; Park, D.J.; Choi, G.H.; Yang, D.-N.; Heo, J.S.; Lee, S.C. PH-Responsive Mineralized Nanoparticles as Stable Nanocarriers for Intracellular Nitric Oxide Delivery. *Colloids Surf. B Biointerfaces* **2016**, *146*, 1–8. [CrossRef] [PubMed]
145. Albright, V.; Zhuk, I.; Wang, Y.; Selin, V.; van de Belt-Gritter, B.; Busscher, H.J.; van der Mei, H.C.; Sukhishvili, S.A. Self-Defensive Antibiotic-Loaded Layer-by-Layer Coatings: Imaging of Localized Bacterial Acidification and pH-Triggering of Antibiotic Release. *Acta Biomater.* **2017**, *61*, 66–74. [CrossRef] [PubMed]
146. Yang, T.; Wu, Y.; Yue, X.; Wang, C.; Zhang, J. Biomimetic Synthesis of Vaterite CaCO$_3$ Microspheres under Threonine for Preparation of pH-Responsive Antibacterial Biofilm. *J. Mater. Res.* **2020**, *35*, 2427–2440. [CrossRef]
147. Ferreira, A.M.; Vikulina, A.; Cave, G.W.V.; Loughlin, M.; Puddu, V.; Volodkin, D. Vaterite-Nanosilver Hybrids with Antibacterial Properties and pH-Triggered Release. *Mater. Today Chem.* **2023**, *30*, 101586. [CrossRef]
148. Lengert, E.; Yashchenok, A.M.; Atkin, V.; Lapanje, A.; Gorin, D.A.; Sukhorukov, G.B.; Parakhonskiy, B.V. Hollow Silver Alginate Microspheres for Drug Delivery and Surface Enhanced Raman Scattering Detection. *RSC Adv.* **2016**, *6*, 20447–20452. [CrossRef]
149. Zhou, Y.; Li, H.; Liu, J.; Xu, Y.; Wang, Y.; Ren, H.; Li, X. Acetate Chitosan with CaCO$_3$ Doping Form Tough Hydrogel for Hemostasis and Wound Healing. *Polym. Adv. Technol.* **2019**, *30*, 143–152. [CrossRef]
150. He, W.; Huang, X.; Zhang, J.; Zhu, Y.; Liu, Y.; Liu, B.; Wang, Q.; Huang, X.; He, D. CaCO$_3$–Chitosan Composites Granules for Instant Hemostasis and Wound Healing. *Materials* **2021**, *14*, 3350. [CrossRef]
151. Park, D.J.; Min, K.H.; Lee, H.J.; Kim, K.; Kwon, I.C.; Jeong, S.Y.; Lee, S.C. Photosensitizer-Loaded Bubble-Generating Mineralized Nanoparticles for Ultrasound Imaging and Photodynamic Therapy. *J. Mater. Chem. B* **2016**, *4*, 1219–1227. [CrossRef]
152. Min, K.H.; Min, H.S.; Lee, H.J.; Park, D.J.; Yhee, J.Y.; Kim, K.; Kwon, I.C.; Jeong, S.Y.; Silvestre, O.F.; Chen, X.; et al. pH-Controlled Gas-Generating Mineralized Nanoparticles: A Theranostic Agent for Ultrasound Imaging and Therapy of Cancers. *ACS Nano* **2015**, *9*, 134–145. [CrossRef]
153. Feng, Q.; Zhang, W.; Yang, X.; Li, Y.; Hao, Y.; Zhang, H.; Hou, L.; Zhang, Z. pH/Ultrasound Dual-Responsive Gas Generator for Ultrasound Imaging-Guided Therapeutic Inertial Cavitation and Sonodynamic Therapy. *Adv. Healthc. Mater.* **2018**, *7*, 1700957. [CrossRef]
154. Manickam, S.; Camilla Boffito, D.; Flores, E.M.M.; Leveque, J.-M.; Pflieger, R.; Pollet, B.G.; Ashokkumar, M. Ultrasonics and Sonochemistry: Editors' Perspective. *Ultrason. Sonochem.* **2023**, *99*, 106540. [CrossRef] [PubMed]
155. Lukes, P.; Fernández, F.; Gutiérrez-Aceves, J.; Fernández, E.; Alvarez, U.M.; Sunka, P.; Loske, A.M. Tandem Shock Waves in Medicine and Biology: A Review of Potential Applications and Successes. *Shock Waves* **2016**, *26*, 1–23. [CrossRef]
156. Cai, A.; Zhu, Y.; Qi, C. Biodegradable Inorganic Nanostructured Biomaterials for Drug Delivery. *Adv. Mater. Interfaces* **2020**, *7*, 2000819. [CrossRef]
157. Ma, M.-G.; Zhu, J.-F. Recent Progress on Fabrication of Calcium-Based Inorganic Biodegradable Nanomaterials. *Recent Pat. Nanotechnol.* **2010**, *4*, 164–170. [CrossRef] [PubMed]
158. Fu, K.; Xu, Q.; Czernuszka, J.; Triffitt, J.T.; Xia, Z. Characterization of a Biodegradable Coralline Hydroxyapatite/Calcium Carbonate Composite and Its Clinical Implementation. *Biomed. Mater.* **2013**, *8*, 065007. [CrossRef]
159. Stengelin, E.; Kuzmina, A.; Beltramo, G.L.; Koziol, M.F.; Besch, L.; Schröder, R.; Unger, R.E.; Tremel, W.; Seiffert, S. Bone Scaffolds Based on Degradable Vaterite/PEG-Composite Microgels. *Adv. Healthc. Mater.* **2020**, *9*, 1901820. [CrossRef]
160. Shors, E.C.; White, E.W.; Kopchok, G. Biocompatibility, Osteoconduction and Biodegradation of Porous Hydroxyapatite, Tricalcium Phosphate, Sintered Hydroxyapatite and Calcium Carbonate in Rabbit Bone Defects. *MRS Proc.* **1987**, *110*, 211. [CrossRef]
161. Fujioka-Kobayashi, M.; Tsuru, K.; Nagai, H.; Fujisawa, K.; Kudoh, T.; Ohe, G.; Ishikawa, K.; Miyamoto, Y. Fabrication and Evaluation of Carbonate Apatite-Coated Calcium Carbonate Bone Substitutes for Bone Tissue Engineering. *J. Tissue Eng. Regen. Med.* **2018**, *12*, 2077–2087. [CrossRef]
162. Bohner, M. Resorbable Biomaterials as Bone Graft Substitutes. *Mater. Today* **2010**, *13*, 24–30. [CrossRef]
163. Lu, J.; Descamps, M.; Dejou, J.; Koubi, G.; Hardouin, P.; Lemaitre, J.; Proust, J.-P. The Biodegradation Mechanism of Calcium Phosphate Biomaterials in Bone. *J. Biomed. Mater. Res.* **2002**, *63*, 408–412. [CrossRef]
164. Tolba, E.; Müller, W.E.G.; Abd El-Hady, B.M.; Neufurth, M.; Wurm, F.; Wang, S.; Schröder, H.C.; Wang, X. High Biocompatibility and Improved Osteogenic Potential of Amorphous Calcium Carbonate/Vaterite. *J. Mater. Chem. B* **2016**, *4*, 376–386. [CrossRef]

165. Unger, R.E.; Stojanovic, S.; Besch, L.; Alkildani, S.; Schröder, R.; Jung, O.; Bogram, C.; Görke, O.; Najman, S.; Tremel, W.; et al. In Vivo Biocompatibility Investigation of an Injectable Calcium Carbonate (Vaterite) as a Bone Substitute Including Compositional Analysis via SEM-EDX Technology. *Int. J. Mol. Sci.* **2022**, *23*, 1196. [CrossRef] [PubMed]
166. Jamalpoor, Z.; Asgari, A.; Lashkari, M.H.; Mirshafiey, A.; Mohsenzadegan, M. Modulation of Macrophage Polarization for Bone Tissue Engineering Applications. *Iran. J. Allergy Asthma Immunol.* **2018**, *17*, 398–408. [CrossRef] [PubMed]
167. Guillemin, G.; Hunter, S.J.; Gay, C.V. Resorption of Natural Calcium Carbonate by Avian Osteoclasts In Vitro. *Cells Mater.* **1995**, *5*, 157–165.
168. Freiwald, A. Bacteria-Induced Carbonate Degradation: A Taphonomic Case Study of Cibicides Lobatulus from a High-Boreal Carbonate Setting. *Palaios* **1995**, *10*, 337. [CrossRef]
169. Iversen, T.-G.; Skotland, T.; Sandvig, K. Endocytosis and Intracellular Transport of Nanoparticles: Present Knowledge and Need for Future Studies. *Nano Today* **2011**, *6*, 176–185. [CrossRef]
170. Tuchin, V.V.; Genina, E.A.; Tuchina, E.S.; Svetlakova, A.V.; Svenskaya, Y.I. Optical Clearing of Tissues: Issues of Antimicrobial Phototherapy and Drug Delivery. *Adv. Drug Deliv. Rev.* **2022**, *180*, 114037. [CrossRef] [PubMed]
171. Svenskaya, Y.I.; Talnikova, E.E.; Parakhonskiy, B.V.; Tuchin, V.V.; Sukhorukov, G.B.; Gorin, D.A.; Utz, S.R. Enhanced Topical Psoralen-Ultraviolet A Therapy via Targeting to Hair Follicles. *Br. J. Dermatol.* **2019**, *182*, 1479–1481. [CrossRef]
172. Utz, S.R.; Sukhorukov, G.B.; Tuchin, V.V.; Gorin, D.A.; Genina, E.A.; Svenskaya, Y.I.; Talnikova, E.E. Targeted Photosensitizer Delivery: A Prospective Approach to Vitiligo Photochemotherapy. *Vestn. Dermatol. Venerol.* **2019**, *95*, 21–29. [CrossRef]
173. Lengert, E.; Verkhovskii, R.; Yurasov, N.; Genina, E.; Svenskaya, Y. Mesoporous Carriers for Transdermal Delivery of Antifungal Drug. *Mater. Lett.* **2019**, *248*, 211–213. [CrossRef]
174. Svenskaya, Y.I.; Genina, E.A.; Tuchin, V.V. Sonophoretic Acceleration of Degradation Process for Vaterite Particles Delivered into the Hair Follicles. *Izv. Saratov Univ. New Ser. Ser. Phys.* **2021**, *21*, 80–85. [CrossRef]
175. Campbell, J.; Ferreira, A.M.; Bowker, L.; Hunt, J.; Volodkin, D.; Vikulina, A. Dextran and Its Derivatives: Biopolymer Additives for the Modulation of Vaterite $CaCO_3$ Crystal Morphology and Adhesion to Cells. *Adv. Mater. Interfaces* **2022**, *9*, 2201196. [CrossRef]
176. Manoli, F.; Kanakis, J.; Malkaj, P.; Dalas, E. The Effect of Aminoacids on the Crystal Growth of Calcium Carbonate. *J. Cryst. Growth* **2002**, *236*, 363–370. [CrossRef]
177. Zhang, Z.; Gao, D.; Zhao, H.; Xie, C.; Guan, G.; Wang, D.; Yu, S.-H. Biomimetic Assembly of Polypeptide-Stabilized $CaCO_3$ Nanoparticles. *J. Phys. Chem. B* **2006**, *110*, 8613–8618. [CrossRef] [PubMed]
178. Trushina, D.B.; Bukreeva, T.V.; Kovalchuk, M.V.; Antipina, M.N. $CaCO_3$ Vaterite Microparticles for Biomedical and Personal Care Applications. *Mater. Sci. Eng. C* **2014**, *45*, 644–658. [CrossRef]
179. Bentov, S.; Weil, S.; Glazer, L.; Sagi, A.; Berman, A. Stabilization of Amorphous Calcium Carbonate by Phosphate Rich Organic Matrix Proteins and by Single Phosphoamino Acids. *J. Struct. Biol.* **2010**, *171*, 207–215. [CrossRef]
180. Kirboga, S.; Oner, M. Effect of the Experimental Parameters on Calcium Carbonate Precipitation. *Chem. Eng. Trans.* **2013**, *32*, 2119–2124. [CrossRef]
181. Huang, S.-C.; Naka, K.; Chujo, Y. A Carbonate Controlled-Addition Method for Amorphous Calcium Carbonate Spheres Stabilized by Poly(Acrylic Acid)S. *Langmuir* **2007**, *23*, 12086–12095. [CrossRef]
182. Kim, I.W.; Robertson, R.E.; Zand, R. Effects of Some Nonionic Polymeric Additives on the Crystallization of Calcium Carbonate. *Cryst. Growth Des.* **2005**, *5*, 513–522. [CrossRef]
183. Nagaraja, A.T.; Pradhan, S.; McShane, M.J. Poly (Vinylsulfonic Acid) Assisted Synthesis of Aqueous Solution Stable Vaterite Calcium Carbonate Nanoparticles. *J. Colloid Interface Sci.* **2014**, *418*, 366–372. [CrossRef]
184. Luo, W.; Hua, J.; Xie, X. Polyethylenimine-CO_2 Adduct-Stabilized Vaterite Hydrocolloidal Particles. *Mater. Chem. Phys.* **2023**, *294*, 127025. [CrossRef]
185. El-Shahate Ismaiel Saraya, M.; Hassan Abdel Latif Rokbaa, H. Preparation of Vaterite Calcium Carbonate in the Form of Spherical Nano-Size Particles with the Aid of Polycarboxylate Superplasticizer as a Capping Agent. *Am. J. Nanomater.* **2016**, *4*, 44–51.
186. Naka, K.; Tanaka, Y.; Chujo, Y. Effect of Anionic Starburst Dendrimers on the Crystallization of $CaCO_3$ in Aqueous Solution: Size Control of Spherical Vaterite Particles. *Langmuir* **2002**, *18*, 3655–3658. [CrossRef]
187. Liu, R.; Huang, S.; Zhang, X.; Song, Y.; He, G.; Wang, Z.; Lian, B. Bio-Mineralisation, Characterization, and Stability of Calcium Carbonate Containing Organic Matter. *RSC Adv.* **2021**, *11*, 14415–14425. [CrossRef] [PubMed]
188. Rodriguez-Navarro, C.; Jimenez-Lopez, C.; Rodriguez-Navarro, A.; Gonzalez-Muñoz, M.T.; Rodriguez-Gallego, M. Bacterially Mediated Mineralization of Vaterite. *Geochim. Cosmochim. Acta* **2007**, *71*, 1197–1213. [CrossRef]
189. Parakhonskiy, B.V.; Abalymov, A.; Ivanova, A.; Khalenkow, D.; Skirtach, A.G. Magnetic and Silver Nanoparticle Functionalized Calcium Carbonate Particles—Dual Functionality of Versatile, Movable Delivery Carriers Which Can Surface-Enhance Raman Signals. *J. Appl. Phys.* **2019**, *126*, 203102. [CrossRef]
190. Parakhonskiy, B.V.; Svenskaya, Y.I.; Yashchenok, A.M.; Fattah, H.A.; Inozemtseva, O.A.; Tessarolo, F.; Antolini, R.; Gorin, D.A. Size Controlled Hydroxyapatite and Calcium Carbonate Particles: Synthesis and Their Application as Templates for SERS Platform. *Colloids Surf. B Biointerfaces* **2014**, *118*, 243–248. [CrossRef] [PubMed]
191. Kozlova, A.A.; German, S.V.; Atkin, V.S.; Zyev, V.V.; Astle, M.A.; Bratashov, D.N.; Svenskaya, Y.; Gorin, D.A. Magnetic Composite Submicron Carriers with Structure-Dependent MRI Contrast. *Inorganics* **2020**, *8*, 11. [CrossRef]

192. Choukrani, G.; Maharjan, B.; Park, C.H.; Kim, C.S.; Kurup Sasikala, A.R. Biocompatible Superparamagnetic Sub-Micron Vaterite Particles for Thermo-Chemotherapy: From Controlled Design to In Vitro Anticancer Synergism. *Mater. Sci. Eng. C* **2020**, *106*, 110226. [CrossRef]
193. Demina, P.A.; Abalymov, A.A.; Voronin, D.V.; Sadovnikov, A.V.; Lomova, M.V. Highly-Magnetic Mineral Protein–Tannin Vehicles with Anti-Breast Cancer Activity. *Mater. Chem. Front.* **2021**, *5*, 2007–2018. [CrossRef]
194. McDermott, J.J.; Kar, A.; Daher, M.; Klara, S.; Wang, G.; Sen, A.; Velegol, D. Self-Generated Diffusioosmotic Flows from Calcium Carbonate Micropumps. *Langmuir* **2012**, *28*, 15491–15497. [CrossRef] [PubMed]
195. Guix, M.; Meyer, A.K.; Koch, B.; Schmidt, O.G. Carbonate-Based Janus Micromotors Moving in Ultra-Light Acidic Environment Generated by HeLa Cells In Situ. *Sci. Rep.* **2016**, *6*, 21701. [CrossRef] [PubMed]
196. Saad, S.; Kaur, H.; Natale, G. Scalable Chemical Synthesis Route to Manufacture pH-Responsive Janus $CaCO_3$ Micromotors. *Langmuir* **2020**, *36*, 12590–12600. [CrossRef] [PubMed]
197. Wu, T.; Nieminen, T.A.; Mohanty, S.; Miotke, J.; Meyer, R.L.; Rubinsztein-Dunlop, H.; Berns, M.W. A Photon-Driven Micromotor Can Direct Nerve Fibre Growth. *Nat. Photonics* **2012**, *6*, 62–67. [CrossRef]
198. Svenskaya, Y.I.; Fattah, H.; Zakharevich, A.M.; Gorin, D.A.; Sukhorukov, G.B.; Parakhonskiy, B.V. Ultrasonically Assisted Fabrication of Vaterite Submicron-Sized Carriers. *Adv. Powder Technol.* **2016**, *27*, 618–624. [CrossRef]
199. Li, W.; Gai, M.; Rutkowski, S.; He, W.; Meng, S.; Gorin, D.; Dai, L.; He, Q.; Frueh, J. An Automated Device for Layer-by-Layer Coating of Dispersed Superparamagnetic Nanoparticle Templates. *Colloid J.* **2018**, *80*, 648–659. [CrossRef]
200. Reactor CR-1 by TetraQuant LLC. Available online: https://www.tetraquant.com/products (accessed on 12 October 2023).

Disclaimer/Publisher's Note: The statements, opinions and data contained in all publications are solely those of the individual author(s) and contributor(s) and not of MDPI and/or the editor(s). MDPI and/or the editor(s) disclaim responsibility for any injury to people or property resulting from any ideas, methods, instructions or products referred to in the content.

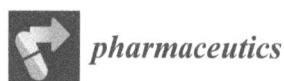

Article

Computational Amendment of Parenteral In Situ Forming Particulates' Characteristics: Design of Experiment and PBPK Physiological Modeling

Nada M. El Hoffy [1,*], Ahmed S. Yacoub [1,2], Amira M. Ghoneim [1], Magdy Ibrahim [3], Hussein O. Ammar [1] and Nermin Eissa [4,*]

[1] Department of Pharmaceutics and Pharmaceutical Technology, Faculty of Pharmacy, Future University in Egypt, New Cairo 11835, Egypt; ahmed.yacoub@fue.edu.eg (A.S.Y.); amiraghoneim@gmail.com (A.M.G.); drhusseinammar@hotmail.com (H.O.A.)
[2] Bone Muscle Research Center, The University of Texas at Arlington, Arlington, TX 76013, USA; asy3317@mavs.uta.edu
[3] Department of Pharmaceutics and Industrial Pharmacy, Faculty of Pharmacy, Cairo University, Giza 11562, Egypt; magdymohamed1@hotmail.com
[4] Department of Biomedical Sciences, College of Health Sciences, Abu Dhabi University, Abu Dhabi P.O. Box 59911, United Arab Emirates
* Correspondence: nada.mohamed@fue.edu.eg or nadahoffi@hotmail.com (N.M.E.H.); nermin.eissa@adu.ac.ae (N.E.); Tel.: +20-10-080202020 (N.M.E.H.); +97-15-09338431 (N.E.)

Abstract: Lipid and/or polymer-based drug conjugates can potentially minimize side effects by increasing drug accumulation at target sites and thus augment patient compliance. Formulation factors can present a potent influence on the characteristics of the obtained systems. The selection of an appropriate solvent with satisfactory rheological properties, miscibility, and biocompatibility is essential to optimize drug release. This work presents a computational study of the effect of the basic formulation factors on the characteristics of the obtained in situ-forming particulates (IFPs) encapsulating a model drug using a $2^1.3^1$ full factorial experimental design. The emulsion method was employed for the preparation of lipid and/or polymer-based IFPs. The IFP release profiles and parameters were computed. Additionally, a desirability study was carried out to choose the optimum formulation for further morphological examination, rheological study, and PBPK physiological modeling. Results revealed that the type of particulate forming agent (lipid/polymer) and the incorporation of structure additives like Brij 52 and Eudragit RL can effectively augment the release profile as well as the burst of the drug. The optimized formulation exhibited a pseudoplastic rheological behavior and yielded uniformly spherical-shaped dense particulates with a PS of 573.92 ± 23.5 nm upon injection. Physiological modeling simulation revealed the pioneer pharmacokinetic properties of the optimized formulation compared to the observed data. These results assure the importance of controlling the formulation factors during drug development, the potentiality of the optimized IFPs for the intramuscular delivery of piroxicam, and the reliability of PBPK physiological modeling in predicting the biological performance of new formulations with effective cost management.

Keywords: in situ forming nanoparticles; parenteral; targeted drug delivery; design of experiment; PDLG; cholesterol; PBPK; lipid; polymer

Citation: El Hoffy, N.M.; Yacoub, A.S.; Ghoneim, A.M.; Ibrahim, M.; Ammar, H.O.; Eissa, N. Computational Amendment of Parenteral In Situ Forming Particulates' Characteristics: Design of Experiment and PBPK Physiological Modeling. *Pharmaceutics* 2023, 15, 2513. https://doi.org/10.3390/pharmaceutics15102513

Academic Editors: Gábor Vasvári and Ádám Haimhoffer

Received: 14 September 2023
Revised: 13 October 2023
Accepted: 16 October 2023
Published: 23 October 2023

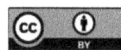

Copyright: © 2023 by the authors. Licensee MDPI, Basel, Switzerland. This article is an open access article distributed under the terms and conditions of the Creative Commons Attribution (CC BY) license (https://creativecommons.org/licenses/by/4.0/).

1. Introduction

Numerous drug candidates who suffer from poor oral bioavailability or minimal half-life now have a higher therapeutic potential, thanks to the development of innovative drug discovery tools, including genetic engineering, combinatorial chemistry, and high-throughput screening [1]. Additionally, these improvements in drug discovery have focused a lot of emphasis on the invention of creative methods to deliver them effectively and efficiently. Long-acting injectable systems are one innovator of such strategies [2].

These systems can sustain therapeutic drug levels for extended periods, offering benefits such as improved bioavailability, consistent plasma concentration, and targeted drug delivery. Furthermore, they are adaptable for various routes of administration, including subcutaneous, intramuscular, and intra-articular, with drug release rates controlled by the formulation's characteristics [3–5]. Both the vehicle and drug characteristics, as well as how the drug interacts with both the tissue and the vehicle, control the drug absorption kinetics and, thus, its duration of action [6].

In systems in which there is positive interaction between the drug and the carrier lipid and/or polymer-yielding implants and/or microparticles, a variety of approaches have been investigated to sustain the drug release. Numerous formulation issues have been observed, including increased process temperature, poor content homogeneity, and the continued requirement for invasive administration in the case of implants in addition to the multi-step manufacturing process and the formulation parameters, which should be closely monitored due to their influence on the scale-up process as well as manufacturing expenses [7].

Initially, approaches that lead to the prolongation of therapeutic activity were examined as viscous oil-based preparations, which could decrease the rate of drug diffusion. Recently, the development of injectable lipid and/or polymer-based particles with biodegradable as well as biocompatible characteristics, exhibiting optimal sizes ranging from 250 nm to 125 nm, has received attention. These particles are used to avoid the discomfort associated with surgical procedures for inserting bulky implants [8]. The latest research focuses on the preparation of a liquid lipid and/or polymer-based formulae containing the drug that solidifies and forms an implant at the site of injection upon contact with body fluids, which represents an effective substitute for conventional solid implants [9]. These formulations are prepared by dissolving polymers as poly(lactide) (PLA) and poly(lactide-co-glycolide) (PLGA) and lipids as cholesterol, phosphatidylcholine, and lecithin in solvents that are miscible with water, such as N-methyl-2-pyrrolidone (NMP) and dimethyl sulfoxide (DMSO). When the lipid and/or polymer solution containing the drug is injected, the lipid and/or polymer converts into an implant by solidification at the injection site [10]. When compared to conventional dosage forms, these cutting-edge formulation technologies have been found to decrease drug clearance and prolong its residence duration. The substantially high initial burst as well as the unfavorable viscosity of these preparations that renders injection inconvenient, are a key disadvantage of such systems. Innovative in situ micro-particles (ISM) were approached after extensive research presenting valid solutions to these issues [11].

ISM dosage forms involve emulsifying the drug-containing internal polymer solution with an external continuous phase of oily or aqueous nature. ISMs are deposited as soon as the emulsified solution comes into contact with the physiological fluids due to the diffusion of the internal phase solvent. These ISM systems greatly minimize the initial burst release as well as the viscosity of the injectable solution, leading to nearly painless injectability and reduced discomfort compared to the outdated polymer solutions. Additionally, ISMs are multi-particulate, which improves the stability as well as the consistency of the release profile of the drug while reducing implant morphological variations [12]. Recently, the application of these multi-particulate systems utilizing lipids as well as non-ionic surfactants is gaining much attention.

Non-steroidal anti-inflammatory drugs (NSAIDs) are the main building block in the treatment of well-known chronic inflammatory disorders via prohibiting cyclo-oxygenase (COX) enzymes. Overdose toxicity is the predominant side effect associated with their clinical usage [13]. While these moieties are mostly administered orally, they cause many systemic drawbacks, which arouses the need for the development of alternative localized formulations [14].

The design of experiments (DOE) is a structured and systematic approach that plays a pivotal role in drug development. In the complex and highly regulated field of pharmaceuticals, DOE is applied to efficiently and comprehensively explore the multifaceted factors affecting drug development processes. It enables scientists and researchers to optimize drug formulations, dosing regimens, and manufacturing processes while minimizing the need for extensive and costly experimentation. By varying and controlling multiple variables simultaneously, DOE can uncover critical interactions and dependencies that impact the safety, efficacy, and quality of drugs. This approach not only accelerates drug development but also enhances the quality of pharmaceutical products, reduces production costs, and ultimately leads to safer and more effective medications for patients. Whether it is the formulation of new drugs, the assessment of potential drug–drug interactions, or the optimization of manufacturing processes, DOE is an indispensable tool in the journey to bring innovative and safe pharmaceuticals to market [15,16].

Physiologically based pharmacokinetic (PBPK) modeling is a vital tool in the realm of drug delivery development. It allows researchers and pharmaceutical scientists to simulate and predict how drugs are absorbed, distributed, metabolized, and eliminated within the human body. Recently, the physiologically based pharmacokinetic (PBPK) modeling approach has grabbed attention in terms of the computational prediction of the different pharmacokinetic parameters of the drug following its administration [17]. PBPK modeling can predict drug concentration–time profiles as well as exposure in blood and specific organs, which are crucial for predicting efficacy/toxicity and risk assessment based on the physicochemical properties of the drug as well as the in vitro and/or ex vivo characterization results [18,19]. In drug delivery, PBPK models are instrumental in designing and optimizing delivery systems to enhance drug effectiveness and minimize side effects. By accounting for factors such as physiological variations, drug properties, and delivery methods, PBPK modeling aids in tailoring drug formulations and dosing regimens for specific patient populations [20]. It guides the development of novel drug delivery systems like nanoparticles, liposomes, and implants, ensuring they reach target tissues or organs effectively. Furthermore, PBPK modeling is indispensable for predicting the pharmacokinetics of sustained-release formulations, intravenous infusions, and transdermal patches, ultimately contributing to safer and more efficient drug delivery strategies, personalized medicine, and the successful translation of drug delivery innovations from the laboratory to clinical practice [21]. The obtained model through PBPK physiological modeling ultimate technological advancement should be validated through its correlation to the published clinical pharmacokinetic data prior to implementation [22]. Pharmaceutical research is currently visualizing PBPK modeling as a useful tool for decision-making at different stages of drug development [23].

The goal of the present work was the computational study of the influence of the various preparation factors on the characteristics of the obtained in situ-forming particulate formulations (IFPs) using the design of experiments (DOE) for the parenteral formulation of a model NSAID (piroxicam). Design Expert® 11 (Stat-Ease, Minneapolis, MN, USA) was used for the creation and analysis of the $2^1 \cdot 3^1$ full factorial experimental design. Furthermore, the release profile of the obtained formulae, as well as their kinetic models, were investigated. The optimum formulation was further investigated morphologically, and the obtained data were correlated to compute their expected biological performance using PK-Sim physiological modeling.

2. Materials and Methods

2.1. Materials

Piroxicam (PX) was kindly gifted from Medical Union Pharmaceutical (MUP) Co., Egypt. Polyethylene sorbitan monooleate (Tween® 80), Freund's complete adjuvant (CFA), Sorbitan monooleate (Span® 80), Cholesterol Brij 52®, and cellulose membrane dialysis bags were obtained from Sigma-Aldrich Chemie GmbH, Steinheim, Germany. Captex® GTO was kindly donated by Abitec Corporation, Janesville, WI, USA. Dimethyl sulfoxide (DMSO) and triacetin were purchased from Merck KGaA, Darmstadt, Germany. Sodium di-hydrogen orthophosphate-1-hydrate (Minimum Assay 98%), di-sodium hydrogen orthophosphate anhydrous (Minimum Assay Acidimetric 98%), and sodium chloride were acquired from ADWIC, Egypt. Eudragit® Rl 100 was bought from Evonik Operations GmbH, Germany. PURASORB® PDLG 7502 was a kind gift From Corbion Co., Amsterdam, The Netherlands.

2.2. Methods

2.2.1. Preparation of Drug-Loaded In Situ-Forming Particulate Formulations (IFPs)

The in situ-forming particulate formulations were prepared using the emulsion method in order to obtain nano-emulsions [24]. The emulsions consisted of two phases: the internal phase, which was prepared by liquifying precise amounts of the particulate-forming agent, and different structural additives in the organic solvent (triacetin), which were incubated in an incubation shaker stirrer (IKA Ks4000ic, Staufen, Germany) at 65 °C ± 0.5 °C (180 stroke/minute) for 12 h (Table 1). Furthermore, a precisely weighed amount of the drug was added to the internal phase, followed by vortexing for one minute. Using a vortex mixer, the accurate and consistent proportions of Captex® GTO and Span® 80 were merged to prepare the external phase. Finally, the emulsion was obtained by simple mixing of the internal and external phases by vertexing for one min.

2.2.2. Design of Experiment (DOE) and Construction of the $2^1.3^1$ Full Factorial Experimental Design

Design of experiments (DOE) is a systematic and structured approach to planning, conducting, and analyzing experiments or tests in order to obtain the most valuable information from the fewest trials. DOE represents a powerful tool that allows researchers to efficiently optimize processes, understand the influence of various factors, and make data-driven decisions, thus augmenting efficiency, data quality, and robustness and minimizing cost and trial and error while allowing for optimization, which leads to a better data-based decision making [25,26]. DOE was utilized for the generation and evaluation of the obtained models for the formulation of IFPs using Design Expert® 11 software (Stat-Ease, USA). A $2^1.3^1$ full factorial experimental design was computed to investigate the joint effect of independent formulation variables on the characteristics of the prepared formulations. One factor at two levels and the other at three levels were the two inputs evaluated as independent variables. The two independent factors were (A) the percentage of a particulate-forming agent and (B) the particulate-forming agent's type. Particle size (PS), Zeta potential, polydispersity index (PDI), mean dissolution time (MDT), percentage drug released after 0.5 h (Q0.5), half-life (T50%), and time required for ninety percent of the drug concentration to be released (T90%) were the computed dependent variables (Table 1).

2.2.3. Characterization of the Prepared IFPs

Particle Size and Polydispersity Index (PDI) Determination

Exactly one ml of the formulation was diluted 1:10 with deionized water, followed by one hour of stirring using a magnetic stirrer (Velp-AREC.T F20500051, Velp Scientifica, Usmate Velate, Italy) to produce IFPs. In order to determine the particle size and polydispersity index (PDI) of the formulated IFPs, the prepared sample was centrifuged for 15 min at 15,000 rpm at 4 °C in a refrigerating ultracentrifuge (3-30KS, Sigma Laborzentrifugen, Germany) just before the oily phase was eliminated. Particle size was determined after 1mL of deionized water was used to suspend the separated particles. The mean PS, as well as the vesicle PDI, were determined utilizing ZetaSizer (Nano Zs, Malvern Instruments Limited, Malvern, UK) (n = 3) SD in a dynamic light scattering (DLS) analysis.

Table 1. Dependent and independent variables of the $2^1.3^1$ full factorial experimental design of the piroxicam loaded in situ-forming particulate formulations.

Formulae	Independent Factors		Dependent Factors *								
	Percentage of Particulate Forming Agent	Type of Particulate Forming Agent	Particle Size Mean ± SD (nm)	PDI Mean ± SD (nm)	Zeta Potential Mean ± SD (mV)	$Q_{0.5}$ ± SD (h)	K ± SD (h^{-1})	$T_{25\%}$ ± SD (h)	$T_{50\%}$ ± SD (h)	$T_{90\%}$ ± SD (h)	MDT ± SD (h)
IFP1	5%	PLGA	1043 ± 98.26	0.854 ± 0.064	−11.6 ± 0.81	58.4 ± 3.31	2.20 ± 0.14	0.13 ± 0.016	0.32 ± 0.017	1.51 ± 0.12	0.46 ± 0.03
IFP2	7.5%	PLGA	951 ± 87.10	0.751 ± 0.041	−11.4 ± 0.92	43.65 ± 2.34	1.53 ± 0.12	0.19 ± 0.013	0.45 ± 0.020	3.60 ± 0.42	0.68 ± 0.04
IFP3	10%	PLGA	569 ± 34.21	0.663 ± 0.036	−18.4 ± 1.56	31.10 ± 2.80	0.50 ± 0.06	0.58 ± 0.041	1.40 ± 0.160	4.66 ± 0.51	1.24 ± 0.14
IFP4	5%	Cholesterol	470.5 ± 23.89	0.452 ± 0.035	−12.6 ± 0.76	71.65 ± 5.42	2.27 ± 0.19	0.13 ± 0.018	0.31 ± 0.024	4.17 ± 0.36	0.48 ± 0.06
IFP5	7.5%	Cholesterol	462 ± 39.74	0.426 ± 0.024	−12.5 ± 1.10	47.70 ± 3.90	0.64 ± 0.08	0.45 ± 0.032	1.10 ± 0.250	1.05 ± 0.16	1.04 ± 0.09
IFP6	10%	Cholesterol	363.5 ± 21.67	0.347 ± 0.017	−12.8 ± 1.07	39.45 ± 1.23	0.55 ± 0.02	0.52 ± 0.047	1.26 ± 0.19	1.02 ± 0.22	1.32 ± 0.28

* n = 3. PDI: polydispersity index; K: release rate constant; T90%, T50%, and T25%: time required for 90, 50, and 25% of the drug to be released, respectively; MDT: mean dissolution time; Q0.5: percentage drug released after 0.5 h. Internal phase contains 2 mg of piroxicam in all formulations stabilized by 0.1% tween 80.

In Vitro Drug Release Profile and Kinetic Modeling of the Prepared IFPs

In order to investigate the drug's release pattern from the designed formulation, the donor compartment was a cellulose membrane dialysis bag with dimensions of 7 cm in length, 2.2 cm in width, and a molecular weight cutoff of 12–14,000 Daltons [27]. The dialysis bag was filled with a precisely measured volume (0.5 mL) of drug-loaded IFPs, while exactly 100 mL of phosphate-buffered saline (pH 7.4) were used to mimic the receiving compartment, and the IFPs were incubated at a constant temperature of 37 °C ± 0.5 °C in an incubation shaker (180 rpm). At regular time intervals, 5 mL of the release medium were collected and replaced with fresh medium to maintain the sink conditions. Spectrophotometric analysis was used to determine the amount of encapsulated drug in the withdrawn samples at the previously determined wavelength. The average cumulative drug released percentage was plotted against time, followed by kinetic analysis of the obtained data by computationally fitting the data into various kinetic models, including the Zero, First, and Higuchi diffusion release models, followed by determining the best fit of the release data utilizing linear regression analysis [28,29]. In order to compare the formulations under investigation, various release parameters were calculated. The examined release metrics included mean dissolution time (MDT), percentage of drug released after 0.5 h ($Q_{0.5}$), time required for 25% of the drug concentration to be released ($T_{25\%}$), half-life ($T_{50\%}$), and time required for 90% of the drug concentration to be released ($T_{90\%}$).

2.2.4. Desirability Study

A selected formulation was chosen for additional research using the Design Expert® 11 software's integrated desirability function. The intended outcomes were to augment MDT, T25%, and T50% and reduce Q0.5 and PS. Only significant models were included.

2.2.5. Investigation of the Effect of Further Variations in Formulation Factors on the Selected Formulation
Effect of Adding Some Structural Additives

The selected formulation was subjected to further modification in order to control the initial drug release and enhance the retention time. Eudragit RL, either alone or in combination with Brij 52, was added to the internal phase, and the obtained formulations were characterized to investigate the significance of the addition of these structure additives on the Q0.5 followed by PS if the Q0.5 value was significantly minimized.

Effect of Solvent Variation

Further adjustments were made to the chosen formulation from the desirability study section to investigate the effect of different organic solvents on the characteristics of the formulation. DMSO and triacetin were investigated individually and as an equal combination (1:1) as the organic solvent in the internal phase. The obtained formulations were re-evaluated in terms of their Q0.5 followed by PS if the Q0.5 value was significantly minimized.

2.2.6. Characterization of the Optimized Formulation

The optimized formulation was chosen based on better control of the initial release with minor changes in PS for additional examinations.

Morphological Study Using Transmission Electron Microscope (TEM)

Using a high-resolution transmission electron microscope (TEM) (HR-TEM)—JEOL2100-USA, Wilmington, DE, USA), optimized IFPs were examined morphologically. To ensure the formation of IFPs, the prepared emulsions were introduced into 10 mL of phosphate buffer of pH 7.4 and then incubated for 24 h in an incubation shaker. The oily phase was separated by centrifugation at 15,000 rpm and 4 °C for fifteen minutes [24]. The morphology of the obtained particulates was examined using TEM with an 80 kV accelerating voltage after they had been dispersed in 1 mL of pH 7.4 phosphate-buffered saline. A drop of the IFPs was positioned on a copper grid that had been coated with carbon, and it was left there for approximately two minutes to adhere. On top of the carbon grid, a drop of phosphotungstic acid solution (2% w/v) was applied. The prepared sample was air-dried first prior to analyzing the IFP film [30].

Rheological Study

A computerized Brookfield rheometer (DV3THB cone/plate rheometer, spindle CPE-40, and RheocalcT software, version 1.1.13 software) (PolyScience model 9006, Niles, IL, USA) was utilized for the viscosity measurement of the chosen IFPs at 25 °C ± 0.2 °C, utilizing a cone and plate setup with a 20 mm diameter/4° angle and a set shear rate (1/s). The rheological characteristics of the prepared formulae were computed by plotting the shear stress versus the shear rate. Farrow's equation was implemented to investigate the flow pattern:

$$\text{Log } D = N \text{ Log } S - \text{Log } \eta,$$

where S stands for the shear stress, and D stands for the shear rate (s^{-1}) (Pa). N is the Farrow constant, and η is the viscosity (Pa·s) [31].

PBPK Physiological Modeling

Physiologically based pharmacokinetic (PBPK) modeling is a mathematical and computational approach used in pharmacology and toxicology to simulate and predict the behavior of drugs, chemicals, and other substances within the human body. It is a crucial tool in drug development, regulatory approval, risk assessment, and various research areas [18,19].

- Construction of the PBPK Model

PX constructed the PBPK model, which was developed and validated using PK-Sim® version 8.0 (Bayer AG, Leverkusen, Germany). Absorption, distribution, metabolism, and excretion (ADME) process data, physicochemical characteristics, and literature-based clinical pharmacokinetic figures for the drug were acquired from former publications and/or drug databases [32]. The software automatically computed the specific intestinal and organ permeabilities. The renal clearance value was computed to simulate the profile of cumulative excretion as an unchanged form within urine following the ranges presented in Ishizaki et al. [33]. Cellular permeabilities and partition coefficients were computed as Schmitt and PK-Sim® standard methods, respectively [34,35]. The PBPK model was developed for the intramuscular administration protocol of a single 10 mg/kg in the adult population.

- PBPK Model Evaluation

The PBPK model was validated through comparison with the observed clinical data by Calvo et al. after simulating the oral administration of a single dose of 20 mg of PX in adults [36]. The numerical evaluation of the model was carried out by comparing observed to predicted AUC0-24, C_{max}, and t_{max} values. The acceptance criterion for the model was set to a two-fold error range. In other words, if the predicted value/observed value (fold error) is in the 0.5–2 range, the PBPK model may be justified [37].

2.2.7. Statistical Analysis of Data

The collected data were displayed as mean ± SD (standard deviation). The computation of the results of the full factorial experimental design was performed using Design-Expert® 11 software (Stat-Ease, Inc., Minneapolis, MN, USA), followed by ANOVA testing to evaluate the statistical significance. The statistical significance level was set at a p-value of 0.05 in each experiment.

3. Results and Discussion

3.1. Preparation of Drug-Loaded In Situ-Forming Particulate Formulations (IFPs)

IFP formulations were prepared using the emulsification method. The resulting nano-emulsions were immiscible liquids that were stabilized with the aid of the appropriate surfactant and/or self-emulsifying oil phase with a typical mean droplet diameter of 500 nm or less. All obtained formulations had a homogenous clear or hazy appearance due to their small droplet size, as opposed to the milky white color of a coarse emulsion [38].

3.2. Statistical Analysis of the $2^1.3^2$ Full Factorial Experimental Design

3.2.1. Effect of Formulation Factors on Average PS and PDI Values of the Prepared IFPs

To determine the level of significance of the examined independent factors on the particle size and PDI of the formulations, an ANOVA test was conducted. The measured response values are presented in Table 1, and the model regression analysis is presented in Table 2. The particle size ranged from 363.5 ± 21.67 to 1043 ± 98.26 nm, and the PDI ranged from 0.347 ± 0.017 to 0.854 ± 0.064. The two models showed good correlation between the values of the R^2 (0.9999 and 0.9891, for PS and PDI, respectively), adjusted R^2 (0.9997 and 0.9728, for PS and PDI, respectively), and predicted R^2 (0.9990 and 0.9022, for PS and PDI, respectively), as well as the adequate precision of values (187.885 and 18.163, for PS and PDI, respectively), which guarantees the adequacy of the constructed model and ensures that the model may be used to investigate the entire design space. The PDI model results were sufficiently satisfactory with no need for further transformation, while the PS model required further transformation, as evident from the Box–Cox diagnostic, as presented in Figure 1B. Results revealed that both the percentage of particulate-forming agent (A) and the type of particulate-forming agent (B) significantly (p = 0.0004 and <0.0001, respectively) influenced the obtained values of particle size. The increase in the percentage of the particulate-forming agent significantly decreased the particle size, as presented in Figure 1A. This can be simply due to the better availability of the particulate building block with the possibility of better crosslinking leading to the formation of denser core smaller particulates. On the other hand, the cholesterol (CHL)-based particulates exhibited a significantly smaller particle size compared to the PDLG particulates. This may be attributed to the CHL imparting rigidity to the obtained particulates and decreasing the fluidization of the particles with a minimization of the surface free energy, all of which results in smaller-sized particulates. Moreover, the increased lipophilicity accompanied by the change in the type of particulate forming agent from PDLG to CHL, which in turn slowed down the diffusion of the internal phase solvent and consequently the deposition of the particles may have resulted in the formation of denser, uniform, and smaller particles. This is consistent with the outcomes that were described by Saberi et al. [39].

Regarding the PDI, only the type of particulate-forming agent significantly (p = 0.0061) influenced the PDI of the resulting particles, as presented in Figure 1C. Changing the particulate-forming agent from PDLG to CHL significantly decreased the PDI. This is in good agreement with the PS results, where the observed decrease in PS was accompanied by better homogeneity in the obtained size distribution, resulting in monodisperse systems with lower PDI values. These results are comparable to the results observed by Kumar et al. [40].

3.2.2. Effect of Formulation Factors on In Vitro Release Parameters

In vitro release study is one of the most fundamental studies for most controlled release systems. It is a great way to eliminate systems with release profiles that are undesirable. The effectiveness of in vitro tests for evaluating the finished systems' quality is extremely important.

Table 2. Model parameters of the $2^1.3^1$ full factorial experimental design of the piroxicam-loaded in situ-forming particulate formulations (IFPs).

Model Parameters	PDI Mean (nm)	Particle Size Mean (nm)	Q0.5 (h)	MDT (h)
Model Type	Main Effects	Main Effects	Main Effects	Main Effects
R^2	0.9891	0.9999	0.9797	0.9868
Adjusted R^2	0.9728	0.9997	0.9492	0.9670
Predicted R^2	0.9022	0.9990	0.8171	0.8811
Adequate Precision	18.163	187.885	14.411	16.929
Final Equation in Terms of Coded Factors	PDI = +0.58 +0.071 * A [1] +6.333 × 10^{-3} * A [2] −0.17 * B	$(P.S)^{\wedge -1.39}$ = +1.585 × 10^{-4} −3.019 × 10^{-5} * A [1] −2.335 × 10^{-5} * A [2] +6.371 × 10^{-5} * B	Q0.5 = +48.66 +16.37 * A [1] −2.98 * A [2] +4.28 * B	$(MDT)^{\wedge -1.68}$ = +1.80 +1.77 * A [1] −0.38 * A [2] −0.29 * B

PDI: polydispersity index; Q0.5: percentage drug released after 0.5 h; MDT: mean dissolution time; R2: squared regression coefficient.

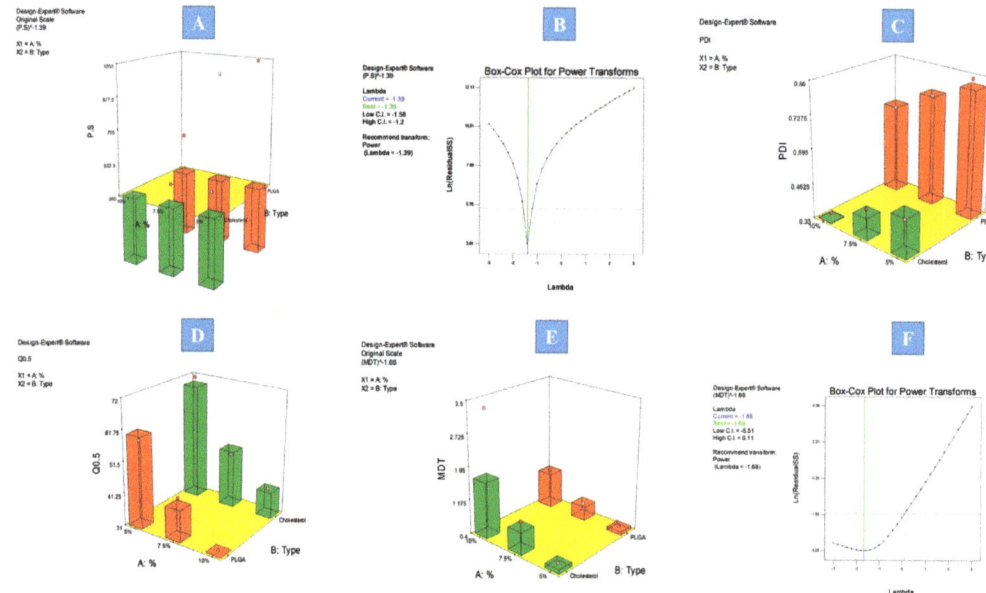

Figure 1. Example of 3D-response surface plots for the effect of formulation factors on (**A**) PS, (**B**) Box–Cox transformation for PS, (**C**) PDI, (**D**) Q0.5, (**E**) MDT, and (**F**) Box–Cox transformation for MDT.

As shown in Figure 2A, all formulations displayed a two-phased release pattern, exhibiting an initial rapid release phase, then a more extended-release stage follows. As soon as the formulation meets the dissolution medium, diffusion of the internal phase solvent takes place through the external oily phase, causing the particulates to deposit and solidify, trapping the drug into its core. The existence of some drug that was not trapped into the core of the produced particulates and is free to be released more rapidly than the drug that is entrapped, is what causes biphasic release [41]. In order to evaluate the distinctions between the prepared formulations, various release parameters were computed. The studied release parameters were mean dissolution time (MDT), percentage of drug released after 0.5 h ($Q_{0.5}$), time required for 25% of the drug concentration to be released ($T_{25\%}$), half-life ($T_{50\%}$), and time required for 90% of the drug concentration to be released

($T_{90\%}$). Only the constructed models for mean dissolution time (MDT) and percentage drug released after 0.5 h ($Q_{0.5}$) proved significant. Insignificant models were excluded from the study.

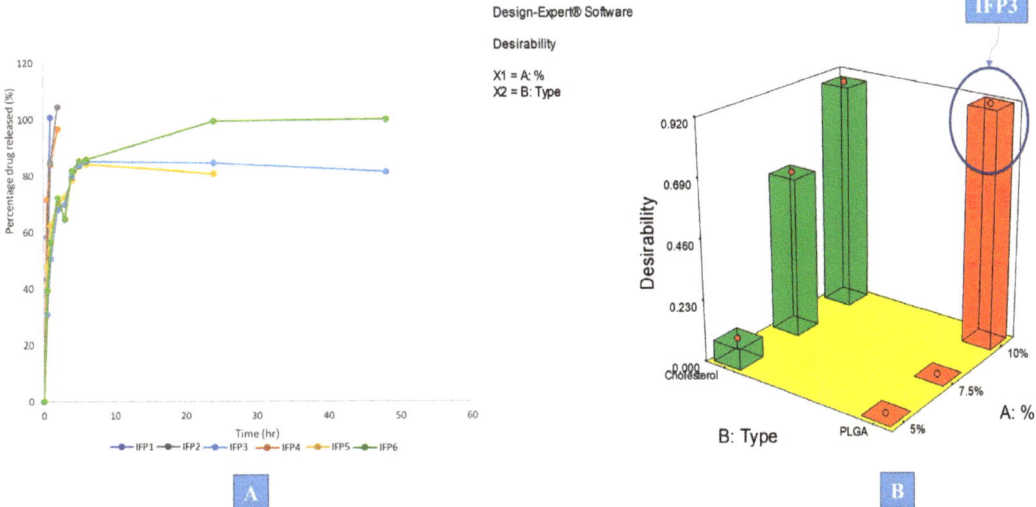

Figure 2. (**A**) Release profile of the prepared IFPs and (**B**) the desirability study marked with the chosen formulation.

The average cumulative drug release percentage was plotted versus time, and the release data were kinetically analyzed by substituting the obtained release data into various kinetic models, including the First, Zero, and Higuchi diffusion release models, utilizing linear regression analysis to find the release data's best fit. Followed by confirmation of the obtained results using the Korsmeyer–Peppas equation. All formulations exhibited first-order release kinetics, which is common in many particulate systems [42].

Effect of Formulation Factors on $Q_{0.5}$

To determine the level of significance of the examined independent variables on $Q_{0.5}$, an ANOVA test was conducted. The values of the measured responses are shown in Table 1, while the model regression analysis is presented in Table 2. The constructed model showed a good correlation between the values of the R^2 (0.9797), adjusted R^2 (0.9492), and predicted R^2 (0.8171), as well as the adequate precision of value 14.411, which assures the adequacy of the model. Results showed that the $Q_{0.5}$ values ranged from (31.10 ± 2.80 to 71.65 ± 5.42) and only the percentage of particulate forming agent (A) significantly (p = 0.0227) influenced the obtained values of ($Q_{0.5}$). The change in the percentage of the particular forming agent from the lower level to the higher level significantly decreased the $Q_{0.5}$ values, which reflects the drug's delayed release and the management of the formulation's well-known burst effect, as shown in Figure 1D. Additionally, since PDLG and cholesterol are the key particle producers, an increase in their percentage results in the formation of more particles; thus, more drug was entrapped within the formed particles. This decrease in the amount of free drug resulted in a significant decrease in $Q_{0.5}$, representing better control of the drug release pattern.

Effect of Formulation Factors on the Mean Dissolution Time (MDT)

Utilizing the ANOVA test, the level of significance of the independent factors on the MDT values was computed as shown in Tables 1 and 2 and ranged from 0.46 ± 0.03 to

3.32 ± 0.28 h. Applying the Box–Cox diagnostic test, power transformation was implemented to augment the sensitivity of the constructed model, as presented in Figure 1F. Results showed that the percentage of particulate forming agent (A) significantly ($p = 0.0138$) augmented the MDT values, as shown in Figure 1E. The previously observed significant control of $Q_{0.5}$ was attributed to the increase in PLGA and cholesterol concentrations, which accelerated the standard rate of IFPs deposition. Subsequently, the significantly increased portion of the entrapped drug reduced the initial release, revealed in the significant minimization in $Q_{0.5}$. All of which adds up to the total delay in medication release and the notable rise in MDT. This facilitated the total delay in the release of the drug and the notable rise in MDT value.

3.3. Desirability Study

IFP3 was recognized as the chosen formulation for additional investigation based on the desirability study implemented using Design® Expert desirability function with the target criteria of minimizing PS, PDI, and $Q_{0.5}$ and maximizing MDT, as shown in Figure 2B. Only significant models were included.

3.4. Further Investigation of the Effect of Formulation Factors on the Selected Formulation

3.4.1. Effect of Some Structural Additives

Further modifications were implemented into the optimized formulation IFP3 in terms of minimizing the initial release of the drug and maximizing the retention time. Eudragit RL was added as a structural additive in the internal phase with a concentration of 2.5% either alone (IFP3-E) or in combination with 2.5% Brij 52 (IFP3-EB). The release profile showed that the combination between Eudragit RL and Brij 52 significantly decreased the initial dug release represented in minimization of $Q_{0.5}$, which was 15.95 ± 1.32 and $13.95 \pm 0.9\%$ for IFP3-E and IFP3-EB, respectively, which are both significantly lower than IFP3, which had a $Q_{0.5}$ value of $31.10 \pm 2.80\%$, as shown in Figure 3A. This may be due to the expected physical interaction of the O–H group of Brij 52 and the C=O group of the drug that may suggest the development of a new hydrogen bond between the PX and Brij 52, which may have augmented the drug encapsulation within the deposition phase of the IFPs. Moreover, the presence of Eudragit RL may have increased the viscosity of the injected solution favorably, slowing down the diffusion of the internal phase into the surrounding medium and the deposition of the particulates allowing the encapsulation of more drug, which has significantly controlled $Q_{0.5}$. This is in correlation with the findings of Yacoub et al. [43]. The PS of IFP3-EB was 573.92 ± 23.5 nm, which was insignificantly ($p > 0.05$) different from IFP3.

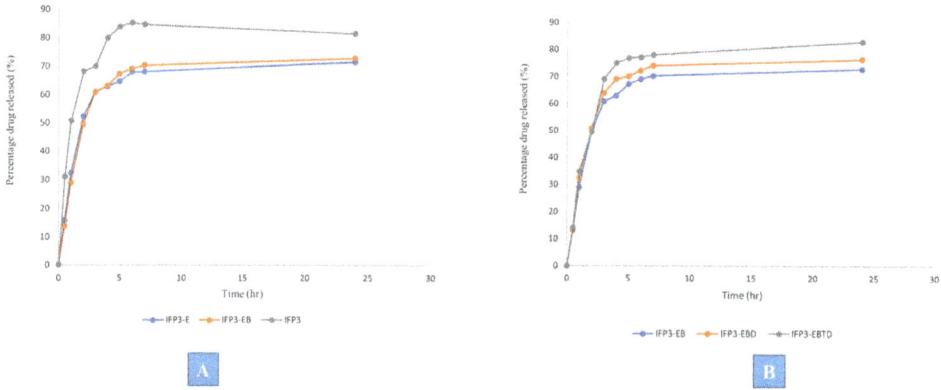

Figure 3. Release profiles of the chosen formulation IFP3 against modified formulations with (**A**) structural additives and (**B**) different solvents.

3.4.2. Effect of Solvent Variation

For many gases, synthetic fibers, paint, hydrocarbons, salts, and natural products, DMSO is a useful industrial and laboratory solvent. It is stable at high temperatures, aprotic, and relatively inert. Furthermore, DMSO has low acute and chronic toxicity. High concentrations of test organisms exposed via contact, ingestion, or inhalation repeatedly show low toxicity. It was noticed that the use of DMSO enhanced the solubility of the particulate-forming agents either alone (IFP3-EBD) or in combination with triacetin in the ratio 1:1 (IFP3-EBTD). The results showed the insignificance ($p > 0.05$) of changing the solvent from triacetin to DMSO in terms of its effect on the release profile of the prepared formulations, as shown in Figure 3B. Therefore, IFP3-EBD was chosen for further investigations based on the proven safety margin of DMSO compared to triacetin [44]. The PS of IFP3-ED was 579.12 ± 13.55, which was insignificantly ($p > 0.05$) different from IFP3-EB in spite of the difference in polarity between DMSO and triacetin. This may be attributed to the presence of Brij 52 with its large hydrophilic head that may have hindered the expected rapid diffusion of DMSO into the surrounding media and conserved the PS.

3.5. Characterization of the Optimized Formulation

3.5.1. Transmission Electron Microscopy (TEM)

The morphological pattern of the optimum formulation IFP3-EBD was identified using TEM. As shown in Figure 4A, the generated photographs demonstrated the deposition of uniformly spherical particulates with a dense core. This may be explained by the particulate formation mechanism, which depends on the solvent diffusing into the aqueous surroundings and the particulates depositing there. The assembly of dense particulates may have occurred as a result of the Brij 52 characteristic large polar head, delaying the diffusion of DMSO into the release medium.

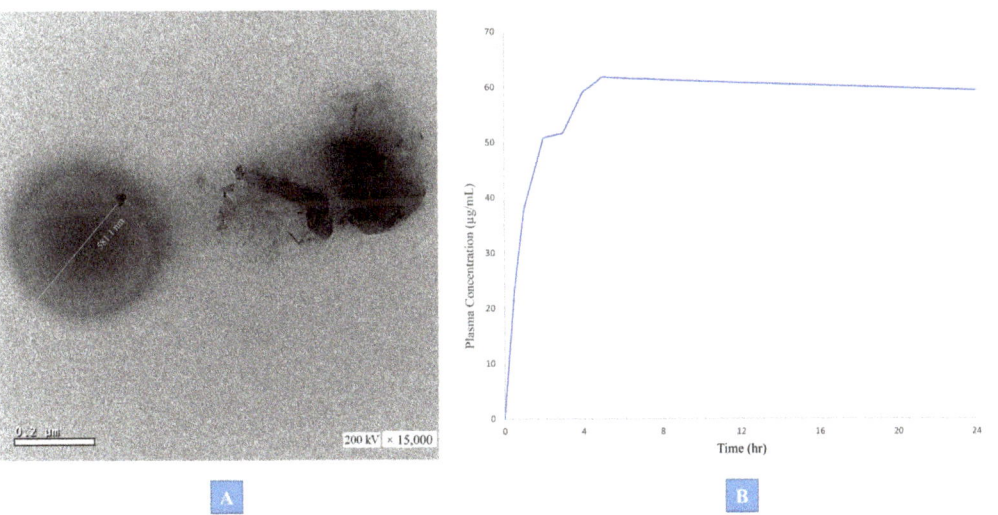

Figure 4. (**A**) Transmission electron micrograph (TEM) of the optimized formulations (IFP3-EBD). (**B**) PBPK simulated PX plasma concentration–time curves following IM application of IFP3-EBD.

3.5.2. Rheological Study

Rheology of the injectable formulation represents a crucial characteristic as it may hinder the ease of administration as well as cause pain upon application. IFP3-EBD exhibited a pseudoplastic flow, proved by the computed n value from Farrow's equation (n = 3.95). This flow ensures ease of application with minimal pain due to its decreased viscosity upon applying shear, which is favored in these types of formulation.

3.5.3. PBPK Physiological Modeling

Prior to the adult PX pharmacokinetic parameters' prediction following the intramuscular (IM) application of the optimum IFP3-EBD formulation, the constructed PBPK model was validated against the reported clinical data by Calvo et al. [36]. The model was verified by contrasting the T_{max}, C_{max}, and AUC_{0-24} of PX after a single oral dosage of 20 mg with the corresponding published pharmacokinetic values by Calvo et al. As shown in Table 3, the findings showed that the mean predicted/observed ratios for T_{max}, C_{max}, and AUC_{0-24} were 1.3, 0.9, and 0.6, respectively. This could verify the accuracy of the model that was selected and the modeling software that was being evaluated.

Table 3. Results for the development and validation of the piroxicam PBPK model.

Reference	AUC_{0-24} (µg·h/mL)			C_{max} (µg/mL)			T_{max} (h)		
	Observed	Predicted	Fold Error *	Observed	Predicted	Fold Error *	Observed	Predicted	Fold Error *
Calvo et al. [36]	78.7	45.4	0.6	2.28	2	0.9	4	5.25	1.3

* Fold error indicates predicted value divided by observed value (predicted/observed). AUC_{0-24}: area under the plasma concentration–time curve; C_{max}: maximum plasma concentration; t_{max}: time required to reach maximum plasma concentration.

The PBPK model-simulated plasma concentration–time curve of PX following the IM application of the optimized formulation in adults is presented in Figure 4B, while the predicted pharmacokinetic parameters are presented in Table 4. Results revealed that the C_{max} value of PX following the IM application of IFP3-EBD (10 µg/mL) was significantly higher than the corresponding mean value (2.28 µg/mL) observed with the reference oral administration (20 mg). At the same time, the AUC_{0-24} of the IFP3-EBD was 1383.03 compared to a value of 78.7 (µg·h/mL) for the observed oral formulation with a relative bioavailability value of 1757%. Finally, the T_{max} was 5 and 4 h for IFP3-EBD and the oral formulation, respectively. This obvious augmentation in the pharmacokinetic profile of IFP3-EBD compared to the oral formulation is attributed to the remarkable components of the IM formulation as well as the nan-range of the obtained particulates upon injection. Brij 52, as a surfactant, has the ability to enhance the biological absorption of the encapsulated drugs via the liquefaction of the biological membranes and the loosening of their tight junctions, allowing for better penetration of the drug into the bloodstream. Moreover, Brij 52 imparts more flexibility to the basically soft lipidic nano-particulates, thus facilitating their penetration. Additionally, these particulate systems serve as nano-reservoir systems that release the drug in a continuous and controlled manner. Finally, the negatively charged particulates are thought to have a lower clearance rate than that of the neutral ones. This is highly reflected by the maximized C_{max} and AUC_{0-24} values of IFP3-EBD. This is in line with the reported observations of Sharma et al. [45]. The comparably higher T_{max} of the IM formulation may be attributed to the sustained release pattern of the drug from the IFP3-EBD nano-particulates.

Table 4. Physiologically based pharmacokinetic model simulating piroxicam pharmacokinetic parameters following intramuscular administration of IFP3-EBD at 10 mg/kg dose in adults.

AUC_{0-24} (µg·h/mL)	C_{max} (µg/mL)	T_{max} (h)
1383.03	61.79	5

AUC: area under the plasma concentration–time curve; C_{max}: maximum plasma concentration; T_{max}: time required to reach maximum plasma concentration; IFP3-EBD: in situ-forming particulate formulation containing Eudragit RL and Brij 52 as structural additives and DMSO as solvent.

4. Conclusions

Design of experiments was adopted for the design, characterization, and optimization of in situ-forming particulates (IFPs) for the IM administration of piroxicam via designing a full factorial experimental approach where the effect of the different formulation variables on the characteristics of the obtained IFPs was studied. The selected formulation was further investigated for the influence of the addition of some structural additives to augment the kinetic profile of the drug release. The optimized formulation (IFP3-EBD) presented favorable rheological features with the formation of spherical dense particulates upon injection showing minimal aggregates. The study of the release profile proved the extended-release behavior of IFP3-EBD endorsed with the virtual investigation of its biological efficacy using PBPK physiological modeling. The adopted physiological model was proved reliable upon its correlation to the literature-based clinical data. The optimized formulation exhibited an augmented biological profile with a relative bioavailability of 1757% compared to the literature data. These results demonstrated the ultimate importance of the close control of the different formulation factors for the significant effect of their variation on the characteristics of the obtained drug delivery systems. The invented IFPs proved their potential for efficient piroxicam IM delivery as well as the reliability of the PBPK physiological modeling in the prediction of the biological performance of novel formulations in a cost-effective, comprehensive manner.

Author Contributions: Conceptualization, A.S.Y., H.O.A., M.I., N.E., A.M.G. and N.M.E.H.; methodology, A.S.Y., H.O.A., M.I., N.E., A.M.G. and N.M.E.H.; software, A.M.G. and N.M.E.H.; validation, A.S.Y., H.O.A., M.I., N.E., A.M.G. and N.M.E.H.; formal analysis, A.S.Y., H.O.A., M.I., N.E., A.M.G. and N.M.E.H.; investigation, A.S.Y., H.O.A., M.I., N.E., A.M.G. and N.M.E.H.; resources, A.S.Y., H.O.A., M.I., N.E., A.M.G. and N.M.E.H.; data curation, A.S.Y., H.O.A., M.I., N.E., A.M.G. and N.M.E.H.; writing—original draft preparation, A.S.Y., H.O.A., M.I., N.E., A.M.G. and N.M.E.H.; writing—review and editing, A.S.Y., H.O.A., M.I., N.E., A.M.G. and N.M.E.H.; visualization, A.S.Y., H.O.A., M.I., N.E., A.M.G. and N.M.E.H.; supervision, H.O.A. and M.I.; project administration, H.O.A. and M.I.; funding acquisition, N.E. All authors have read and agreed to the published version of the manuscript.

Funding: The APC was funded by Abu Dhabi University's Office of Research and Sponsored Programs. Grant number: 19300800.

Institutional Review Board Statement: Not applicable as the study did not involve humans or animals but was performed virtually using physiological modeling software (PK-sim®).

Informed Consent Statement: Not applicable.

Data Availability Statement: The datasets generated during and/or analyzed during the current study are available from the corresponding author upon reasonable request.

Acknowledgments: Nermin Eissa acknowledges financial support from Abu Dhabi University's Office of Research and Sponsored Programs. Grant number: 19300800.

Conflicts of Interest: The authors declare no conflict of interest.

References

1. Hughes, J.P.; Rees, S.; Kalindjian, S.B.; Philpott, K.L. Principles of early drug discovery. *Br. J. Pharmacol.* **2011**, *162*, 1239–1249. [CrossRef] [PubMed]
2. Yun, Y.H.; Lee, B.K.; Park, K. Controlled Drug Delivery: Historical perspective for the next generation. *J. Control. Release* **2015**, *219*, 2–7. [CrossRef] [PubMed]
3. Tiwari, G.; Tiwari, R.; Sriwastawa, B.; Bhati, L.; Pandey, S.; Pandey, P.; Bannerjee, S.K. Drug delivery systems: An updated review. *Int. J. Pharm. Investig.* **2012**, *2*, 2–11. [CrossRef]
4. Trenfield, S.J.; Basit, A.W. Modified Drug Release: Current Strategies and Novel Technologies for Oral Drug Delivery. In *Nanotechnology for Oral Drug Delivery*; Martins, J.P., Santos, H.A., Eds.; Academic Press: Cambridge, MA, USA, 2020; pp. 177–197, Chapter 6.
5. Rahnfeld, L.; Luciani, P. Injectable Lipid-Based Depot Formulations: Where Do We Stand? *Pharmaceutics* **2020**, *12*, 567. [CrossRef] [PubMed]
6. Patrick, M.G.; Vladimir, R.M. Pharmacokinetic and Pharmacodynamic Properties of Drug Delivery Systems. *J. Pharmacol. Exp. Ther.* **2019**, *370*, 570.
7. Quarterman, J.C.; Geary, S.M.; Salem, A.K. Evolution of drug-eluting biomedical implants for sustained drug delivery. *Eur. J. Pharm. Biopharm.* **2021**, *159*, 21–35. [CrossRef]

8. Prasad, S.; Dangi, J.S. Targeting efficacy and anticancer activity of polymeric nanoparticles of SN-38 on colon cancer cell lines. *Futur. J. Pharm. Sci.* **2023**, *9*, 1–9. [CrossRef]
9. Camargo, J.A.; Sapin, A.; Nouvel, C.; Daloz, D.; Leonard, M.; Bonneaux, F.; Six, J.L.; Maincent, P. Injectable PLA-based in situ forming implants for controlled release of Ivermectin a BCS Class II drug: Solvent selection based on physico-chemical characterization. *Drug Dev. Ind. Pharm.* **2013**, *39*, 146–155. [CrossRef]
10. Śmiga-Matuszowicz, M.; Korytkowska-Wałach, A.; Nowak, B.; Pilawka, R.; Lesiak, M.; Sieroń, A.L. Poly(isosorbide succinate)-based in situ forming implants as potential systems for local drug delivery: Preliminary studies. *Mater. Sci. Eng. C* **2018**, *91*, 311–317. [CrossRef]
11. Haider, M.; Elsayed, I.; Ahmed, I.S.; Fares, A.R. In Situ-Forming Microparticles for Controlled Release of Rivastigmine: In Vitro Optimization and In Vivo Evaluation. *Pharmaceuticals* **2021**, *14*, 66. [CrossRef]
12. Wang, X.; Burgess, D.J. Drug release from in situ forming implants and advances in release testing. *Adv. Drug Deliv. Rev.* **2021**, *178*, 113912. [CrossRef]
13. Thakur, S.; Riyaz, B.; Patil, A.; Kaur, A.; Kapoor, B.; Mishra, V. Novel drug delivery systems for NSAIDs in management of rheumatoid arthritis: An overview. *Biomed. Pharmacother.* **2018**, *106*, 1011–1023. [CrossRef] [PubMed]
14. Derry, S.; Massey, T.; Moore, R.A.; McQuay, H.J. Topical NSAIDS for chronic musculoskeletal pain in adults. *Cochrane Database Syst. Rev.* **2008**. [CrossRef]
15. Kasemiire, A.; Avohou, H.T.; De Bleye, C.; Sacre, P.-Y.; Dumont, E.; Hubert, P.; Ziemons, E. Design of experiments and design space approaches in the pharmaceutical bioprocess optimization. *Eur. J. Pharm. Biopharm.* **2021**, *166*, 144–154. [CrossRef] [PubMed]
16. Bowden, G.D.; Pichler, B.J.; Maurer, A. A Design of Experiments (DoE) Approach Accelerates the Optimization of Copper-Mediated 18F-Fluorination Reactions of Arylstannanes. *Sci. Rep.* **2019**, *9*, 11370. [CrossRef]
17. Fairman, K.; Li, M.; Ning, B.; Lumen, A. Physiologically based pharmacokinetic (PBPK) modeling of RNAi therapeutics: Opportunities and challenges. *Biochem. Pharmacol.* **2021**, *189*, 114468. [CrossRef] [PubMed]
18. Zhao, P.; Rowland, M.; Huang, S.-M. Best Practice in the Use of Physiologically Based Pharmacokinetic Modeling and Simulation to Address Clinical Pharmacology Regulatory Questions. *Clin. Pharmacol. Ther.* **2012**, *92*, 17–20. [CrossRef]
19. Zhao, P.; Zhang, L.; Grillo, J.A.; Liu, Q.; Bullock, J.M.; Moon, Y.J.; Song, P.; Brar, S.S.; Madabushi, R.; Wu, T.C.; et al. Applications of Physiologically Based Pharmacokinetic (PBPK) Modeling and Simulation During Regulatory Review. *Clin. Pharmacol. Ther.* **2011**, *89*, 259–267. [CrossRef] [PubMed]
20. Deepika, D.; Kumar, V. The Role of "Physiologically Based Pharmacokinetic Model (PBPK)" New Approach Methodology (NAM) in Pharmaceuticals and Environmental Chemical Risk Assessment. *Int. J. Environ. Res. Public Health* **2023**, *20*, 3473. [CrossRef]
21. Alshawwa, S.Z.; Kassem, A.A.; Farid, R.M.; Mostafa, S.K.; Labib, G.S. Nanocarrier Drug Delivery Systems: Characterization, Limitations, Future Perspectives and Implementation of Artificial Intelligence. *Pharmaceutics* **2022**, *14*, 883. [CrossRef] [PubMed]
22. Sager, J.E.; Yu, J.; Ragueneau-Majlessi, I.; Isoherranen, N. Physiologically Based Pharmacokinetic (PBPK) Modeling and Simulation Approaches: A Systematic Review of Published Models, Applications, and Model Verification. *Drug Metab. Dispos.* **2015**, *43*, 1823. [CrossRef]
23. Smits, A.; De Cock, P.; Vermeulen, A.; Allegaert, K. Physiologically based pharmacokinetic (PBPK) modeling and simulation in neonatal drug development: How clinicians can contribute. *Expert Opin. Drug Metab. Toxicol.* **2019**, *15*, 25–34. [CrossRef]
24. Ammar, H.O.; Ibrahim, M.; Mahmoud, A.A.; Shamma, R.N.; El Hoffy, N.M. Non-ionic Surfactant Based In Situ Forming Vesicles as Controlled Parenteral Delivery Systems. *AAPS PharmSciTech* **2018**, *19*, 1001–1010. [CrossRef]
25. Antony, J. (Ed.) 1—Introduction to Industrial Experimentation. In *Design of Experiments for Engineers and Scientists*, 2nd ed.; Elsevier: Oxford, UK, 2014; pp. 1–6.
26. Muralidharan, K.; Romero, M.; Wüthrich, K. Factorial Designs, Model Selection, and (Incorrect) Inference in Randomized Experiments. *Rev. Econ. Stat.* **2023**, 1–44. [CrossRef]
27. Yu, M.; Yuan, W.; Li, D.; Schwendeman, A.; Schwendeman, S.P. Predicting drug release kinetics from nanocarriers inside dialysis bags. *J. Control. Release* **2019**, *315*, 23–30. [CrossRef] [PubMed]
28. Basak, S.C.; Kumar, K.S.; Ramalingam, M. Planejamento e características de liberação de comprimidos de liberação controlada de cloridrato de metformina. *Rev. Bras. Cienc. Farm.* **2008**, *44*, 477–483. [CrossRef]
29. Onnainty, R.; Granero, G. Chitosan-based nanocomposites: Promising materials for drug delivery applications. In *Biomedical Applications of Nanoparticles*; Grumezescu, A.M., Ed.; William Andrew Publishing: New York, NY, USA, 2019; pp. 375–407, Chapter 14.
30. Buhr, E.; Senftleben, N.; Klein, T.; Bergmann, D.; Gnieser, D.; Frase, C.G.; Bosse, H. Characterization of nanoparticles by scanning electron microscopy in transmission mode. *Meas. Sci. Technol.* **2009**, *20*, 084025. [CrossRef]
31. Blasco-Martinez, A.B.; Mateo-Orobia, A.; Blasco-Alberto, J.; Pablo-Julvez, L. Rheological Behavior Patterns in Artificial Tears. *Optom. Vis. Sci.* **2022**, *99*, 455–462. [CrossRef]
32. Thelen, K.; Coboeken, K.; Willmann, S.; Burghaus, R.; Dressman, J.B.; Lippert, J. Evolution of a detailed physiological model to simulate the gastrointestinal transit and absorption process in humans, Part 1: Oral solutions. *J. Pharm. Sci.* **2011**, *100*, 5324–5345. [CrossRef] [PubMed]
33. Ishizaki, T.; Nomura, T.; Abe, T. Pharmacokinetics of piroxicam, a new nonsteroidal anti-inflammatory agent, under fasting and postprandial states in man. *J. Pharmacokinet. Biopharm.* **1979**, *7*, 369–381. [CrossRef]

34. Schmitt, W. General approach for the calculation of tissue to plasma partition coefficients. *Toxicol. In Vitro* **2008**, *22*, 457–467. [CrossRef] [PubMed]
35. Hindmarsh, A.C.; Brown, P.N.; Grant, K.E.; Lee, S.L.; Serban, R.; Shumaker, D.E.; Woodward, C.S. SUNDIALS: Suite of nonlinear and differential/algebraic equation solvers. *ACM Trans. Math. Softw.* **2005**, *31*, 363–396. [CrossRef]
36. Calvo, A.M.; Santos, G.M.; Dionísio, T.J.; Marques, M.P.; Brozoski, D.T.; Lanchote, V.L.; Fernandes, M.H.R.; Faria, F.A.C.; Santos, C.F. Quantification of piroxicam and 5'-hydroxypiroxicam in human plasma and saliva using liquid chromatography–tandem mass spectrometry following oral administration. *J. Pharm. Biomed. Anal.* **2016**, *120*, 212–220. [CrossRef]
37. Cho, C.; Kang, P.; Park, H.-J.; Ko, E.; Mu, C.Y.; Lee, Y.J.; Choi, C.-I.; Kim, H.S.; Jang, C.-G.; Bae, J.; et al. Physiologically based pharmacokinetic (PBPK) modeling of piroxicam with regard to CYP2C9 genetic polymorphism. *Arch. Pharm. Res.* **2022**, *45*, 352–366. [CrossRef]
38. Porras, M.; Solans, C.; González, C.; Gutiérrez, J. Properties of water-in-oil (W/O) nano-emulsions prepared by a low-energy emulsification method. *Colloids Surf. A Physicochem. Eng. Asp.* **2008**, *324*, 181–188. [CrossRef]
39. Saberi, A.H.; Fang, Y.; McClements, D.J. Fabrication of vitamin E-enriched nanoemulsions: Factors affecting particle size using spontaneous emulsification. *J. Colloid Interface Sci.* **2013**, *391*, 95–102. [CrossRef] [PubMed]
40. Kumar, N.; Goindi, S. Development and Optimization of Itraconazole-Loaded Solid Lipid Nanoparticles for Topical Administration Using High Shear Homogenization Process by Design of Experiments: In Vitro, Ex Vivo and In Vivo Evaluation. *AAPS PharmSciTech* **2021**, *22*, 248. [CrossRef]
41. Ammar, H.O.; Ibrahim, M.; Mahmoud, A.A.; Shamma, R.N.; El Hoffy, N.M. Polymer-Free Injectable In Situ Forming Nanovesicles as a New Platform for Controlled Parenteral Drug Delivery Systems. *J. Pharm. Innov.* **2022**, *17*, 391–398. [CrossRef]
42. Saharan, P.; Bahmani, K. Preparation, Optimization and In vitro Evaluation of Glipizide Nanoparticles Integrated with Eudragit RS-100. *Pharm. Nanotechnol.* **2019**, *7*, 72–85. [CrossRef]
43. Yacoub, A.S.; Ammar, H.O.; Ibrahim, M.; Mansour, S.M.; El Hoffy, N.M. Artificial intelligence-assisted development of in situ forming nanoparticles for arthritis therapy via intra-articular delivery. *Drug Deliv.* **2022**, *29*, 1423–1436. [CrossRef]
44. Galvao, J.; Davis, B.; Tilley, M.; Normando, E.; Duchen, M.R.; Cordeiro, M.F. Unexpected low-dose toxicity of the universal solvent DMSO. *FASEB J.* **2014**, *28*, 1317–1330. [CrossRef] [PubMed]
45. Sharma, M.; Sharma, R.; Jain, D.K. Nanotechnology Based Approaches for Enhancing Oral Bioavailability of Poorly Water Soluble Antihypertensive Drugs. *Scientifica* **2016**, *2016*, 8525679. [CrossRef] [PubMed]

Disclaimer/Publisher's Note: The statements, opinions and data contained in all publications are solely those of the individual author(s) and contributor(s) and not of MDPI and/or the editor(s). MDPI and/or the editor(s) disclaim responsibility for any injury to people or property resulting from any ideas, methods, instructions or products referred to in the content.

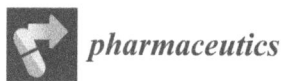

Article

Co-Dispersion Delivery Systems with Solubilizing Carriers Improving the Solubility and Permeability of Cannabinoids (Cannabidiol, Cannabidiolic Acid, and Cannabichromene) from *Cannabis sativa* (Henola Variety) Inflorescences

Anna Stasiłowicz-Krzemień [1], Piotr Szulc [2] and Judyta Cielecka-Piontek [1,3,*]

[1] Department of Pharmacognosy and Biomaterials, Faculty of Pharmacy, Poznan University of Medical Sciences, Rokietnicka 3, 60-806 Poznan, Poland; astasilowicz@ump.edu.pl
[2] Department of Agronomy, Poznań University of Life Sciences, Dojazd 11, 60-632 Poznan, Poland; piotr.szulc@up.poznan.pl
[3] Department of Pharmacology and Phytochemistry, Institute of Natural Fibres and Medicinal Plants, Wojska Polskiego 71b, 60-630 Poznan, Poland
[*] Correspondence: jpiontek@ump.edu.pl

Citation: Stasiłowicz-Krzemień, A.; Szulc, P.; Cielecka-Piontek, J. Co-Dispersion Delivery Systems with Solubilizing Carriers Improving the Solubility and Permeability of Cannabinoids (Cannabidiol, Cannabidiolic Acid, and Cannabichromene) from *Cannabis sativa* (Henola Variety) Inflorescences. *Pharmaceutics* 2023, 15, 2280. https://doi.org/10.3390/pharmaceutics15092280

Academic Editors: Gábor Vasvári and Ádám Haimhoffer

Received: 27 July 2023
Revised: 31 August 2023
Accepted: 1 September 2023
Published: 4 September 2023

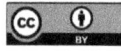

Copyright: © 2023 by the authors. Licensee MDPI, Basel, Switzerland. This article is an open access article distributed under the terms and conditions of the Creative Commons Attribution (CC BY) license (https://creativecommons.org/licenses/by/4.0/).

Abstract: Cannabinoids: cannabidiol (CBD), cannabidiolic acid (CBDA), and cannabichromene (CBC) are lipophilic compounds with limited water solubility, resulting in challenges related to their bioavailability and therapeutic efficacy upon oral administration. To overcome these limitations, we developed co-dispersion cannabinoid delivery systems with the biopolymer polyvinyl caprolactam-polyvinyl acetate-polyethylene glycol (Soluplus) and magnesium aluminometasilicate (Neusilin US2) to improve solubility and permeability. Recognizing the potential therapeutic benefits arising from the entourage effect, we decided to work with an extract instead of isolated cannabinoids. *Cannabis sativa* inflorescences (Henola variety) with a confirming neuroprotective activity were subjected to dynamic supercritical CO_2 (scCO_2) extraction and next they were combined with carriers (1:1 mass ratio) to prepare the co-dispersion cannabinoid delivery systems (HiE). In vitro dissolution studies were conducted to evaluate the solubility of CBD, CBDA, and CBC in various media (pH 1.2, 6.8, fasted, and fed state simulated intestinal fluid). The HiE-Soluplus delivery systems consistently demonstrated the highest dissolution rate of cannabinoids. Additionally, HiE-Soluplus exhibited the highest permeability coefficients for cannabinoids in gastrointestinal tract conditions than it was during the permeability studies using model PAMPA GIT. All three cannabinoids exhibited promising blood-brain barrier (BBB) permeability (P_{app} higher than 4.0×10^{-6} cm/s), suggesting their potential to effectively cross into the central nervous system. The improved solubility and permeability of cannabinoids from the HiE-Soluplus delivery system hold promise for enhancement in their bioavailability.

Keywords: cannabidiol; cannabidiolic acid; cannabichromene; cannabis; solubility; permeability

1. Introduction

Cannabis sativa L. is a plant rich in secondary plant metabolites as it contains cannabinoids, terpenes, flavonoids, amino acids, fatty acids, phytosterols, vitamins, and minerals [1]. Cannabis flowers, also known as inflorescences, possess a range of potential medicinal properties such as analgesic, anti-inflammatory, and antiemetic effects [2–4]. Additionally, cannabis flowers have shown promise in aiding sleep, stimulating appetite, and modulating neurological conditions like epilepsy [5,6]. Academic research is progressively expanding to explore the medicinal capabilities of cannabis flowers and their constituents.

Cannabinoids, such as tetrahydrocannabinol (THC), cannabidiol (CBD), cannabidiolic acid (CBDA), cannabigerol (CBG), or cannabichromene (CBC) are lipophilic constituents of *Cannabis sativa* L. that are poorly soluble in water (2–10 µg/mL) [7], which is the result of their lipophilic nature (log P 6–7) [8]. This is a limitation for cannabinoid oral administration as only dissolved compounds can be absorbed across the gastrointestinal epithelium [9], which results in low bioavailability (THC: 4–12%; CBD: ≈6%) [10,11]. The solubility of a molecule is a key determinant of its gastrointestinal fate and poorly soluble compounds may require formulation strategies, such as micronization, lipid-based formulations, or complexation, to improve their solubility and enhance their oral bioavailability [12,13]. However, findings in the literature in this field focus on work with pure cannabinoids, not extracts, excluding the entourage effect between cannabis plant components. The vast potential of the phenomenon of synergy between biologically active compounds may be reflected in pharmacotherapy or phytotherapy only after they cross biological barriers, which is only possible for dissolved substances. So far, research to improve the solubility of cannabinoids has focused on improving the solubility of CBD as a result of encapsulation, including nano-emulsions, Pickering emulsions, and inclusion complexes [14]. For example, a recently published article by Wang et al. describes zein and whey protein composite nanoparticles of CBD prepared by a modified anti-solvent method in which the water solubility of CBD was increased by 465–505 times and increased pharmacokinetic parameters [14]. Research to improve the solubility of THC included the use of cyclodextrins in the case of Δ^9-THC and Δ^8-THC; for the second substance, it resulted in not only an increase of aqueous solubility but also in the increase of stability and transcorneal permeation [15,16].

Another way to overcome poor cannabinoid solubility in water is by using inhalation as a delivery method in smoking or vaporizing. When a cannabis flower or concentrate is heated to a high enough temperature, the cannabinoids are vaporized and can be inhaled, and they have better bioavailability after inhalation. The value ranges from 10% to 35% for THC and varies among patients due to divergence in number, duration, interval of puffs, breath hold time, inhalation volume, used device, and the site of deposition within the respiratory system; for CBD, the average value is 11–45% [11]. An alternative is to use sublingual drops, which are an extract diluted in a carrier oil to ensure the dissolution of cannabinoids, allowing for rapid absorption through the oral mucosa [17]. The bioavailability of cannabinoids after sublingual administration was assessed for CBD as 13–19%, whilst for THC it was 13–14% [18].

All activities to improve the bioavailability of cannabinoids are aimed at better use of the pharmacological activity of individual cannabinoids—or their mixtures—with a specific potency of individual cannabinoids. Current literature reports confirm neuroprotective, anti-epileptic [19], and sedative effects, which are associated with the achievement of therapeutic goals within the central nervous system. For example, CBD has demonstrated anxiolytic and calming effects in preclinical and clinical studies [20–23]. By interacting with serotonin receptors and enhancing the action of gamma-aminobutyric acid (GABA), CBD may promote relaxation and potentially aid in managing sleep disturbances and insomnia [24]. The modulation of ion channels, neurotransmitter systems, and anti-inflammatory activity are among the proposed mechanisms through which CBD exerts its antiseizure properties [25]. CBD reduces neuronal excitability through functional antagonism of GPR55 receptors, desensitization of TRPV1 receptors, and inhibition of adenosine transport [26]. Neuroimaging investigations have revealed noteworthy changes in brain activity and connectivity patterns during both resting states and while engaging in cognitive tasks following the administration of CBD [27]. CBD has been found to reduce the accumulation of amyloid-beta (Aβ) plaques and decrease the hyperphosphorylation of tau proteins, which are central pathological features of Alzheimer's disease [28]. There are not many studies about CBDA or CBC on the nervous system; rather the majority of studies concern CBD and THC. THC interacts with the endocannabinoid system's CB1 receptors, regulating neurotransmitter release, pain perception, and immune responses [29,30]. However, the use of plant material with a high THC content, even for medicinal purposes, could be deemed illegal in many countries across the globe [31]. The findings indicate that both CBDA and THCA possess properties that may be beneficial in combating Alzheimer's disease. These cannabinoids can alleviate memory impairments and enhance the brain's ability to withstand higher levels of calcium (Ca^{2+}), Aβ, and hyperphosphorylated tau (p-tau) in the hippocampus [32]. Moreover, a substantial concentration of CBDA effectively reduces neurotoxicity induced by rotenone [32]. In the rat maximal electroshock seizure test, it has been observed that CBDA exhibits anticonvulsant properties [33]. CBC interacts with specific TRP cation channels, namely TRPA1, TRPV1, and TRPV8, which play crucial roles in pain relief and inflammation regulation [34]. Upon binding to these receptors, CBC induces an antinociceptive effect within the brain. CBC positively influenced the viability of adult neural stem progenitor cells during in vitro differentiation, upregulating the marker nestin while downregulating the astrocyte marker Glial fibrillary acidic protein, possibly involving adenosine signaling and ATP modulation in the process [35]. CBC might be also a potential neuronal differentiation inducer for NSC-34 cells (a hybridoma between spinal cord cells from the embryos of mice and neuroblastoma) [36]. In addition to the affinity of cannabinoids to selected receptors, there are also non-specific mechanisms of their action within the central nervous system. There are literature reports, including the results published by us, confirming the scavenging of free radicals [37–39]. Recent articles present the variety of antioxidant mechanisms of cannabinoids [38,40,41].

Polyvinyl caprolactam-polyvinyl acetate-polyethylene glycol (Soluplus) is an amphiphilic copolymer composed of hydrophilic and lipophilic segments. This structure allows Soluplus to form micelles or colloidal structures when dispersed in water [42] increasing the solubility of various compounds like curcumin [43], hesperidin [44], pterostilbene [45], or itraconazole [46]. Magnesium aluminometasilicate (Neusilin US2) is an amorphous, porous material with a high surface area and adsorption capacity. Its porous structure can adsorb hydrophobic molecules onto its surface or within its pores and increase the solubility of compounds such as naringenin [47], caffeic acid [48], and celecoxib [49].

In order to justify the need to increase the solubility and, as a result, the bioavailability of phytocannabinoids present in the inflorescences of *Cannabis* sp., we undertook work to improve the solubility of cannabinoids, CBD, CBDA, and CBC whose structures are presented in Figure 1, by preparing delivery systems with biopolymer (Soluplus) and Neusilin US2 to achieve better bioavailability. Limited research regarding the enhancement of solubility for cannabinoids within whole extracts, rather than isolated or synthesized forms, and notably, the lack of data on dissolution profiles and membrane permeability of CBC and CBDA ensures the novelty of the study.

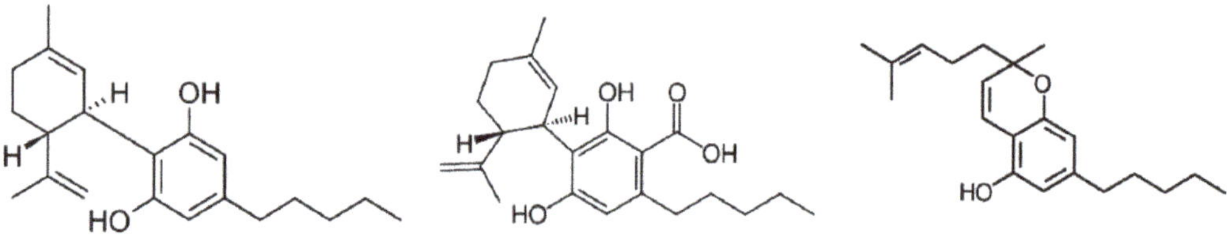

Figure 1. The structure of cannabidiol (**a**), cannabidiolic acid (**b**), and cannabichromene (**c**).

2. Materials and Methods

2.1. Materials

Cannabis sativa plant material, Białobrzeskie, Tygra, Henola varieties, was donated from the Experimental Station for the Cultivar Testing in Chrząstowo, belonging to the Research Centre for Cultivar Testing in Słupia Wielka. The agricultural details are presented in Supplementary Materials. The plant material for the study was collected after hemp plants reached the maturation phase, i.e., from the moment of seed formation to the first seed. Immediately after collection, two samples of 500 g each were separated and dried to an absolutely dry mass. The entire drying period lasted twenty hours. The temperature in the oven was maintained at no higher than 50 °C for the first 6 hours and the oven temperature was maintained at 105 °C for the remaining 14 h of drying.

Food-grade CO_2 was provided by Air Liquide Polska (Cracow, Poland). Soluplus® (polyvinyl caprolactam-polyvinyl acetate-polyethylene glycol graft copolymer), was supplied by BASF SE (Ludwigshafen, Germany). Neusilin US2 (magnesium aluminometasilicate) was kindly provided by Fuji Chemical Industry (Minato, Tokyo). Cannabinoid standards (CBD–CAS: 13956-29-1, CBDA–CAS: 1244-58-2, and CBC–CAS: 20675-51-8) were purchased from Sigma-Aldrich (Poznan, Poland). Trifluoroacetic acid and acetonitrile (high-performance liquid chromatography [HPLC] grade) were provided by Merck (Darmstadt, Germany). The chemicals 2,2-Diphenyl-1-picrylhydrazyl, iron (III) chloride hexahydrate, 2,2′-azino-bis(3-ethylbenzothiazoline-6-sulfonic acid), neocuproine, 2,4,6-Tri(2-pyridyl)-s-triazine, trolox, Trizma® Base, Trizma® hydrochloride, butyrylcholine iodide, acetylcholine iodide, acetylcholinesterase, butyrylcholinesterase, 5,5-dithiobis-2-nitrobenzoic acid, tyrosinase, galantamine, azelaic acid were purchased from Sigma-Aldrich (Schnelldorf, Germany). Sodium chloride, sodium dihydrogen phosphate, sodium hydrogen phosphate, and dimethyl sulfoxide were obtained from Avantor Performance Materials (Gliwice, Poland). Ammonium acetate, an analytical weighed amount of HCl, 1 N, and methanol were supplied by Chempur (Piekary Śląskie, Poland). Cupric chloride dihydrate, acetic acid (99.5%), and ethanol (96%) were supplied by POCH (Gliwice, Poland). Prisma HT, GIT, BBB lipid solution, an acceptor sink buffer, and a brain sink buffer were supplied by Pion Inc. (Forest Row, East Sussex, UK). High-quality pure water was prepared using a Direct-Q 3 UV purification system (Millipore, Molsheim, France; model Exil SA 67120). FaSSIF and FeSSIF were purchased from Biorelevant (London, UK).

2.2. Preparation of the Systems of Cannabis sativa (Henola Variety) Inflorescences Extract-Carriers

The extract of *Cannabis sativa* inflorescences was obtained using the dynamic supercritical CO_2 (scCO$_2$) extraction process (SFT-120, shim-pol, Izabelin, Polska). In total, 6.5 g of dried plant material was placed in the extraction vessel and extracted under 6000 psi at 50 °C with 250 mL of CO_2. The extraction yield was calculated as the mass of extract obtained and subjected to drying (to remove any water from the eventually frozen needle) (g) divided by the mass (g) of plant material placed in the extractor and expressed as a percentage (%). The choice of the Henola extract (HiE) was based on the screening studies on three varieties (Białobrzeskie, Tygra, and Henola) of leaves and inflorescences and their neuroprotective potential (data not presented). After extraction, the antioxidant studies and inhibition of enzymes (acetylcholinesterase, butyrylcholinesterase, and tyrosinase) connected with neurodegeneration were repeated.

Next, the extracts were dried in a vacuum at 50 °C, weighed, and suspended in methanol (if the process was repeated to obtain more extract, at this stage the extracts were combined together), winterized, and filtered (Figure 2). For fluid extracts (HiE), carriers (Neusilin US2, Soluplus, or lactose for apparent solubility study) were added in a 1:1 mass ratio to the earlier weight of the extract. Systems were dried on rota-vapor at 50 °C until dry and grounded in mortar.

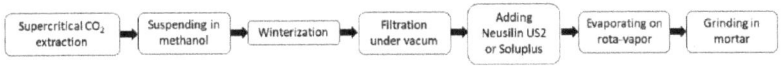

Figure 2. Scheme of preparation of co-dispersion delivery systems of Henola inflorescences extract with Neusilin US2 and Soluplus.

2.3. Chromatographic Analysis

The cannabinoid profile (CBD, CBDA, and CBC) of the extract, and during the apparent solubility and permeability study, was analyzed using the ultra-high-performance liquid chromatography with the diode array detector (HPLC-DAD) method, Shimadzu Corp. (Kyoto, Japan). The previously described method was used [37]. The analysis was conducted on a CORTECS Shield RP18 stationary phase, 2.7 µm; 150 mm × 4.6 mm, with a mobile phase consisting of 0.1% trifluoroacetic acid (41%) and acetonitrile (41:59, v/v). The flow rate was set to 2.0 mL/min, and the column temperature was maintained at 35 °C. The injection volume was 10.0 µL, and the detection wavelength was set at 228 nm, with an analysis time of 50 min. The retention times for each cannabinoid were as follows: CBD at approximately 5.83 min, CBDA at approximately 6.42 min, and CBC at 14.57 min. The LabSolutions LC software (version 1.86 SP2) from Shimadzu Corp. (Kyoto, Japan) was used to obtain chromatograms. The method was validated according to ICH guidelines for current research, the validation parameters are collected in Table S1 (Supplementary Materials).

2.4. Apparent Solubility of Cannabinoids

The dissolution rate was determined in the paddle apparatus (Agilent Technologies, Santa Clara, CA, USA). HiE had a thick, oily consistency, so for the purpose of apparent solubility study it was combined with lactose; the preparation steps were the same as for Neusilin US2 and Soluplus (HiE–control). The systems and control (600 mg) were placed into two gelatin capsules. The capsules were placed into coiled sinkers for floating prevention. The test was carried out in triplicate for 180 min in a pH 1.2 of 0.1 N hydrochloric acid, a pH 6.8 of phosphate buffer, Fasted State Simulated Intestinal Fluid (FaSSIF), and Fed State Simulated Intestinal Fluid (FeSSIF).

FaSSIF and FeSSIF dissolution media are more complex solutions specifically designed to simulate the conditions of the human small intestine under fasted and fed conditions. FaSSIF and FeSSIF contain natural surfactants present in the gut to simulate gastrointestinal fluids much more accurately than conventional dissolution media, and they simulate the conditions of the human intestine in a fasted state and after a meal [50]. Sodium taurocholate is included to replicate the role of bile acids in facilitating lipid absorption and emulsification. Lecithin is incorporated to mimic the presence of phospholipids, which play a vital role in the formation of mixed micelles that enhance the solubilization of lipophilic compounds. The buffer ensures a stable pH in the intestinal fluid (6.5 for FaSSIF and 5.0 for FeSSIF), and sodium chloride is added to ensure physiological osmolarity (a FaSSIF of 270 Osm/L and FeSSIF of 670 Osm/L) [51].

The vessels were filled with 500 mL of media at the temperature set at 310.15 K and the rotation speed of 100 rpm. At specific time intervals, 2.0 mL of the sample was taken out and immediately replaced with an equal amount of fresh medium at the same temperature. The percentage cumulative cannabinoid release (% CBD, CBDA, and CBC) was measured at different time points (5, 10, 15, 30, 45, 60, 90, 120, and 180 min) for each formulation. The samples were then passed through a filter with a pore size of 0.22 µm and analyzed using high-performance liquid chromatography (HPLC). Sample chromatograms from the dissolution study are presented in Figure S1 (Supplementary Materials). The standard deviation (SD) was also calculated for each time point and delivery system.

The differences and similarities between the apparent solubility profiles were determined by the two-factor values, f_1 and f_2, introduced by Moore and Flanner [52] with the use of the following equations:

$$f_1 = \frac{\sum_{j=1}^{n}|R_j - T_j|}{\sum_{j=1}^{n} R_j} \quad (1)$$

$$f_2 = 50 \times \log\left(\left(1 + \left(\frac{1}{n}\right)\sum_{j=1}^{n}|R_j - T_j|^2\right)^{-\frac{1}{2}} \times 100\right) \quad (2)$$

where n is the number of time points, R_j is the percentage of the reference dissolved substance in the medium, T_j is the percentage of the dissolved tested substance, and t is the time point. Dissolution profiles are described as similar when the f_1 value is close to 0, or f_2 is close to 100 (between 50 and 100) [53]. The similarities and dissimilarities between profiles were marked in the figures with letters. If profiles share the same letter, they are similar.

The data from the dissolution studies were graphically correlated to mathematical models: zero-order, first-order, Higuchi's model, and Korsmeyer–Peppas model in MS Excel (version 1808, Microsoft Corporation, Redmond, WA, USA) [54,55]. The mathematical equations of kinetic models are described below:

$$\text{Zero-order model: } F = k \times t$$

$$\text{First-order model: } \ln F = k \times t$$

$$\text{Higuchi model: } F = kt^{1/2}$$

$$\text{Korsmeyer-Peppas model: } F = kt^n$$

where F is the fraction of the released drug, k is the constant associated with the release, and t is the time (h).

2.5. Permeability Study of Cannabinoids

The permeability of cannabinoids through biological membranes was measured using the Parallel Artificial Membrane Permeability Assay (PAMPA) model. The study was conducted in the gastrointestinal (GIT) and blood-brain barrier (BBB) models. The model consists of two 96-well microfilter plates, the donor and the acceptor plate. The wells were separated by a 120 μm thick microfilter disc coated with a 20% (w/v) dodecane solution of a lecithin mixture (Pion Inc., Billerica, MA, USA). The extract was diluted and the systems were dissolved (or suspended, centrifuged, and filtered) in dimethyl sulfoxide (DMSO) and placed in the donor solutions, which were adjusted to 6.8 for GIT application and pH 7.4 for BBB. The BBB permeability was only studied for extract, as Neusilin US2 does not leave the GIT. The plates were incubated at 310.15 K for 3 h for the GIT and BBB assay in a humidity-saturated atmosphere. After incubation, the plates were separated and the concentration of CBD and CBDA, as their concentration in the extract was the highest, was determined using the HPLC-DAD method. Each measurement was repeated six times. CBC was present in a quantifiable concentration only in the BBB study, thus, it was not determined in GIT conditions. The P_{app} was calculated using the following formulas:

$$P_{app} = \frac{-\ln\left(1 - \frac{C_A}{C_{equilibrium}}\right)}{S \times \left(\frac{1}{V_D} + \frac{1}{V_A}\right) \times t} \tag{3}$$

$$C_{equilibrium} = \frac{C_D \times V_D + C_A \times V_A}{V_D + V_A} \tag{4}$$

where V_D is the donor volume, V_A is the acceptor volume, $C_{equilibrium}$ is the equilibrium concentration ($C_{equilibrium} = \frac{C_D \times V_D + C_A \times V_A}{V_D + V_A}$), S is the membrane area, and t is the incubation time (in seconds).

Substances with a P_{app} in the GIT model below 0.1×10^{-6} cm/s are considered to have poor permeability, compounds with 0.1×10^{-6} cm/s $\leq P_{app} < 1 \times 10^{-6}$ cm/s are classified as mediocre permeable, and compounds found as well permeable have a $P_{app} \geq 1 \times 10^{-6}$ cm/s [56]. Compounds whose P_{app} in the BBB model is $<2.0 \times 10^{-6}$ cm/s are known as poorly permeable. Compounds with questionable permeability have P_{app} values in the range of 2.0 to 4.0×10^{-6} cm/s. Substances that have a P_{app} value greater than 4.0×10^{-6} cm/s are regarded as highly permeable [57].

2.6. Biological Activity Studies

The extract and systems antioxidant activity was studied by four assays: DPPH, ABTS, CUPRAC, and FRAP. Two of them determine the ability to scavenge free radicals (DPPH and ABTS), whilst the other assays check the possibility of performing redox reactions (CUPRAC and FRAP). A linear regression equation between the trolox concentration and its scavenging percentage (DPPH and ABTS) or absorbance (CUPRAC and FRAP) was built. Thus, the results, presented as mg trolox/g plant material, were calculated through the equation according to the antioxidant properties of the extracts in all four assays [58,59]. Pure excipients showed no antioxidant potential under test conditions.

To perform the DPPH assay, a 96-well plate was used and the samples were measured spectrophotometrically [60]. The main reagent was a methanol solution of DPPH at a concentration of 0.2 mM. To initiate the assay, 25.0 µL of the system/trolox solution was mixed with 175.0 µL of the DPPH solution. The plate was then incubated in the dark at room temperature while shaking for 30 min. After the incubation period, the absorbances were obtained using a plate reader (Multiskan GO, Thermo Fisher Scientific, Waltham, MA, USA) at 517 nm. The absorbance (A) was also measured for a blank sample, which consisted of a mixture of DPPH solution and solvent at 517 nm. Each sample was tested for its absorbance at 517 nm. The inhibition of DPPH radicals by the studies' systems/trolox was calculated using the equation:

$$\text{DPPH scavenging activity } (\%) = \frac{A_o - A_i}{A_o} \times 100\% \quad (5)$$

where A_o is the absorbance of the control sample and A_i is the absorbance of the test sample. Each measurement was repeated six times.

As another assay to determine the scavenging radical potential, the ABTS study [61], was also performed. This study is based on the production of green cation radicals through the loss of electrons by nitrogen atoms of ABTS caused by potassium persulfate. During the assay, the green ABTS radical can be converted into a colorless neutral form in the presence of an antioxidant. In this assay, 200.0 µL of ABTS$^{\bullet+}$ solution and 10.0 µL of the system/trolox solution were pipetted into 96-well plates and incubated for 10 min in the dark at room temperature while shaking [62]. After incubation, the absorbance values were measured at λ = 734 nm using a plate reader (Multiskan GO, Thermo Fisher Scientific, Waltham, MA, USA). The mixture of solvent and ABTS (control) and the wells filled with system and water (systems' absorbance) at 734 nm were also studied. The inhibition of ABTS$^{\bullet+}$ was calculated using the following equation:

$$\text{ABTS scavenging activity } (\%) = \frac{A_0 - A_1}{A_0} \times 100\% \quad (6)$$

where:

A_0—The absorbance of the control;

A_1—The absorbance of the sample.

To determine the reducing potential of the systems, the CUPRAC assay [63] was used. In this assay, the antioxidants' phenolic groups undergo oxidation to form quinones, while the bluish neocuproine and copper (II) ion complex is reduced to the yellow neocuproine and copper (I) ion complex. To perform this study, a mixture of 50.0 µL of the system/trolox solution and 150.0 µL of the CUPRAC reagent was added to the plate and then incubated for 30 min at room temperature while shaking in the dark [62]. The control and systems' own absorbance were also measured simultaneously. The absorbance was measured at a wavelength of 450 nm using a plate reader (Multiskan GO, Thermo Fisher Scientific, Waltham, MA, USA) after the 30 min incubation period. The analysis was performed using six replicates.

The FRAP technique was also used to determine the reducing properties of the systems, which involves reducing colorless Fe^{3+} ion to Fe^{2+} to form a dark blue complex with 2,4,6-

tris(2-pyridyl)-1,3,5-triazine (TPTZ) [62]. In this method, 25.0 μL of the system/trolox solution and 175.0 μL of the FRAP mixture (consisting of 25 mL acetate buffer, 2.5 mL TPTZ solution, and 2.5 mL of $FeCl_3 \cdot 6H_2O$ solution) were applied to the plate and incubated in dark conditions at 37 °C for 30 min. The control and systems' absorbance were also measured. Subsequently, the absorbance was measured at λ = 593 nm using a plate reader (Multiskan GO, Thermo Fisher Scientific, Waltham, MA, USA). The analysis was performed using six replicates.

The neuroprotective effect of cannabinoids was assessed against the possibility of inhibiting enzymes whose expression is associated with neurodegenerative changes.

As a standard inhibitor of esterases, galantamine was chosen, while for tyrosinase, azelaic acid was selected [64,65]. A linear regression equation that relates the standard concentration of a substance to its ability to inhibit an enzyme, as measured by the percentage of potential inhibition was created. An equation to calculate the standard equivalent for each extract based on its inhibitory properties in all three assays was obtained. The results were presented as a galantamine equivalent (GALAE) (mg galantamine/g plant material) for AChe and BChE assays and as an azelaic acid equivalent (AzAE) (mg azelaic acid/g plant material) [66–71].

The inhibition of acetylcholinesterase (AChE) and butyrylcholinesterase (BChE) was carried out using a colorimetric Ellman et al. modified assay [72]. This method requires artificial substrates (thiocholine esters). Thiocholine is liberated during the enzymatic reactions with 5,5′-dithio-bis-(2-nitrobenzoic) acid (DTNB), and the 3-carboxy-4-nitrothiolate anion (TNB anion) is formed. The potential to inhibit AChE and BChe was measured according to the increase in the thiocholine color in a 96-well plate. In total, 60.0 μL of 0.05 M Tris-HCl buffer (pH of 8.0), 10.0 μL of test solution, and 30.0 μL of AChE/BChE solution at a concentration of 0.2 U/mL were added to the wells. Subsequently, the plate was incubated for 5 min at 37 °C while shaking. Next, 30.0 μL acetylthiocholine iodide (ATCI)/butyrylthiocholine iodide (BTCI) at a concentration of 1.5 mM and 125.0 μL of 0.3 mM DTNB solution (5,5′-dithiobis-(2-nitrobenzoic acid)) were added to the wells. The plate was then incubated for another 20 min under the same conditions. A blank sample (the reaction mixture without the enzyme, with an increase in the volume of Tris-HCl buffer), a control sample (the solvent instead of the test sample), and a blank sample for the control sample (the reaction mixture without the enzyme, with an increase in the volume of Tris-HCl buffer) were also prepared. The measurements were performed at a wavelength of 405 nm. The analysis was performed using six replicates. The percentage of inhibition of AChE and BChE by the test samples was calculated using the following formula:

$$\text{AChE/BChE inhibition (\%)} = \frac{1 - (A_1 - A_{1b})}{(A_0 - A_{0b})} \times 100\% \tag{7}$$

where:

A_1—The absorbance of the test sample;
A_{1b}—The absorbance of the blank of the test sample;
A_0—The absorbance of control;
A_{0b}—The absorbance of the blank of control.

The tyrosinase inhibition assay measures the activity of an inhibitor to prevent L-DOPA from accessing the tyrosinase active site. This leads to a decrease in the color intensity of the solution, which indicates enzyme inhibition [73]. To conduct the assay, 75.0 μL of 0.1 M phosphate buffer (pH 6.8) was added to each well of a 96-well plate, followed by 25.0 μL of the extract and 50.0 μL of enzyme solution (192 U/mL). The plate was shaken at room temperature for 10 min, after which 50 μL of 2.0 mM L-DOPA was added to each well and incubated for an additional 20 min under the same conditions. In addition to the test sample, a blank for the test sample (without enzyme, the volume of phosphate buffer was elevated), a control sample (with solvent instead of the test sample), and a blank sample for the control (without enzyme) were also prepared. The absorbance of the samples was measured at 475 nm. Each measurement was repeated six times. The percentage inhibition of the tyrosinase by the samples was calculated using an equation:

$$\text{Tyrosinase inhibition } (\%) = \frac{1 - (A_1 - A_{1b})}{(A_0 - A_{0b})} \times 100\% \tag{8}$$

where:
- A_1—The absorbance of the test sample;
- A_{1b}—The absorbance of the blank of the test sample;
- A_0—The absorbance of control;
- A_{0b}—The absorbance of the blank of control.

2.7. Statistical Analysis

Statistical analysis of results obtained in permeability assay, and in antioxidant activity study, was performed with the use of Statistica 13.3 software (StatSoft Poland, Krakow, Poland). Data are presented as mean values ± standard deviations. Experimental data were analyzed using the skewness and kurtosis tests to determine the normality of each distribution, and Levene's test assessed the equality of variances. Statistical significance was determined using a one-way analysis of variance (ANOVA), followed by the Bonferroni post hoc test (to compare the experimental results acquired for cannabinoids in extract and in the systems). Differences were considered significant at $p < 0.05$.

3. Results

3.1. Preparation and Characterization of Co-Dispersion Delivery Systems

Using extracts obtained from inflorescences with the $scCO_2$ extraction technique (the extraction yield was ~16.74%), cannabinoid delivery systems with increased solubility and permeability were obtained. As model carriers, biopolymer Soluplus and Neusilin US2 were applied. The systems of cannabinoids with carriers (Figure 2) were prepared using a solvent-evaporation method which enables the incorporation of a wide range of active ingredients into the resulting systems [74,75].

The extracts and systems have undergone the HPLC-DAD analysis to determine the cannabinoid content. In HiE, CBD was at the level of 6042.76 ± 82.19 µg/g plant material, CBDA at 2033.01 ± 67.98 µg/g plant material, whilst for CBC, 238.71 ± 11.20 µg/g plant material. The results of the systems analysis are presented in Table 1.

Table 1. The content of cannabinoids in the prepared systems described as mg cannabinoid/g system.

System	CBD	CBDA	CBC
	mg Cannabinoid/g System		
HiE-Neusilin US2	8.73 ± 0.08	2.85 ± 0.02	0.379 ± 0.004
HiE-Soluplus	10.77 ± 0.06	3.60 ± 0.02	0.323 ± 0.004

3.2. Apparent Solubility of Cannabinoids

Two systems of the HiE with Neusilin US2, and Sol prepared in a 1:1 mass ratio (extract weight: carrier) using a solvent-evaporation technique, were enrolled in the dissolution study. The percentage cumulative cannabinoid release (% CBD, CBDA, and CBC) was measured at different time points (5, 10, 15, 30, 45, 60, 90, 120, and 180 min) for each system.

In 0.1 M hydrochloric acid, at pH 1.2 (Figure 3a), CBD was dissolved to the smallest extent compared to other media. After 60 min of the study, the percentage of dissolved CBD is only in HiE-Soluplus 4.08% ± 0.21%, in HiE-Neusilin US2 0.44% ± 0.09%, and even less in HiE. In the phosphate buffer at pH 6.8 (Figure 3b), the dissolution rate of CBD was overall greater for CBD in the co-dispersion delivery systems than in pH 1.2; however, CBD from HiE did not dissolve. After 60 min, the % CBD values were as follows:

HiE-Soluplus at 39.83% ± 0.23% and HiE-Neusilin US2 at 33.21% ± 1.09%. CBD had the highest dissolution rate in HiE-Soluplus at pH 6.8 throughout the whole study.

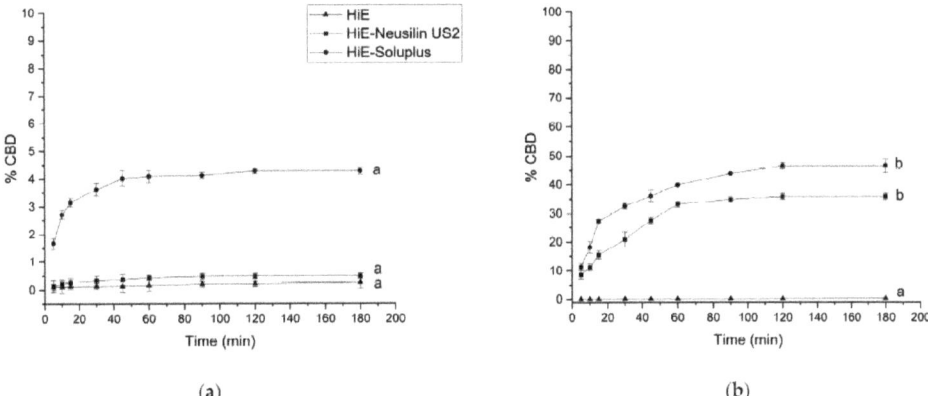

Figure 3. The dissolution profiles of CBD from HiE, HiE-Neusilin US2, and HiE-Soluplus systems at pH 1.2 (**a**) and 6.8 (**b**). Profiles with the same superscript letters were similar (according to f_1 or f_2 values). Profiles with different superscript letters differ significantly (according to f_1 and f_2 values).

The apparent solubility of CBD was also studied in FaSSIF and FeSSIF (Figure 4a,b). The dissolution profile of CBD was greater in FaSSIF and FeSSIF than in pharmacopeial media at pH 1.2 and 6.8. It is observed that in both advanced media, CBD was rapidly released from co-dispersion delivery systems. After 60 min, in FaSSIF, CBD was dissolved in HiE-Soluplus at 77.40% ± 1.15%, in HiE-Neusilin US2 at 75.47% ± 2.91%, and in HiE at 17.92% ± 1.79%. In FeSSIF (Figure 4b), CBD was released to the greatest extent, reaching after 60 min in HiE-Soluplus 99.25% ± 3.23%, in HiE-Neusilin US2 98.37% ± 1.82%, and in HiE 24.76% ± 2.48%. Co-dispersion delivery system HiE-Soluplus provided the best dissolution rate of CBD at each time point, which was statistically significantly different than CBD dissolution profiles in HiE-Neusilin US2 and HiE.

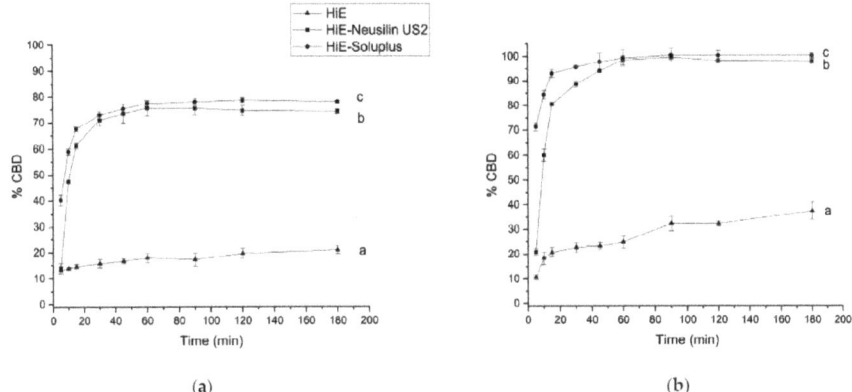

Figure 4. The dissolution profiles of CBD from HiE, HiE-Neusilin US2, and HiE-Soluplus systems in FaSSIF (**a**) and FeSSIF (**b**). Profiles with different superscript letters (a–c) differ significantly (according to f_1 and f_2 values).

The dissolution of CBD is a complex process influenced by various factors. The dissolution kinetics of CBD were investigated using various mathematical models under different media conditions and in extract and co-dispersion delivery systems with Neusilin US2 and Soluplus (Table 2) [76–79]. Four mathematical models, namely zero-order kinetics, first-order kinetics, Higuchi kinetics, and Korsmeyer–Peppas kinetics were employed to analyze the dissolution data [80–82]. CBD in HiE displayed high R^2 values for zero-order and first-order kinetics, indicating a reliable and predictable release mechanism. The Higuchi model also showed notable correlations, suggesting diffusion-driven release. Moreover, the Korsmeyer–Peppas model displayed moderate to high correlations, and the n values indicated a Fickian diffusion. For both HiE-Soluplus and HiE-Neusilin US2, the Higuchi model consistently revealed diffusion-driven release mechanisms across pH conditions and biorelevant media. The Korsmeyer–Peppas model, which was also dominating for CBD in co-dispersion delivery systems, indicated the involvement of Fickian transport based on the n values (n < 0.5) [83].

Table 2. Mathematical models of release kinetics of cannabidiol in pH 1.2, pH 6.8, FaSSIF, and FeSSIF.

	CBD	Mathematical Model								
		Zero-Order Kinetics		First-Order Kinetics		Higuchi Kinetics		Korsmeyer–Peppas Kinetics		
		R^2	k	R^2	k	R^2	k	R^2	k	n
pH 1.2	HiE	0.980	0.054	0.980	2.350×10^{-4}	0.945	0.107	0.863	0.176	0.236
	HiE-Neusilin US2	0.708	0.111	0.708	4.845×10^{-4}	0.874	0.249	0.938	0.395	0.356
	HiE-Soluplus	0.525	0.659	0.528	2.962×10^{-3}	0.712	1.546	0.819	3.839	0.236
pH 6.8	HiE	0.985	0.075	0.985	3.269×10^{-4}	0.975	0.151	0.959	0.194	0.332
	HiE-Neusilin US2	0.709	9.520	0.731	5.508×10^{-2}	0.871	21.254	0.948	27.542	0.443
	HiE-Soluplus	0.693	10.654	0.744	6.981×10^{-2}	0.859	23.900	0.906	37.182	0.380
FaSSIF	HiE	0.904	2.516	0.910	1.321×10^{-2}	0.961	5.223	0.949	17.489	0.126
	HiE-Neusilin US2	0.331	12.107	0.403	1.229×10^{-1}	0.506	30.172	0.603	68.325	0.357
	HiE-Soluplus	0.413	8.387	0.503	1.107×10^{-1}	0.596	20.291	0.745	73.871	0.158
FeSSIF	HiE	0.682	6.715	0.721	4.000×10^{-2}	0.737	14.056	0.724	27.930	0.263
	HiE-Neusilin US2	0.376	16.443	0.542	5.556×10^{-1}	0.556	40.260	0.644	89.267	0.340
	HiE-Soluplus	0.412	6.380	0.844	1.349	0.593	15.408	0.772	102.742	0.083

The CBDA dissolution rate was also monitored under the same conditions. In hydrochloric acid, at pH 1.2, the overall results were the poorest (Figure 5a), it practically did not dissolve from HiE. After 60 min of the assay, CBDA was dissolved in HiE-Soluplus and HiE-Neusilin US2 at the level of 1.58% ± 0.21% and 1.88% ± 0.21%, respectively. The co-dispersion delivery system HiE-Soluplus provided the greatest dissolution rate of CBDA at pH 1.2. However, the overall results are poor and the profiles are statistically similar. The apparent solubility of CBDA was also studied in a phosphate buffer at pH 6.8 (Figure 5b). Similarly, to pH 1.2, CBDA in HiE practically did not dissolve during the study. After 60 min, HiE-Soluplus had a CBDA dissolution rate of 59.56% ± 0.23%, while HiE-Neusilin US2 was 49.64% ± 1.09%.

As for CBD, CBDA was also studied in FaSSIF (Figure 6a). The most noticeable differences are noted at the beginning of the study. After one hour of the assay, the dissolution percentages for CBDA in HiE-Soluplus, HiE-Neusilin US2, and HiE were 76.05% ± 2.91%, 60.20% ± 0.96%, and 23.25% ± 1.87% respectively. The results indicate that CBDA was dissolved to the greatest extent in HiE-Soluplus, which was statistically better than in HiE-Neusilin US2 and HiE. In the FeSSIF medium, the CBDA dissolution profile in HiE-Soluplus reaches the highest dissolution rate values and it differs significantly from the CBDA profile in HiE-Neusilin US2 and HiE (Figure 6b). The first time point, 5 min, shows the biggest variability in CBDA dissolution rate, where the percentage of CBDA released was 66.56% ± 1.09% for HiE-Soluplus, 30.13% ± 1.68% for HiE-Neusilin US2, and 11.52% ± 0.65% for HiE. The maximum dissolution rates are higher in FeSSIF than in FaSSIF.

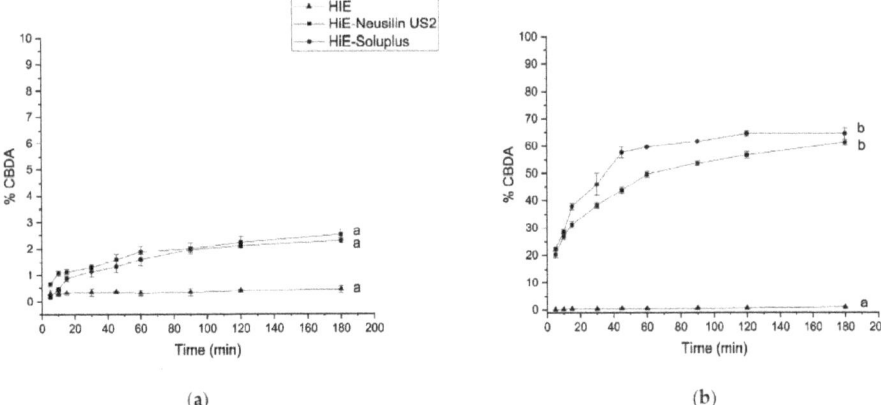

Figure 5. The dissolution profiles of CBDA from HiE, HiE-Neusilin US2, and HiE-Soluplus systems at pH 1.2 (**a**) and 6.8 (**b**). Profiles with the same superscript letters were similar (according to f_1 or f_2 value). Profiles with different superscript letters differ significantly (according to f_1 and f_2 values).

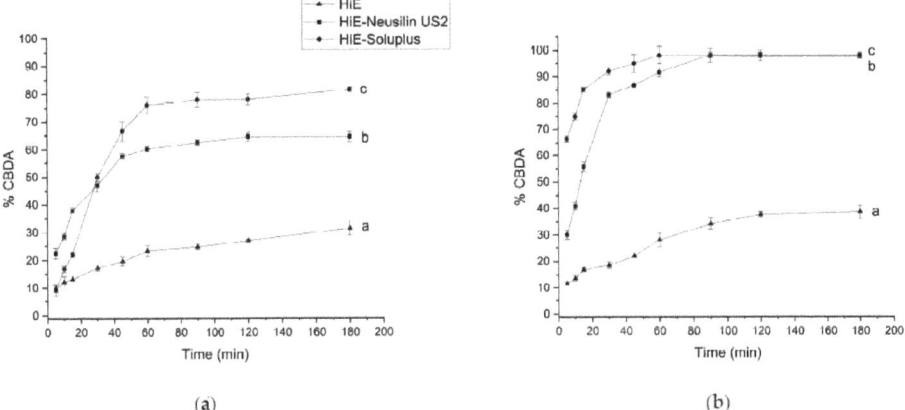

Figure 6. The dissolution profiles of CBDA from HiE, HiE-Neusilin US2, and HiE-Soluplus systems in FaSSIF (**a**) and FeSSIF (**b**). Profiles with different superscript letters (a–c) differ significantly (according to f_1 and f_2 values).

The dissolution kinetics of CBDA was also studied (Table 3). CBDA consistently displayed the highest R^2 values in the Korsmeyer–Peppas and Higuchi models. The n values, fluctuating mostly from below 0.45 to three values below 0.89, suggest a potential dominance of Fickian diffusion. In three cases, the n values between 0.45 and 0.89 indicated the non-Fickian diffusion release mechanism which shows the relative complexity of the prepared co-dispersion delivery systems and may indicate that the CBDA release is controlled by more than one mechanism.

Following the methodology used for the apparent solubility study of CBD and CBDA, the dissolution profiles for CBC were determined in the same media and time points. In the study conducted at pH 1.2 (Figure 7a), the dissolution rate was similar for CBD and CBDA (the lowest). CBC did not dissolve in HiE during the study. At the last time point, 180 min, HiE-Soluplus showed the highest percentage of CBC released at 5.89%, whilst in HiE-Neusilin US2, CBC was dissolved in 5.18% ± 0.28%. CBC profiles were similar due to f_1 and f_2 factors. In the study where vessels were filled with phosphate buffer at pH 6.8

(Figure 7b), CBC in HiE was not dissolved, and the most noticeable differences were noted in the first minutes of the study. The CBC reached in HiE-Soluplus (120 min) of the study was 10.30% ± 1.36%. Whilst in HiE-Neusilin US2, it was 22.75% ± 1.00%. Both dissolution profiles of CBC in co-dispersion delivery systems were similar.

Table 3. Mathematical models of release kinetics of cannabidiolic acid in pH 1.2, pH 6.8, FaSSIF, and FeSSIF.

CBDA		Mathematical Model								
		Zero-Order Kinetics		First-Order Kinetics		Higuchi Kinetics		Korsmeyer–Peppas Kinetics		
		R^2	k	R^2	k	R^2	k	R^2	k	n
pH 1.2	HiE	0.837	0.046	0.837	1.984×10^{-4}	0.797	0.089	0.727	0.357	0.097
	HiE-Neusilin US2	0.884	0.584	0.886	2.581×10^{-3}	0.971	1.233	0.969	1.766	0.350
	HiE-Soluplus	0.830	0.686	0.832	3.022×10^{-3}	0.950	1.479	0.905	1.465	0.666
pH 6.8	HiE	0.908	0.243	0.908	1.061×10^{-3}	0.930	0.495	0.892	0.491	0.566
	HiE-Neusilin US2	0.822	13.118	0.886	1.036×10^{-1}	0.950	28.396	0.986	46.652	0.310
	HiE-Soluplus	0.651	13.299	0.712	1.142×10^{-1}	0.829	30.228	0.927	54.067	0.312
FaSSIF	HiE	0.907	7.126	0.927	3.942×10^{-2}	0.986	14.965	0.994	21.800	0.328
	HiE-Neusilin US2	0.640	13.290	0.699	1.143×10^{-1}	0.821	30.325	0.924	54.393	0.313
	HiE-Soluplus	0.649	24.294	0.753	2.473×10^{-1}	0.823	55.120	0.908	58.247	0.647
FeSSIF	HiE	0.913	10.484	0.933	6.294×10^{-2}	0.974	21.816	0.973	27.257	0.374
	HiE-Neusilin US2	0.579	20.645	0.822	6.125×10^{-1}	0.768	47.898	0.885	83.584	0.344
	HiE-Soluplus	0.484	8.266	0.643	4.122×10^{-1}	0.679	19.713	0.854	93.645	0.108

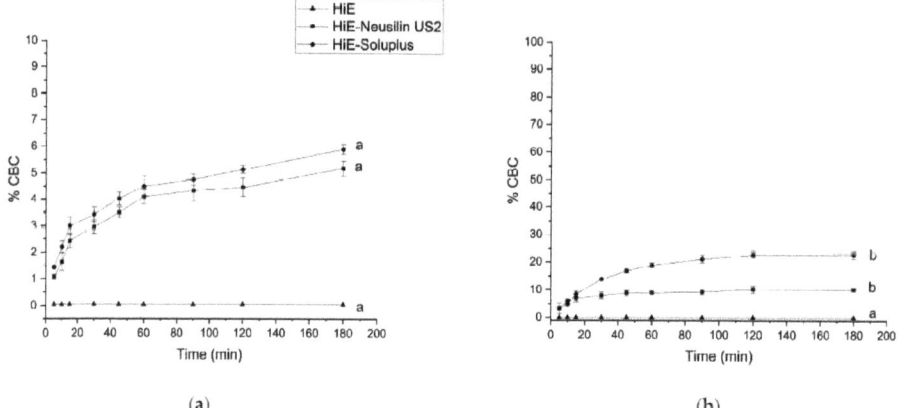

Figure 7. The dissolution profiles of CBC from HiE-Neusilin US2 and HiE-Soluplus systems at pH 1.2 (a) and 6.8 (b). Profiles with the same superscript letters were similar (according to f_1 or f_2 value). Profiles with different superscript letters differ significantly (according to f_1 and f_2 values).

In fasted state intestinal conditions, the most dynamic changes, take place at 5 min of the study, where CBC is dissolved in HiE-Soluplus at 56.63% ± 2.80%, in HiE-Neusilin US2 at 12.28% ± 2.11%, and in HiE at 10.26% ± 0.81% (Figure 8a). After 30 min, CBC reached a plateau. The CBC profile in HiE-Soluplus is significantly better than in HiE-Neusilin US2 and HiE. The last environment in which the CBC dissolution rate was studied was

FeSSIF (Figure 8b), where the greatest dissolution rate of CBC was obtained. After 15 min of the study, CBC was dissolved in 79.32% ± 2.30%, 58.68% ± 0.57%, and 26.25% ± 2.79% in HiE-Soluplus, HiE-Neusilin US2, and HiE, respectively. The CBC dissolution profile in HiE-Soluplus was significantly better than in HiE-Neusilin US2 and HiE.

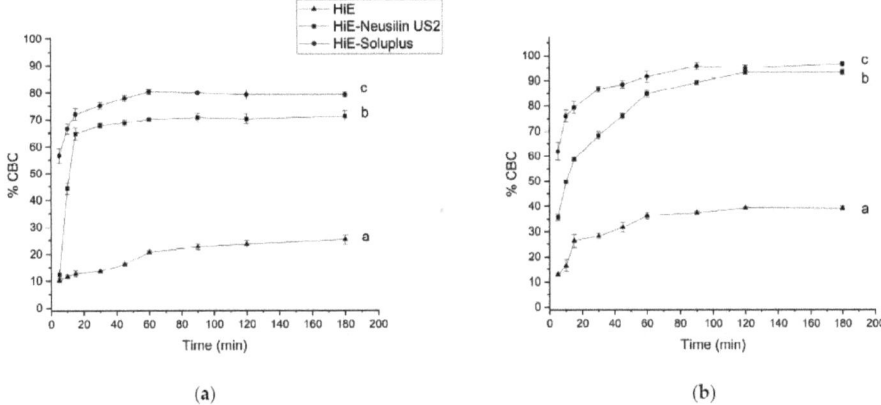

(a)   (b)

Figure 8. The dissolution profiles of CBC from HiE-Neusilin US2 and HiE-Soluplus systems in FaSSIF (**a**) and FeSSIF (**b**). Profiles with the same superscript letters were similar (according to f_1 or f_2 value). Profiles with different superscript letters (a–c) differ significantly (according to f_1 and f_2 values).

The Higuchi and Korsmeyer–Peppas models consistently yield higher R^2 values compared to the zero-order and first-order models across different CBC formulations and pH conditions (Table 4). The release exponent (n) values are consistently below 0.5 across formulations and pH conditions, suggesting the release approximated the Fickian diffusion release mechanism indicative of controlled release predominantly driven by diffusion.

Table 4. Mathematical models of release kinetics of cannabichromene in pH 1.2, pH 6.8, FaSSIF, and FeSSIF.

	CBC	Mathematical Model								
		Zero-Order Kinetics		First-Order Kinetics		Higuchi Kinetics		Korsmeyer–Peppas Kinetics		
		R^2	k	R^2	k	R^2	k	R^2	k	n
pH 1.2	HiE	N/D	N/D	N/D	N/D	N/D	N/D	N/D	N/D	N/D
	HiE-Neusilin US2	0.800	1.264	0.804	5.679×10^{-3}	0.930	2.745	0.950	3.662	0.424
	HiE-Soluplus	0.825	1.340	0.830	6.056×10^{-3}	0.943	2.885	0.954	4.227	0.370
pH 6.8	HiE	N/D	N/D	N/D	N/D	N/D	N/D	N/D	N/D	N/D
	HiE-Neusilin US2	0.642	1.810	0.651	8.519×10^{-3}	0.808	4.091	0.863	8.712	0.265
	HiE-Soluplus	0.733	6.657	0.753	3.393×10^{-2}	0.892	14.795	0.929	16.368	0.578
FaSSIF	HiE	0.868	5.442	0.878	2.895×10^{-2}	0.949	11.466	0.950	18.890	0.276
	HiE-Neusilin US2	0.304	11.161	0.371	1.037×10^{-1}	0.464	27.770	0.568	64.899	0.362
	HiE-Soluplus	0.427	5.302	0.475	8.281×10^{-2}	0.618	12.850	0.804	76.888	0.087
FeSSIF	HiE	0.640	8.272	0.676	5.052×10^{-2}	0.809	18.736	0.877	32.411	0.331
	HiE-Neusilin US2	0.703	17.658	0.878	3.545×10^{-1}	0.870	39.559	0.946	78.768	0.267
	HiE-Soluplus	0.605	9.119	0.845	3.415×10^{-1}	0.780	20.870	0.902	89.911	0.115

The results showed that HiE-Soluplus consistently provided the highest dissolution rate of cannabinoids compared to HiE-Neusilin US2 and HiE. The dissolution rate of CBD, CBDA, and CBC was highest in FeSSIF, followed by FaSSIF and the phosphate buffer at pH 6.8, while the lowest dissolution rate was observed in 0.1 M hydrochloric acid at pH 1.2. At pH 1.2, all three cannabinoids showed poor solubility. In a phosphate buffer with a pH of 6.8, the greatest improvement in solubility was observed for CBDA. CBDA, being the acidic precursor of CBD, might have some advantages in solubility compared to CBD and CBC. In FaSSIF, the maximum dissolution rate was similar for CBD, CBDA, and CBC. However, the fastest increase in dissolution rate was noted for CBC. In FeSSIF, the dissolution profiles for CBD, CBDA, and CBC were again similar, but the fastest increase in dissolution rate was observed for CBD. FaSSIF and FeSSIF provided a more similar composition to intestinal fluid than the pharmacopoeial media, containing surfactants that helped significantly increase the solubility of cannabinoids.

3.3. Permeability Study

Increasing gastrointestinal permeability is important to obtain higher bioavailability as it allows for more efficient absorption into the bloodstream from the GI tract. Thus, a PAMPA study was performed.

The permeability coefficients of CBD in pH 6.8 were analyzed in HiE and co-dispersion delivery systems: HiE-Neusilin US2 and HiE-Soluplus (Table 5). The highest permeability coefficient was observed in HiE-Soluplus ($3.09 \times 10^{-7} \pm 1.07 \times 10^{-8}$ cm/s), followed by HiE-Neusilin US2 ($2.73 \times 10^{-7} \pm 9.75 \times 10^{-9}$ cm/s), and the CBD permeability was statistically the worst in the pure extract ($1.86 \times 10^{-7} \pm 2.24 \times 10^{-8}$ cm/s).

Table 5. Gastrointestinal permeability of CBD and CBDA from HiE, HiE-Neusilin US2, and HiE-Soluplus systems at pH 6.8. Results in columns with different superscript letters (a, b) differ significantly.

	P_{app} (cm/s)	
	CBD	CBDA
HiE	$1.86 \times 10^{-7} \pm 2.24 \times 10^{-8}$ [a]	$7.57 \times 10^{-6} \pm 1.21 \times 10^{-7}$ [a]
HiE-Neusilin US2	$2.73 \times 10^{-7} \pm 9.75 \times 10^{-9}$ [b]	$7.56 \times 10^{-6} \pm 2.69 \times 10^{-7}$ [a]
HiE-Soluplus	$3.09 \times 10^{-7} \pm 1.07 \times 10^{-8}$ [b]	$9.51 \times 10^{-6} \pm 4.66 \times 10^{-8}$ [b]

CBDA was better permeable than CBD through membranes in the study under the same conditions (Table 5). Its permeability coefficient reached $7.57 \times 10^{-6} \pm 1.21 \times 10^{-7}$ cm/s in HiE, while the most noticeable and statistically significant increase was found in HiE-Soluplus, where CBDA reached $9.51 \times 10^{-6} \pm 4.66 \times 10^{-8}$ cm/s and $7.56 \times 10^{-6} \pm 2.69 \times 10^{-7}$ cm/s in HiE-Neusilin US2.

The BBB permeability was assessed for CBD, CBDA, and CBC in HiE. All P_{app} values were determined as higher than 4.0×10^{-6} cm/s, meaning that both cannabinoids cross the blood-brain barrier well.

3.4. Biological Activity Studies

HiE extract and the systems showed antioxidant activity (Table 6). In the DPPH model, the best result was obtained for Hi-Soluplus (0.97 ± 0.02 mg trolox/g plant material), while for HiE (0.85 ± 0.01 mg trolox/g plant material), however, these results are statistically similar. In the other scavenging radicals assay, ABTS, the HiE (17.04 ± 0.08 mg trolox/g plant material) antioxidant potential was improved the most by HiE-Soluplus (18.69 ± 0.17 mg trolox/g plant material). In the CUPRAC redox study, the greatest result was obtained for HiE-Soluplus (7.81 ± 0.22 mg trolox/g plant material). In FRAP, the most noticeable improvement in HiE antioxidant activity (11.58 ± 0.03 mg trolox/g plant material) was shown also for HiE-Soluplus (1.65 ± 0.03 mg trolox/g plant material). In general, the results show statistically significant improvement in ABTS and FRAP assays in antioxidant potential in the systems when compared to HiE, but the changes are subtle.

Table 6. Antioxidant activity of HiE, HiE-Neusilin US2, HiE-Soluplus in DPPH, ABTS, CUPRAC, and FRAP assay expressed as mg trolox/g plant material in the systems. Columns with different superscript letters (a, b) differ significantly.

Extract/System	DPPH	ABTS	CUPRAC	FRAP
	mg Trolox/g Plant Material			
HiE	0.85 ± 0.01 [a]	17.04 ± 0.08 [a]	7.03 ± 0.02 [a]	1.58 ± 0.03 [a]
HiE-Neusilin US2	0.86 ± 0.03 [a]	17.30 ± 0.09 [a]	7.65 ± 0.42 [a]	1.56 ± 0.03 [a]
HiE-Soluplus	0.97 ± 0.02 [a]	18.69 ± 0.17 [b]	7.81 ± 0.22 [a]	1.65 ± 0.03 [b]

The inhibition of the enzymes connected to the development of neurodegeneration was also studied for the extract (Table 7). HiE inhibited an AChE of 20.78 ± 0.56 mg galantamine/g, while BChE was 17.49 ± 0.47 mg galantamine/g. Tyrosinase was also inhibited by the HiE 165.21 ± 7.11 mg azelaic acid/g. Preparation of the systems increased the inhibitory activity of the cannabinoids. The greatest enhancement was noted for HiE-Soluplus (AChE 21.06 ± 0.19 mg galantamine/g, BChE 17.54 ± 0.09 mg galantamine/g, and tyrosinase 171.30 ± 2.13 mg azelaic acid/g). The changes in biological activity are subtle, but there is a visible trend that the neuroprotective potential is increasing.

Table 7. Inhibitory activity of HiE, HiE-Neusilin US2, HiE-Soluplus of acetylcholinesterase (presented as mg galantamine/g plant material), butyrylcholinesterase (presented as mg galantamine/g plant material), and tyrosinase (presented as mg azelaic acid/g plant material). Results with the same superscript letters in the columns are similar.

Extract/System	AChE	BChE	Tyrosinase
	mg Galantamine/g		mg Azelaic Acid/g
HiE	20.23 ± 0.43 [a]	17.49 ± 0.16 [a]	164.25 ± 4.44 [a]
HiE-Neusilin US2	20.82 ± 0.44 [a]	17.32 ± 0.24 [a]	170.76 ± 1.86 [a]
HiE-Soluplus	21.06 ± 0.19 [a]	17.54 ± 0.09 [a]	171.30 ± 2.13 [a]

4. Discussion

Henola inflorescences were extracted with $scCO_2$. $scCO_2$ extraction is widely recognized as a green extraction method. CO_2 functions as a non-polar solvent, and in its supercritical state, it is a good choice for efficiently extracting lipophilic compounds like cannabinoids from plant material [84]. Its selectivity, safety, and environmentally friendly characteristics further contribute to its suitability for this purpose [85,86]. Furthermore, the use of CO_2 as a solvent eliminates the need for harsh organic solvents, resulting in a pure extract without the risk of residual solvent contamination [87–89]. $scCO_2$ extraction is particularly advantageous for extracting cannabinoids from cannabis plant material due to the lipophilic character of these compounds. In its supercritical state, CO_2 exhibits both gas-like diffusion and liquid-like solvency, allowing it to penetrate the plant matrix efficiently and dissolve target compounds [90]. Alcohol extraction is a common method for cannabinoids, extracting a wide range of compounds, but it may also pull undesirable components like chlorophyll and is considered a less environmentally friendly method than $scCO_2$ [91]. Hydrocarbon extraction offers high yields due to its strong solvent power, yet it poses safety risks due to flammable solvents and requires extensive post-extraction purification [91]. Unlike solvent-based techniques, such as ethanol or hydrocarbon extraction, $scCO_2$ is a non-toxic solvent that leaves no residual solvents in the final product, ensuring the purity and safety of extracted cannabinoids. Co-dispersion delivery systems of HiE with Neusilin US2 and Soluplus were prepared with a solvent-evaporation technique, which is a relatively simple, cost-effective, and scalable method [92]. The straightforward nature of the method allows for efficient and cost-effective production of bulk quantities of the desired systems, making it suitable for various industrial applications including pharmaceuticals, cosmetics, and materials engineering. An important aspect was obtaining co-dispersions in powder form for a future oral formulation, which was provided by both Neusilin US2 and Soluplus.

CBD, CBDA, and CBC from HiE did not dissolve in the pharmacopeial media (pH 1.2 and 6.8) as 1% of dissolution was not exceeded in any case within 180 min of the study. Considering CBDA's approximate pKa value of 2.9 [93], CBDA primarily exists in its acidic form under both acidic (pH 1.2) and neutral (pH 6.8) conditions. The improved dissolution rate at pH 6.8 suggests that the neutral environment favors CBDA solubility and release. The approximate pKa value of CBC is around 9.5–10.3 [94], and it is similar to CBD (pKa 9.3–10.3 [94,95]). In the highly acidic environment of pH 1.2, CBC exhibited a similarly low dissolution rate compared to CBD and CBDA. These results suggest that CBC, like CBD and CBDA, has limited solubility and dissolution in highly acidic conditions, which may be attributed to its weakly basic nature. In a phosphate buffer at pH 6.8, CBC demonstrated improved dissolution rates compared to pH 1.2, suggesting enhanced solubility in more neutral environments. In view of the literature reports, the decomposition of cannabinoids in an acidic environment during this study cannot be ruled out [96]. It can, therefore, be assumed that such a low percentage of cannabinoid release in acidic conditions might be due to the poor solubility in the stomach environment, but also due to the degradation of the CBD, CBDA, or CBC.

The solubility and dissolution behavior of cannabinoids, such as CBD, CBDA, and CBC, can vary significantly depending on the pH of the surrounding environment and the presence of specific surfactants. This is visible in the case of the dissolution of cannabinoids from HiE before co-dispersion delivery systems preparation in FaSSIF and FeSSIF as they reached 20–31% and 37–40%, respectively. The dissolution profile of cannabinoids was notably higher in both FaSSIF and FeSSIF compared to the pharmacopeial media. This indicates that the presence of natural surfactants present in FaSSIF and FeSSIF better simulates the complex environment of the gut, leading to a more efficient release of CBD, CBDA, and CBC. Surfactants are amphiphilic molecules, meaning they have both hydrophobic and hydrophilic regions. The presence of surfactants in the solution can help solubilize cannabinoids by forming micelles or emulsions. What is more important, the better solubility of cannabinoids in post-meal conditions was indicated, which was also proven in other studies [97]. The increase in the bioaccessibility of CBD with food could be explained by the fact that micelle formation from hydrolyzed lipids aids in the bioaccessibility of hydrophobic molecules [98]. How cannabinoids are administered, as well as the meal with which they are taken, is a very important aspect to receive the appropriate pharmacological response.

An increase in apparent solubility of cannabinoids was obtained due to co-dispersion delivery systems with Neusilin US2 and Soluplus. Neusilin US2 is a type of synthetic magnesium aluminosilicate which is a porous material with a significant surface area, porosity, and adsorption capacity. Its structure consists of a three-dimensional network of interconnected particles with numerous pores and channels. When Neusilin US2 is in contact with water, its porous structure can adsorb hydrophobic molecules like cannabinoids onto its surface or within its pores [99]. This adsorption effectively increases the apparent solubility of the cannabinoids by creating a reservoir of the drug in a more readily available form. The layered structure allows the material to have both hydrophilic and hydrophobic regions [100]. This dual nature is advantageous for its adsorption capabilities. The hydrophilic regions can interact with water molecules, while the hydrophobic regions can interact with hydrophobic compounds such as cannabinoids (CBD, CBDA, and CBC). Neusilin might also form complexes as a result of acid–base reactions, ion–dipole interactions, and hydrogen bonding [101].

The greatest results were, however, obtained for the co-dispersion delivery systems with Soluplus, which has an amphiphilic graft copolymer structure comprising three main components: polyvinyl caprolactam, polyvinyl acetate, and polyethylene glycol [102]. The polyvinyl caprolactam and polyvinyl acetate segments contribute to the polymer's lipophilic properties, while the PEG segment imparts hydrophilicity [42]. This arrangement allows Soluplus to self-assemble into micelles when placed in an aqueous environment, effectively encapsulating hydrophobic cannabinoids within the micellar core [103]. The polyethylene glycol component in the structure also has a steric stabilizing effect on the micelles [104]. The hydrophilic segments of Soluplus might face outward, interacting with the surrounding water molecules, while the lipophilic segments interact with the cannabinoids, promoting their dispersion within the micelles. Cannabinoids might interact with Soluplus by the formation of hydrogen bonds with their hydroxyl groups [44].

In the literature, in vitro release profiles of CBD and zein and zein-WP nanoparticles in simulated gastric fluid (SGF) and simulated intestinal fluid (SIF) are provided [105]. The free CBD has low bioaccessibility, and only 29% of CBD was detected after SIF digestion. CBD, zein, and zein-WP nanoparticles showed lower sustained release during simulated gastric fluid. Pure CBD has a low solubility profile in both SIF and SGF, with less than 3% within 1 h and less than 10% of CBD released in 48 h [106]. CBD-Silica cast in PVA films show a significantly increased dissolution profile of SIF and SGF, with about 3–7% of CBD released in 1 h and about 40–45% of released CBD in 48 h. Poor solubility of CBD from hemp oil products like oral drops, capsules, and tablets in an acidic medium was also confirmed as 0% of CBD released in FaSSGF, besides one beverage enhancer [107]. Koch et al. [108] conducted a study on the dissolution properties of CBD formulations in a phosphate buffer with a pH of 6.8 and 0.5% sodium lauryl sulfate. They discovered that CBD-cyclodextrin formulations processed through freeze-drying or spray-drying, as well as CBD-mesoporous silica formulations processed through subcritical CO_2 or atmospheric impregnation exhibited a considerable increase in their ability to dissolve in water. The study highlighted Kollidon® VA64 as the excipient that displayed the greatest improvement in aqueous solubility. However, these studies are based on pure CBD, not on extracts, where there is no possible entourage effect between components of the extract. To the best of the authors' knowledge, the release profiles for CBDA and CBC were studied for the first time.

In the current study, the differences in CBD, CBDA, and CBC profiles were mostly noticeable at the beginning of the studies, determining the speed of dissolution of cannabinoids, as well as increasing their dissolution rate, which is very important as orally administered preparations have the latest onset of action compared to other routes of administration, which can be accelerated by orally administered systems with e.g., Soluplus.

Delivery systems are also prepared to enhance the solubility and permeability of various compounds as it is presented in the literature [109–111]. The higher solubility of CBD and CBDA led to more efficient absorption and permeability across the gastrointestinal tract. The improved dissolution rate, increased concentration gradient, and enhanced transport contribute to the higher permeability coefficient observed in the systems compared to the pure extract in the PAMPA study. Achieving higher gastrointestinal permeability is crucial for obtaining higher oral bioavailability as it allows for more efficient absorption into the bloodstream from the gastrointestinal tract.

Oxidative stress occurs when there is an imbalance between the production of reactive oxygen species (ROS) and the body's ability to detoxify them. While some ROS play important roles in cellular signaling and immune function, excess ROS can damage cellular components such as proteins, lipids, and DNA. Oxidative damage has been linked to several chronic diseases such as cancer, cardiovascular disease, and neurodegenerative disorders. Antioxidants neutralize harmful free radicals in the body and reduce inflammation, support the immune system, protect the brain, slow down the aging process, and improve cardiovascular health. These compounds can help protect neurons from oxidative damage, reduce inflammation, and promote cell survival, which can slow down or prevent the progression of neurodegenerative diseases. Cannabinoids exhibit various mechanisms of antioxidant properties [112]. The phenolic hydroxyl groups present in cannabinoid structures play a role in scavenging free radicals [113]. HiE antioxidant activity was slightly improved after preparing co-dispersion delivery systems; however, the changes were often not statistically significant. Similar results were observed for the inhibition of the enzymes related to neuroprotection. The increased solubility of secondary plant metabolites might have influenced their biological activity; however, this phenomenon does not always occur [114].

5. Conclusions

Co-dispersion delivery systems with solubilizing carriers improve the dissolution of cannabinoids: CBD, CBDA, and CBC. Particular improvement was noted for systems co-dispersed with Soluplus. It is also worth noting that the environment of the intestinal contents is the place of optimal dissolution of cannabinoids. Under these conditions, correlations between improved dissolution and better permeability of cannabinoids from co-dispersion delivery systems with solubilizing carriers were also noted. Improved dissolution of cannabinoids (CBD, CBDA, and CBC) induces better permeability through membranes simulating the walls of the digestive system as well as the blood-brain barrier, in view of their confirmed neuroprotective activity, it suggests that the developed co-dispersion delivery systems derived from *Cannabis sativa* (Henola variety) inflorescences may be valuable solutions in preventive and therapeutic procedures.

Supplementary Materials: The following supporting information can be downloaded at: https://www.mdpi.com/article/10.3390/pharmaceutics15092280/s1, Figure S1: Exemplary chromatograms of HiE-Soluplus system in apparent solubility study in pH 1.2 (a), and pH 6.8 (b); Table S1: HPLC method validation parameters.

Author Contributions: Conceptualization, A.S.-K. and J.C.-P.; methodology, A.S.-K., P.S. and J.C.-P.; software, A.S.-K.; validation, A.S.-K. and J.C.-P.; formal analysis, A.S.-K. and J.C.-P.; investigation, A.S.-K. and P.S.; resources, A.S.-K.; data curation, A.S.-K.; writing—original draft preparation, A.S.-K. and J.C.-P.; writing—review and editing, A.S.-K. and J.C.-P.; visualization, A.S.-K.; supervision, J.C.-P.; project administration, A.S.-K. and J.C.-P.; funding acquisition, A.S.-K. and J.C.-P. All authors have read and agreed to the published version of the manuscript.

Funding: This research was funded in whole by the National Science Centre, Poland, the grant Preludium nr UMO-2021/41/N/NZ7/01125. For the purpose of Open Access, the author has applied a CC-BY public copyright license to any Author Accepted Manuscript (AAM) version arising from this submission.

Institutional Review Board Statement: Not applicable.

Informed Consent Statement: Not applicable.

Data Availability Statement: Data are available in a publicly accessible repository.

Conflicts of Interest: The authors declare no conflict of interest. The funders had no role in the design of the study; in the collection, analyses, or interpretation of data; in the writing of the manuscript; or in the decision to publish the results.

References

1. Fordjour, E.; Manful, C.F.; Sey, A.A.; Javed, R.; Pham, T.H.; Thomas, R.; Cheema, M. Cannabis: A Multifaceted Plant with Endless Potentials. *Front. Pharmacol.* **2023**, *14*, 1200269. [CrossRef] [PubMed]
2. Sinclair, J.; Collett, L.; Abbott, J.; Pate, D.W.; Sarris, J.; Armour, M. Effects of Cannabis Ingestion on Endometriosis-Associated Pelvic Pain and Related Symptoms. *PLoS ONE* **2021**, *16*, e0258940. [CrossRef] [PubMed]
3. Calapai, F.; Cardia, L.; Calapai, G.; Di Mauro, D.; Trimarchi, F.; Ammendolia, I.; Mannucci, C. Effects of Cannabidiol on Locomotor Activity. *Life* **2022**, *12*, 652. [CrossRef]
4. Anil, S.M.; Peeri, H.; Koltai, H. Medical Cannabis Activity Against Inflammation: Active Compounds and Modes of Action. *Front. Pharmacol.* **2022**, *13*, 908198. [CrossRef]
5. Kuhathasan, N.; Minuzzi, L.; MacKillop, J.; Frey, B.N. The Use of Cannabinoids for Insomnia in Daily Life: Naturalistic Study. *J. Med. Internet Res.* **2021**, *23*, e25730. [CrossRef]
6. Zaheer, S.; Kumar, D.; Khan, M.T.; Giyanwani, P.R.; Kiran, F. Epilepsy and Cannabis: A Literature Review. *Cureus* **2018**, *10*, e3278. [CrossRef]
7. Bruni, N.; Della Pepa, C.; Oliaro-Bosso, S.; Pessione, E.; Gastaldi, D.; Dosio, F. Cannabinoid Delivery Systems for Pain and Inflammation Treatment. *Molecules* **2018**, *23*, 2478. [CrossRef] [PubMed]
8. Grifoni, L.; Vanti, G.; Donato, R.; Sacco, C.; Bilia, A.R. Promising Nanocarriers to Enhance Solubility and Bioavailability of Cannabidiol for a Plethora of Therapeutic Opportunities. *Molecules* **2022**, *27*, 6070. [CrossRef]

9. Gao, S.; Hu, M. Bioavailability Challenges Associated with Development of Anti-Cancer Phenolics. *Mini Rev. Med. Chem.* **2010**, *10*, 550–567. [CrossRef]
10. Lucas, C.J.; Galettis, P.; Schneider, J. The Pharmacokinetics and the Pharmacodynamics of Cannabinoids. *Br. J. Clin. Pharmacol.* **2018**, *84*, 2477–2482. [CrossRef]
11. Chayasirisobhon, S. Mechanisms of Action and Pharmacokinetics of Cannabis. *Perm. J.* **2020**, *25*, 1–3. [CrossRef] [PubMed]
12. Subramanian, N.; Ghosal, S.K. Enhancement of Gastrointestinal Absorption of Poorly Water Soluble Drugs via Lipid Based Systems. *Indian J. Exp. Biol.* **2004**, *42*, 1056–1065. [PubMed]
13. Buya, A.B.; Beloqui, A.; Memvanga, P.B.; Préat, V. Self-Nano-Emulsifying Drug-Delivery Systems: From the Development to the Current Applications and Challenges in Oral Drug Delivery. *Pharmaceutics* **2020**, *12*, 1194. [CrossRef] [PubMed]
14. Wang, C.; Wang, J.; Sun, Y.; Freeman, K.; Mchenry, M.A.; Wang, C.; Guo, M. Enhanced Stability and Oral Bioavailability of Cannabidiol in Zein and Whey Protein Composite Nanoparticles by a Modified Anti-Solvent Approach. *Foods* **2022**, *11*, 376. [CrossRef]
15. Hippalgaonkar, K.; Gul, W.; ElSohly, M.A.; Repka, M.A.; Majumdar, S. Enhanced Solubility, Stability, and Transcorneal Permeability of Delta-8-Tetrahydrocannabinol in the Presence of Cyclodextrins. *AAPS PharmSciTech* **2011**, *12*, 723–731. [CrossRef]
16. Jarho, P.; Pate, D.W.; Brenneisen, R.; Järvinen, T. Hydroxypropyl-Beta-Cyclodextrin and Its Combination with Hydroxypropyl-Methylcellulose Increases Aqueous Solubility of Delta9-Tetrahydrocannabinol. *Life Sci.* **1998**, *63*, PL381–PL384. [CrossRef]
17. Robinson, D.; Ritter, S.; Yassin, M. Comparing Sublingual and Inhaled Cannabis Therapies for Low Back Pain: An Observational Open-Label Study. *Rambam Maimonides Med. J.* **2022**, *13*, e0026. [CrossRef]
18. Millar, S.A.; Stone, N.L.; Yates, A.S.; O'Sullivan, S.E. A Systematic Review on the Pharmacokinetics of Cannabidiol in Humans. *Front. Pharmacol.* **2018**, *9*, 1365. [CrossRef] [PubMed]
19. Abu-Sawwa, R.; Scutt, B.; Park, Y. Emerging Use of Epidiolex (Cannabidiol) in Epilepsy. *J. Pediatr. Pharmacol. Ther.* **2020**, *25*, 485–499. [CrossRef]
20. Shannon, S.; Lewis, N.; Lee, H.; Hughes, S. Cannabidiol in Anxiety and Sleep: A Large Case Series. *Perm. J.* **2019**, *23*, 18-041. [CrossRef]
21. Blessing, E.M.; Steenkamp, M.M.; Manzanares, J.; Marmar, C.R. Cannabidiol as a Potential Treatment for Anxiety Disorders. *Neurotherapeutics* **2015**, *12*, 825–836. [CrossRef] [PubMed]
22. Wright, M.; Di Ciano, P.; Brands, B. Use of Cannabidiol for the Treatment of Anxiety: A Short Synthesis of Pre-Clinical and Clinical Evidence. *Cannabis Cannabinoid Res.* **2020**, *5*, 191–196. [CrossRef] [PubMed]
23. Souza, J.D.S.; Zuardi, A.W.; Guimarães, F.S.; de Osório, F.L.; Loureiro, S.R.; Campos, A.C.; Hallak, J.E.C.; Dos Santos, R.G.; Machado Silveira, I.L.; Pereira-Lima, K.; et al. Maintained Anxiolytic Effects of Cannabidiol after Treatment Discontinuation in Healthcare Workers during the COVID-19 Pandemic. *Front. Pharmacol.* **2022**, *13*, 856846. [CrossRef]
24. Peng, J.; Fan, M.; An, C.; Ni, F.; Huang, W.; Luo, J. A Narrative Review of Molecular Mechanism and Therapeutic Effect of Cannabidiol (CBD). *Basic Clin. Pharmacol. Toxicol.* **2022**, *130*, 439–456. [CrossRef] [PubMed]
25. Silvestro, S.; Mammana, S.; Cavalli, E.; Bramanti, P.; Mazzon, E. Use of Cannabidiol in the Treatment of Epilepsy: Efficacy and Security in Clinical Trials. *Molecules* **2019**, *24*, 1459. [CrossRef] [PubMed]
26. Gray, R.A.; Whalley, B.J. The Proposed Mechanisms of Action of CBD in Epilepsy. *Epileptic Disord.* **2020**, *22*, S10–S15. [CrossRef]
27. Batalla, A.; Bos, J.; Postma, A.; Bossong, M.G. The Impact of Cannabidiol on Human Brain Function: A Systematic Review. *Front. Pharmacol.* **2021**, *11*, 618184. [CrossRef]
28. Watt, G.; Karl, T. In Vivo Evidence for Therapeutic Properties of Cannabidiol (CBD) for Alzheimer's Disease. *Front. Pharmacol.* **2017**, *8*, 20. [CrossRef]
29. Zou, S.; Kumar, U. Cannabinoid Receptors and the Endocannabinoid System: Signaling and Function in the Central Nervous System. *Int. J. Mol. Sci.* **2018**, *19*, 833. [CrossRef]
30. Lu, H.-C.; Mackie, K. Review of the Endocannabinoid System. *Biol. Psychiatry Cogn. Neurosci. Neuroimaging* **2021**, *6*, 607–615. [CrossRef]
31. Simiyu, D.C.; Jang, J.H.; Lee, O.R. Understanding *Cannabis sativa* L.: Current Status of Propagation, Use, Legalization, and Haploid-Inducer-Mediated Genetic Engineering. *Plants* **2022**, *11*, 1236. [CrossRef] [PubMed]
32. Echeverry, C.; Prunell, G.; Narbondo, C.; de Medina, V.S.; Nadal, X.; Reyes-Parada, M.; Scorza, C. A Comparative In Vitro Study of the Neuroprotective Effect Induced by Cannabidiol, Cannabigerol, and Their Respective Acid Forms: Relevance of the 5-HT1A Receptors. *Neurotox. Res.* **2021**, *39*, 335–348. [CrossRef] [PubMed]
33. Goerl, B.; Watkins, S.; Metcalf, C.; Smith, M.; Beenhakker, M. Cannabidiolic Acid Exhibits Entourage-like Improvements of Anticonvulsant Activity in an Acute Rat Model of Seizures. *Epilepsy Res.* **2021**, *169*, 106525. [CrossRef] [PubMed]
34. Zagožen, M.; Čerenak, A.; Kreft, S. Cannabigerol and Cannabichromene in *Cannabis sativa* L. *Acta Pharm.* **2021**, *71*, 355–364. [CrossRef]
35. Shinjyo, N.; Di Marzo, V. The Effect of Cannabichromene on Adult Neural Stem/Progenitor Cells. *Neurochem. Int.* **2013**, *63*, 432–437. [CrossRef]
36. Valeri, A.; Chiricosta, L.; D'Angiolini, S.; Pollastro, F.; Salamone, S.; Mazzon, E. Cannabichromene Induces Neuronal Differentiation in NSC-34 Cells: Insights from Transcriptomic Analysis. *Life* **2023**, *13*, 742. [CrossRef]
37. Stasiłowicz-Krzemień, A.; Sip, S.; Szulc, P.; Cielecka-Piontek, J. Determining Antioxidant Activity of Cannabis Leaves Extracts from Different Varieties-Unveiling Nature's Treasure Trove. *Antioxidants* **2023**, *12*, 1390. [CrossRef]

38. Pagano, C.; Savarese, B.; Coppola, L.; Navarra, G.; Avilia, G.; Laezza, C.; Bifulco, M. Cannabinoids in the Modulation of Oxidative Signaling. *Int. J. Mol. Sci.* **2023**, *24*, 2513. [CrossRef]
39. dos-Santos-Pereira, M.; Guimarães, F.S.; Del-Bel, E.; Raisman-Vozari, R.; Michel, P.P. Cannabidiol Prevents LPS-Induced Microglial Inflammation by Inhibiting ROS/NF-KB-Dependent Signaling and Glucose Consumption. *Glia* **2020**, *68*, 561–573. [CrossRef]
40. Pereira, S.R.; Hackett, B.; O'Driscoll, D.N.; Sun, M.C.; Downer, E.J. Cannabidiol Modulation of Oxidative Stress and Signalling. *Neuronal Signal.* **2021**, *5*, NS20200080. [CrossRef]
41. Jîtcă, G.; Ősz, B.E.; Vari, C.E.; Rusz, C.-M.; Tero-Vescan, A.; Pușcaș, A. Cannabidiol: Bridge between Antioxidant Effect, Cellular Protection, and Cognitive and Physical Performance. *Antioxidants* **2023**, *12*, 485. [CrossRef] [PubMed]
42. Sofroniou, C.; Baglioni, M.; Mamusa, M.; Resta, C.; Doutch, J.; Smets, J.; Baglioni, P. Self-Assembly of Soluplus in Aqueous Solutions: Characterization and Prospectives on Perfume Encapsulation. *ACS Appl. Mater. Interfaces* **2022**, *14*, 14791–14804. [CrossRef] [PubMed]
43. Al-Akayleh, F.; Al-Naji, I.; Adwan, S.; Al-Remawi, M.; Shubair, M. Enhancement of Curcumin Solubility Using a Novel Solubilizing Polymer Soluplus®. *J. Pharm. Innov.* **2022**, *17*, 142–154. [CrossRef]
44. Rosiak, N.; Wdowiak, K.; Tykarska, E.; Cielecka-Piontek, J. Amorphous Solid Dispersion of Hesperidin with Polymer Excipients for Enhanced Apparent Solubility as a More Effective Approach to the Treatment of Civilization Diseases. *Int. J. Mol. Sci.* **2022**, *23*, 15198. [CrossRef]
45. Rosiak, N.; Tykarska, E.; Cielecka-Piontek, J. Amorphous Pterostilbene Delivery Systems Preparation—Innovative Approach to Preparation Optimization. *Pharmaceutics* **2023**, *15*, 1231. [CrossRef] [PubMed]
46. Darwich, M.; Mohylyuk, V.; Kolter, K.; Bodmeier, R.; Dashevskiy, A. Enhancement of Itraconazole Solubility and Release by Hot-Melt Extrusion with Soluplus®. *J. Drug Deliv. Sci. Technol.* **2023**, *81*, 104280. [CrossRef]
47. Jha, D.K.; Shah, D.S.; Amin, P.D. Thermodynamic Aspects of the Preparation of Amorphous Solid Dispersions of Naringenin with Enhanced Dissolution Rate. *Int. J. Pharm.* **2020**, *583*, 119363. [CrossRef] [PubMed]
48. Stasiłowicz-Krzemień, A.; Rosiak, N.; Miklaszewski, A.; Cielecka-Piontek, J. Screening of the Anti-Neurodegenerative Activity of Caffeic Acid after Introduction into Inorganic Metal Delivery Systems to Increase Its Solubility as the Result of a Mechanosynthetic Approach. *Int. J. Mol. Sci.* **2023**, *24*, 9218. [CrossRef]
49. Jo, K.; Cho, J.M.; Lee, H.; Kim, E.K.; Kim, H.C.; Kim, H.; Lee, J. Enhancement of Aqueous Solubility and Dissolution of Celecoxib through Phosphatidylcholine-Based Dispersion Systems Solidified with Adsorbent Carriers. *Pharmaceutics* **2019**, *11*, 1. [CrossRef]
50. Józsa, L.; Nemes, D.; Pető, Á.; Kósa, D.; Révész, R.; Bácskay, I.; Haimhoffer, Á.; Vasvári, G. Recent Options and Techniques to Assess Improved Bioavailability: In Vitro and Ex Vivo Methods. *Pharmaceutics* **2023**, *15*, 1146. [CrossRef]
51. Simancas-Herbada, R.; Fernández-Carballido, A.; Aparicio Blanco, J.; Slowing, K.; Rubio Retama, J.; López-Cabarcos, E.; Torres-Suarez, A. Controlled Release of Highly Hydrophilic Drugs from Novel Poly(Magnesium Acrylate) Matrix Tablets. *Pharmaceutics* **2020**, *12*, 174. [CrossRef] [PubMed]
52. Hens, B.; Tsume, Y.; Bermejo Sanz, M.; Paixao, P.; Koenigsknecht, M.; Baker, J.; Hasler, W.; Lionberger, R.; Fan, J.; Dickens, J.; et al. Low Buffer Capacity and Alternating Motility Along the Human Gastrointestinal Tract: Implications for In Vivo Dissolution and Absorption of Ionizable Drugs. *Mol. Pharm.* **2017**, *14*, 4281–4294. [CrossRef] [PubMed]
53. Prior, A.; Frutos, P.; Correa, C. Comparison of Dissolution Profiles: Current Guidelines. In Proceedings of the VI Congreso SEFIG, Granada, Spain, 9–11 February 2003; Volume 3, pp. 507–509.
54. Haimhoffer, Á.; Vasvári, G.; Budai, I.; Béresová, M.; Deák, Á.; Németh, N.; Váradi, J.; Sinka, D.; Bácskay, I.; Vecsernyés, M.; et al. In Vitro and In Vivo Studies of a Verapamil-Containing Gastroretentive Solid Foam Capsule. *Pharmaceutics* **2022**, *14*, 350. [CrossRef] [PubMed]
55. Szekalska, M.; Wróblewska, M.; Czajkowska-Kośnik, A.; Sosnowska, K.; Misiak, P.; Wilczewska, A.Z.; Winnicka, K. The Spray-Dried Alginate/Gelatin Microparticles with Luliconazole as Mucoadhesive Drug Delivery System. *Materials* **2023**, *16*, 403. [CrossRef] [PubMed]
56. Fischer, H.; Kansy, M.; Avdeef, A.; Senner, F. Permeation of Permanently Positive Charged Molecules through Artificial Membranes—Influence of Physico-Chemical Properties. *Eur. J. Pharm. Sci.* **2007**, *31*, 32–42. [CrossRef]
57. Di, L.; Kerns, E.H.; Fan, K.; McConnell, O.J.; Carter, G.T. High Throughput Artificial Membrane Permeability Assay for Blood-Brain Barrier. *Eur. J. Med. Chem.* **2003**, *38*, 223–232. [CrossRef]
58. Liao, H.; Dong, W.; Shi, X.; Liu, H.; Yuan, K. Analysis and Comparison of the Active Components and Antioxidant Activities of Extracts from *Abelmoschus esculentus* L. *Pharmacogn. Mag.* **2012**, *8*, 156. [CrossRef]
59. Muzykiewicz, A.; Florkowska, K.; Nowak, A.; Zielonka-Brzezicka, J.; Klimowicz, A. Antioxidant Activity of St. John's Wort Extracts Obtained with Ultrasound-Assisted Extraction. *Pomeranian J. Life Sci.* **2019**, *65*, 89–93. [CrossRef]
60. Stasiłowicz, A.; Tykarska, E.; Lewandowska, K.; Kozak, M.; Miklaszewski, A.; Kobus-Cisowska, J.; Szymanowska, D.; Plech, T.; Jenczyk, J.; Cielecka-Piontek, J. Hydroxypropyl-β-Cyclodextrin as an Effective Carrier of Curcumin—Piperine Nutraceutical System with Improved Enzyme Inhibition Properties. *J. Enzym. Inhib. Med. Chem.* **2020**, *35*, 1811–1821. [CrossRef]
61. Re, R.; Pellegrini, N.; Proteggente, A.; Pannala, A.; Yang, M.; Rice-Evans, C. Antioxidant Activity Applying an Improved ABTS Radical Cation Decolorization Assay. *Free Radic. Biol. Med.* **1999**, *26*, 1231–1237. [CrossRef]
62. Stasiłowicz-Krzemień, A.; Rosiak, N.; Płazińska, A.; Płaziński, W.; Miklaszewski, A.; Tykarska, E.; Cielecka-Piontek, J. Cyclodextrin Derivatives as Promising Solubilizers to Enhance the Biological Activity of Rosmarinic Acid. *Pharmaceutics* **2022**, *14*, 2098. [CrossRef] [PubMed]

63. Apak, R.; Güçlü, K.; Ozyürek, M.; Karademir, S.E.; Altun, M. Total Antioxidant Capacity Assay of Human Serum Using Copper(II)-Neocuproine as Chromogenic Oxidant: The CUPRAC Method. *Free Radic. Res.* **2005**, *39*, 949–961. [CrossRef] [PubMed]
64. Pohanka, M. Inhibitors of Acetylcholinesterase and Butyrylcholinesterase Meet Immunity. *Int. J. Mol. Sci.* **2014**, *15*, 9809–9825. [CrossRef] [PubMed]
65. Chen, W.-C.; Tseng, T.-S.; Hsiao, N.-W.; Lin, Y.-L.; Wen, Z.-H.; Tsai, C.-C.; Lee, Y.-C.; Lin, H.-H.; Tsai, K.-C. Discovery of Highly Potent Tyrosinase Inhibitor, T1, with Significant Anti-Melanogenesis Ability by Zebrafish in Vivo Assay and Computational Molecular Modeling. *Sci. Rep.* **2015**, *5*, 7995. [CrossRef]
66. Tang, G.-Y.; Zhao, C.-N.; Xu, X.-Y.; Gan, R.-Y.; Cao, S.-Y.; Liu, Q.; Shang, A.; Mao, Q.-Q.; Li, H.-B. Phytochemical Composition and Antioxidant Capacity of 30 Chinese Teas. *Antioxidants* **2019**, *8*, 180. [CrossRef]
67. Stojkovic, D.; Drakulic, D.; Dias, M.I.; Zengin, G.; Barros, L.; Ivanov, M.; Gašic, U.; Rajcevic, N.; Stevanovic, M.; Ferreira, I.C.F.R.; et al. *Phlomis fruticosa* L. Exerts in Vitro Antineurodegenerative and Antioxidant Activities and Induces Prooxidant Effect in Glioblastoma Cell Line. *EXCLI J.* **2022**, *21*, 387–399. [CrossRef]
68. Angelini, P.; Venanzoni, R.; Angeles Flores, G.; Tirillini, B.; Orlando, G.; Recinella, L.; Chiavaroli, A.; Brunetti, L.; Leone, S.; Di Simone, S.C.; et al. Evaluation of Antioxidant, Antimicrobial and Tyrosinase Inhibitory Activities of Extracts from *Tricholosporum goniospermum*, an Edible Wild Mushroom. *Antibiotics* **2020**, *9*, 513. [CrossRef]
69. Zhang, L.; Zengin, G.; Rocchetti, G.; Şenkardeş, İ.; Jugreet, S.; Mahomoodally, F.; Behl, T.; Rouphael, Y.; Lucini, L. Phytochemical Constituents and Biological Activities of the Unexplored Plant *Rhinanthus angustifolius* subsp. *grandiflorus*. *Appl. Sci.* **2021**, *11*, 9162. [CrossRef]
70. Kobenan, K.C.; Bini, K.K.N.; Kouakou, M.; Kouadio, I.S.; Zengin, G.; Ochou, G.E.C.; Boka, N.R.K.; Menozzi, P.; Ochou, O.G.; Dick, A.E. Chemical Composition and Spectrum of Insecticidal Activity of the Essential Oils of *Ocimum gratissimum* L. and *Cymbopogon citratus* Stapf on the Main Insects of the Cotton Entomofauna in Côte d'Ivoire. *Chem. Biodivers.* **2021**, *18*, e2100497. [CrossRef]
71. Ferreira, J.; Santos, S.; Pereira, H. In Vitro Screening for Acetylcholinesterase Inhibition and Antioxidant Activity of Quercus Suber Cork and Corkback Extracts. *Evid. Based Complement. Altern. Med.* **2020**, *2020*, 3825629. [CrossRef]
72. Ellman, G.L.; Courtney, K.D.; Andres, V.; Featherstone, R.M. A New and Rapid Colorimetric Determination of Acetylcholinesterase Activity. *Biochem. Pharmacol.* **1961**, *7*, 88–95. [CrossRef]
73. Lim, T.Y.; Lim, Y.Y.; Yule, C.M. Evaluation of Antioxidant, Antibacterial and Anti-Tyrosinase Activities of Four Macaranga Species. *Food Chem.* **2009**, *114*, 594–599. [CrossRef]
74. Garbiec, E.; Rosiak, N.; Tykarska, E.; Zalewski, P.; Cielecka-Piontek, J. Sinapic Acid Co-Amorphous Systems with Amino Acids for Improved Solubility and Antioxidant Activity. *Int. J. Mol. Sci.* **2023**, *24*, 5533. [CrossRef]
75. da Costa, N.F.; Daniels, R.; Fernandes, A.I.; Pinto, J.F. Amorphous and Co-Amorphous Olanzapine Stability in Formulations Intended for Wet Granulation and Pelletization. *Int. J. Mol. Sci.* **2022**, *23*, 10234. [CrossRef]
76. Ullah, M.; Ullah, H.; Murtaza, G.; Mahmood, Q.; Hussain, I. Evaluation of Influence of Various Polymers on Dissolution and Phase Behavior of Carbamazepine-Succinic Acid Cocrystal in Matrix Tablets. *BioMed Res. Int.* **2015**, *2015*, 870656. [CrossRef] [PubMed]
77. Patnaik, S.; Chunduri, L.A.A.; Akilesh, M.S.; Bhagavatham, S.S.; Kamisetti, V. Enhanced Dissolution Characteristics of Piroxicam–Soluplus® Nanosuspensions. *J. Exp. Nanosci.* **2016**, *11*, 916–929. [CrossRef]
78. Nandi, U.; Ajiboye, A.L.; Patel, P.; Douroumis, D.; Trivedi, V. Preparation of Solid Dispersions of Simvastatin and Soluplus Using a Single-Step Organic Solvent-Free Supercritical Fluid Process for the Drug Solubility and Dissolution Rate Enhancement. *Pharmaceuticals* **2021**, *14*, 846. [CrossRef]
79. Krupa, A.; Szlęk, J.; Jany, B.R.; Jachowicz, R. Preformulation Studies on Solid Self-Emulsifying Systems in Powder Form Containing Magnesium Aluminometasilicate as Porous Carrier. *AAPS PharmSciTech* **2015**, *16*, 623–635. [CrossRef]
80. Costa, P.; Sousa Lobo, J.M. Modeling and Comparison of Dissolution Profiles. *Eur. J. Pharm. Sci.* **2001**, *13*, 123–133. [CrossRef] [PubMed]
81. Dash, S.; Murthy, P.N.; Nath, L.; Chowdhury, P. Kinetic Modeling on Drug Release from Controlled Drug Delivery Systems. *Acta Pol. Pharm.* **2010**, *67*, 217–223. [PubMed]
82. Baishya, H. Application of Mathematical Models in Drug Release Kinetics of Carbidopa and Levodopa ER Tablets. *J. Dev. Drugs* **2017**, *6*, 171. [CrossRef]
83. Andriotis, E.G.; Chachlioutaki, K.; Monou, P.K.; Bouropoulos, N.; Tzetzis, D.; Barmpalexis, P.; Chang, M.-W.; Ahmad, Z.; Fatouros, D.G. Development of Water-Soluble Electrospun Fibers for the Oral Delivery of Cannabinoids. *AAPS PharmSciTech* **2021**, *22*, 23. [CrossRef] [PubMed]
84. de Aguiar, A.C.; Vardanega, R.; Viganó, J.; Silva, E.K. Supercritical Carbon Dioxide Technology for Recovering Valuable Phytochemicals from *Cannabis sativa* L. and Valorization of Its Biomass for Food Applications. *Molecules* **2023**, *28*, 3849. [CrossRef] [PubMed]
85. Qamar, S.; Manrique, Y.J.; Parekh, H.S.; Falconer, J.R. Development and Optimization of Supercritical Fluid Extraction Setup Leading to Quantification of 11 Cannabinoids Derived from Medicinal Cannabis. *Biology* **2021**, *10*, 481. [CrossRef] [PubMed]
86. Rochfort, S.; Isbel, A.; Ezernieks, V.; Elkins, A.; Vincent, D.; Deseo, M.A.; Spangenberg, G.C. Utilisation of Design of Experiments Approach to Optimise Supercritical Fluid Extraction of Medicinal Cannabis. *Sci. Rep.* **2020**, *10*, 9124. [CrossRef] [PubMed]

87. Tzima, S.; Georgiopoulou, I.; Louli, V.; Magoulas, K. Recent Advances in Supercritical CO_2 Extraction of Pigments, Lipids and Bioactive Compounds from Microalgae. *Molecules* **2023**, *28*, 1410. [CrossRef]
88. Villacís-Chiriboga, J.; Voorspoels, S.; Uyttebroek, M.; Ruales, J.; Van Camp, J.; Vera, E.; Elst, K. Supercritical CO_2 Extraction of Bioactive Compounds from Mango (*Mangifera indica* L.) Peel and Pulp. *Foods* **2021**, *10*, 2201. [CrossRef]
89. Nagybákay, N.E.; Syrpas, M.; Vilimaitė, V.; Tamkutė, L.; Pukalskas, A.; Venskutonis, P.R.; Kitrytė, V. Optimized Supercritical CO_2 Extraction Enhances the Recovery of Valuable Lipophilic Antioxidants and Other Constituents from Dual-Purpose Hop (*Humulus lupulus* L.) Variety Ella. *Antioxidants* **2021**, *10*, 918. [CrossRef]
90. Uwineza, P.A.; Waśkiewicz, A. Recent Advances in Supercritical Fluid Extraction of Natural Bioactive Compounds from Natural Plant Materials. *Molecules* **2020**, *25*, 3847. [CrossRef]
91. Lazarjani, M.P.; Young, O.; Kebede, L.; Seyfoddin, A. Processing and Extraction Methods of Medicinal Cannabis: A Narrative Review. *J. Cannabis Res.* **2021**, *3*, 32. [CrossRef]
92. Safari, H.; Adili, R.; Holinstat, M.; Eniola-Adefeso, O. Modified Two-Step Emulsion Solvent Evaporation Technique for Fabricating Biodegradable Rod-Shaped Particles in the Submicron Size Range. *J. Colloid Interface Sci.* **2018**, *518*, 174–183. [CrossRef] [PubMed]
93. Anderson, L.L.; Low, I.K.; Banister, S.D.; McGregor, I.S.; Arnold, J.C. Pharmacokinetics of Phytocannabinoid Acids and Anticonvulsant Effect of Cannabidiolic Acid in a Mouse Model of Dravet Syndrome. *J. Nat. Prod.* **2019**, *82*, 3047–3055. [CrossRef] [PubMed]
94. Vacek, J.; Vostalova, J.; Papouskova, B.; Skarupova, D.; Kos, M.; Kabelac, M.; Storch, J. Antioxidant Function of Phytocannabinoids: Molecular Basis of Their Stability and Cytoprotective Properties under UV-Irradiation. *Free Radic. Biol. Med.* **2021**, *164*, 258–270. [CrossRef]
95. Stella, B.; Baratta, F.; Della Pepa, C.; Arpicco, S.; Gastaldi, D.; Dosio, F. Cannabinoid Formulations and Delivery Systems: Current and Future Options to Treat Pain. *Drugs* **2021**, *81*, 1513–1557. [CrossRef] [PubMed]
96. Jeong, M.; Lee, S.; Seo, O.; Kwon, E.; Rho, S.; Cho, M.; Kim, M.Y.; Lee, W.; Lee, Y.S.; Hong, J. Chemical Transformation of Cannabidiol into Psychotropic Cannabinoids under Acidic Reaction Conditions: Identification of Transformed Products by GC-MS. *J. Food Drug Anal.* **2023**, *31*, 165–176. [CrossRef] [PubMed]
97. Zgair, A.; Wong, J.C.; Lee, J.B.; Mistry, J.; Sivak, O.; Wasan, K.M.; Hennig, I.M.; Barrett, D.A.; Constantinescu, C.S.; Fischer, P.M.; et al. Dietary Fats and Pharmaceutical Lipid Excipients Increase Systemic Exposure to Orally Administered Cannabis and Cannabis-Based Medicines. *Am. J. Transl. Res.* **2016**, *8*, 3448–3459. [PubMed]
98. Mozaffari, K.; Willette, S.; Lucker, B.F.; Kovar, S.E.; Holguin, F.O.; Guzman, I. The Effects of Food on Cannabidiol Bioaccessibility. *Molecules* **2021**, *26*, 3573. [CrossRef]
99. Park, H.; Cha, K.-H.; Hong, S.H.; Abuzar, S.M.; Lee, S.; Ha, E.-S.; Kim, J.-S.; Baek, I.-H.; Kim, M.-S.; Hwang, S.-J. Pharmaceutical Characterization and In Vivo Evaluation of Orlistat Formulations Prepared by the Supercritical Melt-Adsorption Method Using Carbon Dioxide: Effects of Mesoporous Silica Type. *Pharmaceutics* **2020**, *12*, 333. [CrossRef]
100. Jadhav, B.V.; Gawali, V.B.; Badadhe, S.G.; Bhalsing, M.D. Study of Neusiln UFL2 and β-Cyclodextrin as Solid Carriers in Solid Self-Microemulsifying Drug Delivery System of Atorvastatin Calcium Prepared by Spray Drying. Available online: https://www.asianpharmtech.com/abstract/study-of-neusiln-ufl2-and-cyclodextrin-as-solidrncarriers-in-solid-selfmicroemulsifying-drugrndelivery-system-of-atorvas-14677.html (accessed on 18 August 2023).
101. Azad, M.; Moreno, J.; Davé, R. Stable and Fast-Dissolving Amorphous Drug Composites Preparation via Impregnation of Neusilin® UFL2. *J. Pharm. Sci.* **2018**, *107*, 170–182. [CrossRef]
102. Cespi, M.; Casettari, L.; Palmieri, G.; Perinelli, D.; Bonacucina, G. Rheological Characterization of Polyvinyl Caprolactam-Polyvinyl Acetate-Polyethylene Glycol Graft Copolymer (SoluplusA (R)) Water Dispersions. *Colloid Polym. Sci.* **2014**, *292*, 235–241. [CrossRef]
103. Alopaeus, J.F.; Hagesæther, E.; Tho, I. Micellisation Mechanism and Behaviour of Soluplus®–Furosemide Micelles: Preformulation Studies of an Oral Nanocarrier-Based System. *Pharmaceuticals* **2019**, *12*, 15. [CrossRef] [PubMed]
104. Piazzini, V.; D'Ambrosio, M.; Luceri, C.; Cinci, L.; Landucci, E.; Bilia, A.R.; Bergonzi, M.C. Formulation of Nanomicelles to Improve the Solubility and the Oral Absorption of Silymarin. *Molecules* **2019**, *24*, 1688. [CrossRef] [PubMed]
105. Wang, C.; Cui, B.; Sun, Y.; Wang, C.; Guo, M. Preparation, Stability, Antioxidative Property and in Vitro Release of Cannabidiol (CBD) in Zein-Whey Protein Composite Nanoparticles. *LWT* **2022**, *162*, 113466. [CrossRef]
106. Khabir, Z.; Partalis, C.; Panchal, J.V.; Deva, A.; Khatri, A.; Garcia-Bennett, A. Enhanced Skin Penetration of Cannabidiol Using Organosilane Particles as Transdermal Delivery Vehicles. *Pharmaceutics* **2023**, *15*, 798. [CrossRef]
107. Analakkattillam, S.; Langsi, V.K.; Hanrahan, J.P.; Moore, E. Comparative Study of Dissolution for Cannabidiol in EU and US Hemp Oil Products by HPLC. *J. Pharm. Sci.* **2021**, *110*, 3091–3098. [CrossRef]
108. Koch, N.; Jennotte, O.; Gasparrini, Y.; Vandenbroucke, F.; Lechanteur, A.; Evrard, B. Cannabidiol Aqueous Solubility Enhancement: Comparison of Three Amorphous Formulations Strategies Using Different Type of Polymers. *Int. J. Pharm.* **2020**, *589*, 119812. [CrossRef]
109. Paczkowska-Walendowska, M.; Miklaszewski, A.; Cielecka-Piontek, J. Improving Solubility and Permeability of Hesperidin through Electrospun Orange-Peel-Extract-Loaded Nanofibers. *Int. J. Mol. Sci.* **2023**, *24*, 7963. [CrossRef]
110. Mahmood, A.; Khan, L.; Ijaz, M.; Nazir, I.; Naseem, M.; Tahir, M.A.; Aamir, M.N.; Rehman, M.U.; Asim, M.H. Enhanced Intestinal Permeability of Cefixime by Self-Emulsifying Drug Delivery System: In-Vitro and Ex-Vivo Characterization. *Molecules* **2023**, *28*, 2827. [CrossRef]

111. Taechalertpaisarn, J.; Ono, S.; Okada, O.; Johnstone, T.C.; Lokey, R.S. A New Amino Acid for Improving Permeability and Solubility in Macrocyclic Peptides through Side Chain-to-Backbone Hydrogen Bonding. *J. Med. Chem.* **2022**, *65*, 5072–5084. [CrossRef]
112. Atalay, S.; Jarocka-Karpowicz, I.; Skrzydlewska, E. Antioxidative and Anti-Inflammatory Properties of Cannabidiol. *Antioxidants* **2019**, *9*, 21. [CrossRef]
113. Zhang, Y.; Li, H.; Jin, S.; Lu, Y.; Peng, Y.; Zhao, L.; Wang, X. Cannabidiol Protects against Alzheimer's Disease in C. Elegans via ROS Scavenging Activity of Its Phenolic Hydroxyl Groups. *Eur. J. Pharmacol.* **2022**, *919*, 174829. [CrossRef] [PubMed]
114. Paczkowska-Walendowska, M.; Szymanowska, D.; Cielecka-Piontek, J. Mechanochemical Properties of Mucoadhesive Tablets Based on PVP/HPβCD Electrospun Nanofibers as Local Delivery of Polygoni Cuspidati Extract for Treating Oral Infections. *Pharmaceuticals* **2023**, *16*, 579. [CrossRef] [PubMed]

Disclaimer/Publisher's Note: The statements, opinions and data contained in all publications are solely those of the individual author(s) and contributor(s) and not of MDPI and/or the editor(s). MDPI and/or the editor(s) disclaim responsibility for any injury to people or property resulting from any ideas, methods, instructions or products referred to in the content.

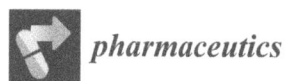

Review

Recent Options and Techniques to Assess Improved Bioavailability: In Vitro and Ex Vivo Methods

Liza Józsa [1], Dániel Nemes [1], Ágota Pető [1], Dóra Kósa [1], Réka Révész [1], Ildikó Bácskay [1,2], Ádám Haimhoffer [1,*,†] and Gábor Vasvári [1,*,†]

1 Department of Pharmaceutical Technology, Faculty of Pharmacy, University of Debrecen, Nagyerdei St. 98, H-4032 Debrecen, Hungary
2 Institute of Healthcare Industry, University of Debrecen, Nagyerdei St. 98, H-4032 Debrecen, Hungary
* Correspondence: haimhoffer.adam@pharm.unideb.hu (Á.H.); vasvari.gabor@pharm.unideb.hu (G.V.)
† These authors contributed equally to this work.

Abstract: Bioavailability assessment in the development phase of a drug product is vital to reveal the disadvantageous properties of the substance and the possible technological interventions. However, in vivo pharmacokinetic studies provide strong evidence for drug approval applications. Human and animal studies must be designed on the basis of preliminary biorelevant experiments in vitro and ex vivo. In this article, the authors have reviewed the recent methods and techniques from the last decade that are in use for assessing the bioavailability of drug molecules and the effects of technological modifications and drug delivery systems. Four main administration routes were selected: oral, transdermal, ocular, and nasal or inhalation. Three levels of methodologies were screened for each category: in vitro techniques with artificial membranes; cell culture, including monocultures and co-cultures; and finally, experiments where tissue or organ samples were used. Reproducibility, predictability, and level of acceptance by the regulatory organizations are summarized for the readers.

Keywords: in vitro methods; cell culture; ex vivo methods; bioavailability

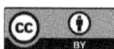

1. Introduction

Over the past decade, efforts have been made to develop reliable in vitro and ex vivo models that mimic all relevant biological barriers in the preclinical drug testing [1]. This phenomenon was stimulated by the need to rationalize drug development and research processes and make the results more reproducible [2]. In addition, significant scientific efforts have been made to discover alternative methods of drug development and testing for ethical reasons, as animal welfare has become a major concern, not only in society but also in the scientific field [3]. In 1959, Russell and Burch defined the "3R" rule (Replace, Reduce, Refine), which sets out the principles for the more ethical use of animals in product testing and scientific research [4]. Animal experiments are often carried out to determine the pharmacokinetics and toxicological data of drugs before the clinical trials; however, the regulatory authorities (e.g., EMA, FDA) enforce the replacement of animal testing and suggest the use of in vitro or ex vivo models because of ethical reasons. The use of these non-animal methods makes it possible to reduce the number of animals involved in animal experiments, refine the methods, and even replace the animals, thereby contributing to the implementation of the 3R principles and giving the potential to further minimize animal testing in preclinical research [2]. Furthermore, many animal tests are simply too costly, take too long, and provide misleading results.

Many techniques and models are successfully used at different stages of drug discovery and development, including in silico, in vitro, ex vivo, and in vivo methods [5]. The present review provides an overview of the characterization and application of novel in vitro and ex vivo methods and cell cultures used in the development and evaluation of new oral, dermal, nasal, and ocular formulations. The development of technology provided the opportunity for in vitro and ex vivo methods to become increasingly widespread. The correlation between the human data and the preclinical data obtained from these models is critical for drug design and development. The accuracy of predicting clinical outcomes is largely determined by the extent to which these models mimic the given part of the human body. Therefore, significant efforts were made to create an environment as close to humans as possible [2,6].

The use of the novel in vitro methods described in this review may lead to better in vitro-in vivo extrapolation (IVIVE) outcomes. Several models are available to screen and predict oral, transdermal, nasal, and even ocular bioavailability of an active pharmaceutical ingredient (API) at different stages of drug discovery and development. Among the latest in vitro assays for the investigation of drug permeability are the parallel artificial membrane permeability assays (PAMPA), which can be used to study both oral and transdermal (skin-PAMPA) dosage forms [7]. PAMPA assays are cost-effective, reliable, robust, quick, reproducible, and high-throughput experiments that predict the passive transcellular permeability of the APIs. According to the type of investigation, the biomimetic membranes can be tailored in terms of their phospholipid compositions, support filter, and type of solvent to successfully predict gastrointestinal or transdermal absorption.

Although many types of in vitro methods are applied during drug discovery and development, the use of cell cultures can be more reliable. Assessment of in vitro absorption, distribution, metabolism, and excretion, as well as drug-drug interaction studies, are mostly performed using various cell culture-based assays. For years, two-dimensional (2D) cell cultures have played a significant role in the testing of various active substances; however, with the appearance of three-dimensional (3D) cell cultures and co-cultures, their importance is decreasing. This is because 3D cultures show protein expression patterns and intercellular junctions, which lead to better IVIVE outcomes as they closely mimic human conditions. Moreover, with the help of co-cultures, it is possible to examine the mutual influence of different cell types [2,8,9].

Compared to in vitro models, ex vivo models are much more complex and therefore closer to human conditions, as these experiments are performed on tissues extracted from humans or animals in a controlled external environment, which allows for higher interplay and cross-talk among the cellular components. They have advantages such as faster and more systematic testing, robustness, and compatibility with high-throughput processes [10]. Therefore, we can consider these models as the tradeoff between in vitro and in vivo methods.

2. Oral Route

2.1. In Vitro Methods

When discussing the oral bioavailability of drugs, basic factors such as key characteristics of the chemical substance and the dosage form should be considered. The solubility and permeability of drug substances were selected to serve as the basis of the Biopharmaceutics Classification System. The solubility of the active ingredient in the digestive juices should be determined, and the affecting factors must be revealed. Following the suggested strategies of the licensing drug authorities, different buffer solutions are recommended. Buffer solutions mimic the environment of the GI tract; therefore, the pH range of 1.2–6.8 at $37 \pm 1\ °C$ is used in most cases. Recent guidelines recommend evaluating drug solubility in buffers at pH 1.2, 4.5, and 6.8. However, several factors could affect the outcome of the solubility investigations. Firstly, the nature of the crystallinity of the substance; compared to the apparent solubility of the crystalline material, amorphous materials possess an increased solubility [11]. Lacking order in their 3D structure, these solid particles form a supersaturated solution; therefore, the drug's rate and extent of dissolution are increased [12]. The ratio of dissolved drug to total drug content is also important because permeation through the enterocytes' membrane is aided when the API is molecularly dispersed. On the other hand, supersaturated solutions are thermodynamically unstable. Several factors in the GI environment could contribute to crystallization, but micelles of bile and polymeric excipients could stabilize the solution [13].

Pharmacopoeias contain detailed guidelines to standardize dissolution studies. The purposes of the dissolution test are performed to serve as drug development and quality assurance tools or to provide evidence for adequate similarity or bioequivalence. Pharmacopeial methods and apparatuses must be chosen, but only in cases where modifications are necessary to reveal minor differences in the formulation or the production. Extensive research was initiated to develop biorelevant dissolution tests and biorelevant media. It is well known that simulated gastric and intestinal fluids contain components such as pepsin or pancreas powder at concentrations that are non-physiologically relevant. Volumes and agitation rate rather provide sink conditions and appropriate mixing of the dissolution media than a biorelevant, dynamic environment. Firstly, the media selection should be considered. Empty and fed states of the stomach are good examples to develop biorelevant dissolution fluids. Everyday life habits were summarized when the Fasted-State Simulated Gastric Fluid (FaSSGF) was published [14]. This dissolution media (pH 1.6) mimics the basal, average gastric juice (including sodium taurocholate and lecithin) plus the so-called glass of water used to swallow the dosage form [15]. Consumed food is temporarily stored and digested in the stomach before being passed in smaller portions. It is evident that the artificial fed-stomach media required a more complex composition. Fed-State Simulated Gastric Fluid (FeSSGF) is an acetic acid/sodium acetate buffer with a pH of 5.0. The ionic strength is set with sodium chloride, and the buffer is mixed in a 1:1 ratio with full fat (3.5%) UHT milk as the food part [16]. Along with the gastric media, their intestinal counterparts were created. It is quite interesting that the Fasted-State Simulated Intestinal Fluid (FaSSIF) and the Fed-State Simulated Intestinal Fluid (FeSSIF) were published earlier [17], but their scientific revision and update resulted in a novel version. The second versions of the FaSSIF and FeSSIF are maleate buffers with pH values of 6.5 and 5.8, respectively. The FaSSIF-V2 contains sodium taurocholate and lecithin as surfactants, while the fed-state media is supplemented with glyceryl monooleate and sodium oleate. These two components were meant to mimic the fatty components of the digested food [15].

The digestive and enzymatic functions of the digestive tracts cannot be skipped when improved bioavailability of the formulation is studied [18]. Enzymatic degradation of lipid-based formulations is often mentioned in publications as lipolysis tests. In vitro lipolysis tests are carried out by adding lipid-based formulations (LBFs) to aqueous media (similar to FaSSIF) containing pancreas powder [19–21].

It is logical to assume that such formulations, delivering the drug in its lipid-based carrier, are preferred to increase bioavailability. However, when the lipid formulation undergoes enzymatic degradation, drug precipitation may occur, resulting in a negligible effect on drug absorption [22,23]. Enzymatic degradation might be due to colonic fermentation as well. Drugs such as polyphenols possess low upper GI tract absorption, and these xenobiotics could accumulate in the colon, where bacteria metabolize them [21]. Therefore, no consistent data is available to establish a rock-hard correlation, especially in vitro and in vivo correlation [24].

Precipitation is also an important factor, not only in the digestion or degradation of the formulation but also when it is transferred from one digestive compartment to another. The pH-dependent solubility of the drug is also important when such transfer dissolution tests are performed. A basic setup is when two compartments of paddle-type dissolution apparatuses are connected with a peristaltic pump. The donor compartment is acidic (pH 1.2–2.0) with a smaller volume compared to the acceptor or intestinal compartment, where the buffer is almost neutral (pH 5.0–6.5). The transfer rates are varied, and zero- or first-order kinetic approaches were used. In the case of the zero-order kinetic transfer model, a constant volume is pumped, while in the first-order model, the transfer speed (mL/min) decreases over time. These experiments were used to successfully describe the precipitation rates of marketed formulations of drugs with pH-dependent solubility [25,26].

The previously detailed dissolution studies (with biorelevant and transfer experiments) could be integrated into systems where the permeability of active ingredients could be measured. In vitro drug permeability is often screened in parallel artificial membrane permeability assays (PAMPA). PAMPA assays are high-throughput experiments predicting the passive transcellular permeability of active ingredients. Biomimetic membranes, separating the donor and acceptor phases, can be tailored regarding their phospholipid compositions, support filters, and type of organic solvent [27,28]. Combined in vitro dissolution and membrane transport experiments were carried out in a modified paddle apparatus where the absorption chamber was submerged into the dissolution vessel. The dissolution compartment or donor compartment was separated by the hydrophobic membrane, resulting in an integrated in vitro dissolution-absorption system where the temperature was maintained at 37 °C and drug concentrations in both chambers were detected using fiber optic probes. In Pion's MacroFLUX™ system, the hydrophobic membrane was made by placing n-dodecane or 20% lecithin dissolved in n-dodecane on the hydrophobic polyvinylidene fluoride filter. To mimic the pH changes during indigestion of the drug formulation, the initial acidic solution (artificial gastric fluid) was converted to FaSSIF. This method was successfully used to detect pH-limited drug dissolution and its effect on the membrane flux. On the other hand, the effect of excipients was revealed among different marketed drug products in terms of drug absorption [29,30].

2.2. Cell Culture

Studying the biorelevant permeability of the drug or formulation requires cell lines, namely the Caco-2 cell culture model, besides artificial membrane assays. Originally, cells were isolated from a human colon adenocarcinoma [31]. They were proven to be an excellent cell culture model for investigating the cellular uptake or the transepithelial permeability through the monolayer they form [32]. When cultivated under certain conditions, they polarize and form monolayer-expressing receptors of the human enterocytes, thus mimicking the absorptive properties of the small intestine [33]. In vivo, the polarized enterocytes face toward the intestinal lumen with their apical surface. This surface is directly exposed to the content of the intestinal lumen [34], and the contact is enormously increased due to the presence of the microvilli [32]. The standard method used to differentiate Caco-2 cells is to seed them on a microporous surface, such as polycarbonate cell culture inserts. On the supporting surface, the cells grow and form a monolayer with tight junctions among the neighboring cells; therefore, an apical and basal compartment is created (Figure 1) [35,36]. Permeability or transport studies are performed by adding the drug or formulation to the apical chamber and detecting its concentration in the basal chamber. The integrity of the monolayer is a vital factor for transport studies, especially when the passive transport of drug or formulation through tight junctions can be expected. To check the high confluency, besides confocal microscopy, fluorescently-labeled markers such as fluorescein [33,37], lucifer yellow [38], or radiolabeled markers like C^{14} mannitol [24] are used. Additionally, the transepithelial electrical resistance (TEER) should be monitored on a regular basis using a volt-ohmmeter equipped with a "chopstick" electrode [38,39]. The integrity of the Caco-2 monolayer can be considered sufficient if the TEER values are at least 800–900 Ω cm^2 [35,36]. This must be checked before and after the transport experiment well by well [38]. A sudden drop in the TEER values indicates a breakdown in the cellular barrier integrity [40].

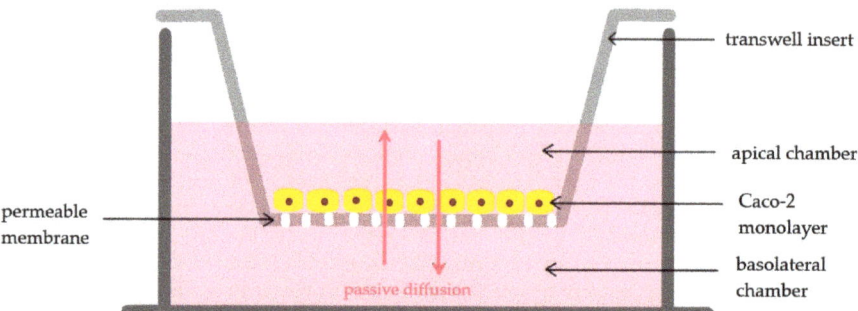

Figure 1. Schematic diagram of a conventional Transwell plate with the Caco-2 cell monolayer for the investigation of oral bioavailability.

Transport experiments can be performed not only with the Caco-2 cells; intracellular uptake or drug internalization could be investigated by fluorescent microscopy or flow cytometry as well. These studies are also important to reveal a possible transcellular pathway of drug absorption [40,41]. The in vitro cytotoxicity or cell viability assays are also extensively used and are cost-effective methods to screen excipients to ensure biocompatibility in their applied concentration. Simple colorimetric assays, such as MTT or neutral red assays, are used to measure the viability of the Caco-2 cells [42,43]. On the other hand, the kinetics of epithelial cell reaction to excipients or formulations can be monitored by impedance measurement with a real-time cell analyzer. This method is non-invasive and label-free, and it linearly correlates with the growth, adherence, and viability of cells [38].

Since cultivated cells are living systems, there is variability in the reproducibility and stability of these models. As an example, decreased TEER values have been detected over time. This problem often extends to cell culture studies and could cause an increase in expenses. Additionally, the transporter proteins are expressed at a different level than in vivo and tiny changes in the cell culture media have a considerable effect on the cell's phenotype. Unfortunately, the results obtained in the Caco-2 cell model may vary among different laboratories [32,37].

2.3. Ex Vivo

Ex vivo methods provide a theoretical means of estimating absorption and bioavailability. They include three main methods: diffusion chambers with separated tissue, everted gut sac, and intestinal perfusion. Ex vivo models have adequate paracellular permeability, mucus layer [44], transport protein expression [45], microbiome [10], and metabolizing properties [46] that separate them from the in vitro Caco-2 model. Ex vivo methods are simple and widely used in the design and testing of potential new drugs or new formulations [47,48].

Diffusion cells can be divided into two major methods, considering the used tissue. In the case of the Ussing chamber, mainly animal or possibly human biopsy intestinal samples are used for the transport model, and the intestinal segment is placed between the two compartments [49,50]. The physiological medium (Krebs, Ringer, PBS, Hank's solution) [51] is circulated separately in both compartments, and the needed gases are ensured by bubbling carbogen gas. The model is suitable to investigate mouse, rat, rabbit, dog, rat, and monkey tissues, which show a very good correlation with the human in vivo results [50]. Furthermore, the method can be used to study differential absorption in pediatrics [52] and to investigate the absorption windows [53]. There are many references in which ex vivo results are well correlated with in vivo results [54–58], but this method requires very expensive equipment, and we cannot ignore the fact that the tissue maintains its integrity for only 2–3 h [5].

Franz cells are similar to the Ussing chamber, but the tissue sections are placed horizontally compared to the above-mentioned method. This diffusion cell model was used for just buccal permeation studies in the oral route because it has limitations for intestinal permeability due to the uncontrolled donor temperature [5]. The continuous mixing effect can lead to higher permeation as observed for standard permeability markers than in the case of the Ussing chamber; therefore, it is beneficial for examining thicker tissues such as skin, avoiding tissue damage [59]. During oral drug administration, the first anatomical site is the buccal tissue, where the active substance can be absorbed. The Franz diffusion cell is most suitable for examining this ex vivo absorption [60,61]. The dog buccal mucosa is similar to human morphology and immunohistology; it shows high drug permeability with moderate correlation with the human study [62,63]. The most common tissue type is porcine, which shows a high correlation; meanwhile, the cost is low and easy to obtain [64]. The thickness is large, so the permeability is low [65]. The rat tissue can be obtained easily at a low cost; nevertheless, due to keratinization, it is not widespread and less correlated with the human surface [61,66]. It is also possible to use rabbit, monkey, or chicken tissue, but these are not very common, either due to the difficulty of obtaining and handling them or the size of the tissue.

The everted rat and hamster intestinal sac models were published first by Wilson and Wiseman [67]. The intestinal sections (duodenum, jejunum, ileum) are cut into small tubes and everted. The mucosal surface is opened towards the API-containing buffer solution, and the serosal layer forms the inside of the sac, which is filled with buffers and solubilizing agents (SLS, Macrogol, Tween). In the case of careful handling of the extracted tissues, the tissue life can be extended up to 2 h from 30 min, which makes it suitable for examinations. Proper handling of the tissue includes keeping it on ice until the test begins and bubbling carbogen gas in the buffers [5,47,68,69]. Standard molecules (mannitol, antipyrine, and digoxin) showed excellent correlation with the everted sac model [70].

The flow through cells can be used to perfuse the API-containing medium through the evacuated intestinal segment, allowing the study of uptake in several intestinal segments simultaneously. The method involves circulating the drug solution in the intestinal segments while measuring the change in concentration. In this case, the media described above and an adequate gas supply are also necessary for the tissue to survive. Although the method is not widespread because of its difficulty, it shows reproducible results because several samples are tested under the same conditions [71].

In Table 1, we have summarized the recent regulatory statuses of the above-mentioned techniques or methods when the bioavailability assessments are performed.

Table 1. Cont.

Study Type	Regulatory Acceptance or Opinion
Solubility	• At least three pH values (pH 1.2, 4.5, and 6.8) should be evaluated. A drug substance is classified as highly soluble if the highest single therapeutic dose is completely soluble in aqueous media not more than 250 mL [72]. • If the drug substance is not stable with >10% degradation during the solubility assessment, the drug substance cannot be classified for BCS Class [73]. • Solubility is a vital factor for immediate-release (IR) products, especially when they are considered for biowaiver during drug approval [74].

Table 1. Regulatory opinions and acceptance of in vitro solubility and dissolution studies, permeability studies, cell culture models, and ex vivo models on the bioavailability of oral drugs.

Study Type	Regulatory Acceptance or Opinion
Dissolution	• Drug dissolution studies are elementary to prove the immediate release of the drug when applying for a BCS-based biowaiver (BCS I and III only) [73]. • Well-defined apparatus with agitation speeds [73]. • The prolonged-release formulation should therefore be evaluated in vitro under various conditions, namely media, pH (normally pH range 1–7.5; if needed up to 8), and the use of biorelevant media is encouraged [75]. • When drug release from MR formulations is investigated, in vitro studies of the release in alcohol solutions should be performed if the drug has higher solubility in ethanolic solutions than in water [76]. • For authorization of MR products with several strengths (in the case of multi-particulate dosage forms/proportional tablets), if their release profiles are similar, the highest strength should be tested in vivo for food effect [76].
Permeability on artificial membrane	• Up to date, no guideline enlists or describes permeability studies for oral products involving artificial membranes.
Cell culture models	• Validation of Caco-2 permeability assay by markers with zero, low, moderate, and high permeability. Markers are enlisted in the guidelines. • BCS classification of test drug is possible; a drug is considered BCS I or II when its permeability value is equal to or greater than that of the highly-permeable internal standard. • The BCS classification by the Caco-2 cell line can be used only for drugs with passive transport [73].
Ex vivo models	• Currently, FDA guidelines enlist permeation studies using excised human or animal intestinal tissues [74].

3. Nasal or Inhalation

3.1. In Vitro

Nasal and inhalation drug delivery has become a common administration route in the last decades for local and even systemic therapies, and there is a growing interest in developing new formulations as well. For these drug delivery routes, the main challenge is to characterize the nasal and/or lung deposition pattern in vivo [77]. Although the recommended in vitro tests, for example, particle size distribution, spray pattern, or emitted dose, are useful to characterize or compare nasal dosage forms and ensure the required quality of the product, they provide limited information about nasal deposition, pharmacokinetics, or pharmacodynamics [78]. Nasal casts offer a cost-effective and rapid method for addressing this issue before the beginning of complex in vivo studies. Even though studies with nasal casts are not a regulatory requirement, the results may provide beneficial information for further development. Targeting the deposition in the nasal cavity has a great impact on the efficiency of local, systemic, and central nervous system drug delivery as well. With the help of anatomically correct in vitro nasal models, the deposition pattern of different nasal preparations can be compared [79]. First nasal casts have evolved from cadavers' heads as they strongly represent human nasal anatomy. To avoid the limitations of tissue preservation issues, the water and lipids were replaced by silicone plastination, resulting in a much more representative structure [80]. Recently, nasal casts are mainly obtained from computed tomography scans with the help of 3D printing since this technology has gained great interest. Most commonly, they are made of plastic, silicone, resin, and acrylonitrile butadiene styrene (ABS) [81–83]. Depending on the specific nasal pathway targeted, the cast model can be divided into 2–3 or 5–7 anatomically relevant regions. Shah et al. designed a seven-section nylon nasal cast according to the computed tomography images of healthy humans. The casts were coated with a glycerol/Brij-35 solution in order to mimic the mucus [84]. Hartigan et al. designed a 3D-printed in vitro tissue model using

ABS filament with a fused deposition modeling 3D printer for preclinical validation of experimental swabs. To mimic the soft human tissue of the nasal cavity, they used aqueous silk sponges; thus, it does not require any cellular material, and the physiological nasal fluid was replaced with synthetic mucus. This model may provide a reproducible, safe, and cost-effective tool for the development of newly designed devices [85]. In order to obtain further information about biological aspects such as permeation, mucoadhesion, and ciliary clearance, in vitro anatomical models can be used in combination with both primary and immortalized cell cultures as well [86].

As for inhalation drug delivery, particle size and in vitro dissolution are the main in vitro parameters that determine the bioavailability of inhaled drugs. The most important aspect that must be taken into consideration is that only a fine fraction of the aerosol (particles <5 μm) reaches the deep lung, and thus, is available for in vitro dissolution testing. This means that the commonly used dissolution protocols for oral dosage forms require adaptations. Mixing forces in the lung are minimal; thus, agitation is questionable during dissolution. As the temperature in the respiratory tract is usually lower than that in the gastrointestinal tract, the testing temperature should be 32.5–33.5 °C according to measurements in healthy volunteers [87]. Since there are no available guidelines provided by regulatory agencies, several dissolution protocols have been described in the literature and developed by researchers. With the help of the UniDose aerosol collection system, the whole powder mass accumulates on a glass microfiber filter membrane and is placed into a disk cassette in the USP2 apparatus (Figure 2). Other methods disperse particles in phosphate-buffered saline, a salt solution with a similar composition to the human hypophysis, or PBS with 0.1% Tween 80. Reproducible and stable physiological dissolution fluids are yet to be identified and standardized. USP1, USP2, USP4, transwells, and Franz diffusion cell systems are all used to expose solid particles to the dissolution fluid, as there is still no adequate in vitro exposure system that can mimic dissolution in vivo [88].

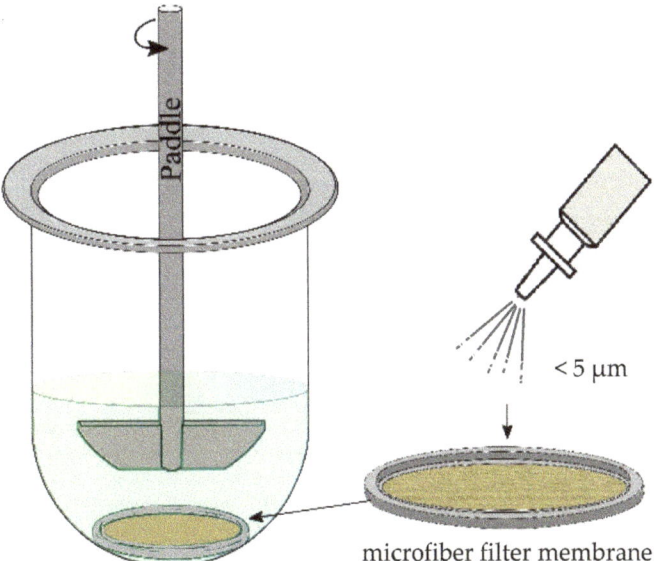

Figure 2. Schematic of paddle-over-disc USP 5 apparatus with a microfiber membrane accumulated with powder mass for the investigation of nasal drug delivery.

3.2. Cell Culture

The respiratory tract is promising as an alternate site of drug delivery because of fast absorption and quick onset of drug action; by avoiding the first-pass metabolism, it is highly beneficial compared to the oral route. Currently, the pharmaceutical industry extensively relies on suitable in vitro models for the faster evaluation of drug absorption and metabolism as an alternative to animal testing. In vitro cell culture models of the respiratory system can decrease the development time for new medicinal products. In the pre-clinical phase, they can be utilized as an alternative to pricey and time-consuming animal testing. Consequently, the information on absorption mechanisms gained from in vitro studies allows for the directed and cost-effective performance of clinical studies and the safety evaluation of new active substances and chemicals [89].

Primary cells and cell lines differ from each other by the time they can be kept in culture. Primary cells must be freshly isolated; thus, they originate from a different individual each time. Primary cultures have some significant limitations, such as the difficult accessibility of suitable human airway tissue and the limited number of cells. On the other hand, they provide the closest in vitro representation of the epithelium [90].

Immortalized cell lines are derived from different tumors, and their advantages over primary cultures are the purity of the cell types and their unlimited lifespan, which enables prolonged experiments. These cell lines are easy to maintain, and they exclude many difficulties, e.g., reproducibility or high costs. The epithelial cells coating the respiratory system play an important role in the protection of the host from different stimuli, including chemicals and pathogens. Human airway epithelial cell cultures are essential for studying aspects of respiratory tract biology, disease, and therapy [91].

Immortalization can cause the occurrence of undesired morphological changes in the cells. Nowadays, the only immortalized nasal cell line of human origin is the RPMI 2650.

RPMI 2650 cells were first isolated from anaplastic squamous cell carcinoma in the nasal septum. The main differences between the nasal mucosa are the absence of ciliary movements and the multilayer cell growth. Despite these few differences, RPMI 2650 cells have shown a similar permeability to nasal mucosa for hydrophilic, lipophilic, and high molecular weight compounds. To perform transport studies, the tight junctions and cell monolayer are crucial points. Furthermore, the cells should be in a high differentiation state. As RPMI 2650 cells are not able to form a monolayer and they lack tight junctions, they are not suitable for transport studies. However, they can be co-cultured with fibroblasts or endothelial cells, which can form a confluent monolayer and develop tight junctions as well. Thus, RPMI 2650 in a co-culture can be a reliable in vitro method for nasal drug absorption [92–94].

16HBE14o- cells are normal human airway epithelial cell lines. They can form polarized cell monolayers and display many properties of bronchial cells, e.g., showing lectin-binding patterns and expressing the intercellular adhesion molecule. The confluent monolayers show extensive tight junctions, which are similar in appearance to those exhibited in intact human tissue. A great disadvantage of the cell line is that it does not secrete mucus that protects the epithelium in vivo, in contrast to Calu-3. 16HBE14o- cell line is assessed with great potential as a bronchial drug absorption model [95,96].

Calu-3 is a human sub-bronchial gland cell line; it was derived from bronchial adenocarcinoma. Calu-3 expresses mRNA and proteins specific to the native epithelium. The cells can form confluent monolayers with tight junctions; the cell line can be an appropriate tool for studying tight junction regulation in the bronchial epithelium [89]. Due to their origin, Calu-3 cells can produce mucus as well. The presence of tight junctions and the secretory activity highlight the potential of this cell line as a suitable in vitro model for studying the pulmonary drug absorption [97,98].

The in vitro cell culture modeling of the respiratory system is not an easy process, but in recent years several solutions have been developed to address the problem. It is crucial to take into consideration the characteristics and limitations of the selected cell culture when designing the experiment and to ensure that the cells are suitable. It is important to compare the properties of the selected cell line with those of the relevant intact tissue, as it is demonstrated above that cell cultures may have shortcomings. For the respiratory system's cell cultures, such important factors may include mucosal secretion, modeling of ciliary activity, the presence of tight junctions, protein expression, or monolayer formation. Primary cells are a lot similar to intact tissue; however, they have several limitations as well.

3.3. Ex Vivo

The isolated and perfused lung model (IPL) was developed and used in the physiological investigation to advance lung transplantation. However, in the last 20 years, it has been used in the investigation of the absorption of inhaled drugs [99,100].

Another method to investigate lung permeability is the precision-cut lung (PCL) method, which truly represents the lung's structural and functional cellular interaction. However, the disadvantages of the method include its inability to mimic ventilation, mechanical stretch, and perfusion [101–103]. To determine the in vivo toxicities, drug permeabilities, and therapeutic efficacies in ex vivo, the PCL model is clinically relevant [104]. Table 2 serves as a representation of the current regulatory acceptance statuses for the in vitro methods and ex vivo opportunities used for evaluating the bioavailability of drugs after intranasal or pulmonary administration.

Table 2. Regulatory opinions and acceptance of in vitro solubility and dissolution studies, permeability studies, cell culture models, and ex vivo models on the bioavailability of nasal/inhalation drugs.

Study Type	Regulatory Acceptance or Opinion
Solubility	• No guidelines are available about solubility studies. However, particle size, morphic form, and the state of solvation of the active substance can affect the bioavailability of a drug product as a result of different solubilities and/or rates of dissolution. Comparable data about particle size distribution, the morphic form of the particles, and the size and number of drug aggregates in the dosage form are recommended [105].
Dissolution	• Availability to the sites of action depends on the particle sizes and distribution patterns, as well as drug dissolution in the case of suspension products, absorption across mucosal barriers to nasal receptors, and rate of removal from the nose. The critical factors are drug release from the product and delivery to the mucosa [105]. • For suspension products, drug particle size is important for the rate of dissolution and availability to sites of action within the nose. Therefore, drug particle size distribution and extent of aggregates should be characterized in formulation before actuation, and in the spray following actuation [105]. • To assess the delivery profile of the product used in in vivo studies, the drug delivery rate and total drug delivered results should be provided for the batches used in these studies. A validated method (e.g., breath simulator), should be employed [106].
Permeability on artificial membrane	• No guidelines describe permeability studies for nasal or inhalation products.
Cell culture models	• No guidelines are available about cell culture models. The most frequently used cell lines for in vitro cell culture studies include RPMI2650, Calu-3, and 16HBE14o.
Ex vivo models	• No guidelines are available.

4. Transdermal

4.1. In Vitro

The dissolution test of semi-solid preparations is a constantly controversial topic because none of the pharmacopoeias have an appropriate section on the dissolution test without a membrane. The Pharmacopoeia recommends three different methods only for patch testing, namely disc assembly (Ph. Eur. 2.9.4.1./USP Apparatus 5), cell (Ph. Eur. 2.9.4.2), and rotating cylinder (Ph. Eur. 2.9.4.3/USP Apparatus 6) [107]. In each case, the active substance is released freely, and the patches are fixed with a 125-mesh net, which keeps the preparation in place and does not affect the way of diffusion. These dissolution studies can be used to compare preparations, but less so for true in vivo correlation [108–111].

In the literature, there are various in vitro release and penetration studies, that can be used to predict in vivo bioavailability [112]. In vitro penetration studies usually use some type of diffusion cell, where passive diffusion is tested on various types of synthetic membranes [113]. The flowthrough cell, vertical diffusion cell, and immersion cell methods were published to describe the dissolution profiles of formulations; nevertheless, the vertical diffusion cell method is the most widely accepted.

The vertical diffusion cells include the same basic parts as a donor and an acceptor compartment and a membrane between the two compartments (Figure 3), but in the literature, a different semantic structure is available to avoid the entrapping bubble or minimize human intervention [114–116]. The acceptor compartment usually contains a buffer and a magnetic stirrer at the bottom of the device, which helps to ensure homogeneous distribution. At various intervals, the acceptor phase is sampled and replaced with a fresh acceptor solution. The limitation of the method and its in vivo correlation are determined by the acceptor buffer and the used membranes. The Start-M membrane and the Tuffryn membrane show a good correlation with in vivo results. The Strat-M membrane is a synthetic, non-animal-based model membrane made from polyether sulfone and polyolefin, which are predictive of diffusion in human skin. The Tuffryn membrane is a polysulfone membrane with low protein binding; hence, it is suitable for the permeation study of biological markers. In most cases, they are used with a buffer and solubilizer agent, such as SLS, Volpo, Tween 80, and PEG 10000 [117–120].

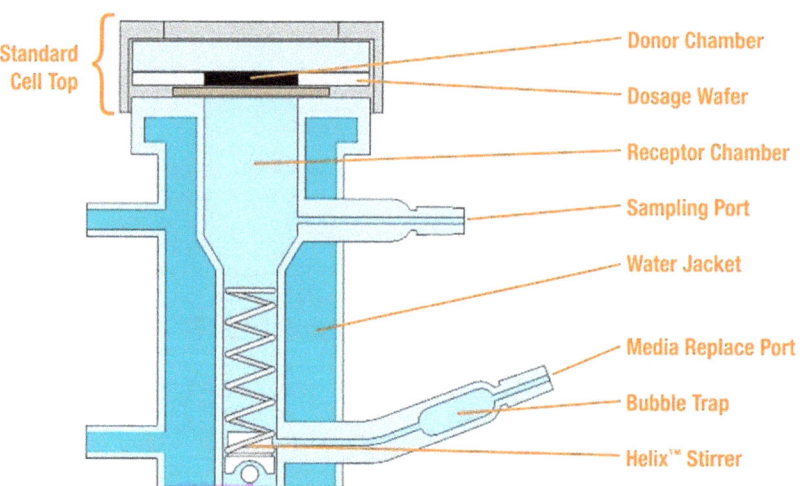

Figure 3. Schematic of a vertical Franz-type in vitro diffusion cell.

A horizontal diffusion cell, also known as a side-by-side diffusion cell [121], also consists of two compartments, but they are smaller in volume and have a smaller diffusion area than vertical cells. Its use is appropriate for small quantities of materials, and it also eliminates the shortcomings of vertical systems, such as the fact that the donor phase is not heated. However, their use is nowadays declining.

The flow-through diffusion cell works similarly to the diffusion cells described above, but with this device, the sampling can be automated [119], as a fraction can be collected from the flowing acceptor phase [122]. Moreover, by setting the parameters of this device, such as the acceptor volume and flow rate, better in vitro-in vivo correlation can be achieved. An important aspect of these measurements is the in vitro-in vivo correlation, which is a new method that has been developed nowadays. This is a bio-predictive IVPT method using a flow-through diffusion cell with the Strat-M membrane mentioned above [117].

Nowadays, a wide range of complex membrane systems is available to simulate human skin. Based on the aforementioned parallel artificial membrane permeability assay (PAMPA), Ottaviani et al. were the first to publish the use of a skin PAMPA. In this case, the membrane was filled with an optimized mixture of silicone (70%) and isopropyl myristate (30%) to reduce skin permeability, thus making it even more similar to human skin [7,123,124].

Lately, a new skin PAMPA model has become available, where the membrane contains special components of the skin barrier, such as cholesterol, free fatty acids, and ceramides that mimic the properties of the lipid matrix [125]. Another advantage is that this skin PAMPA is a 96-well plate-based method, so it can be a relatively quick and low-cost model and an effective high-throughput assessment technique [7].

4.2. Cell Culture

The skin tissue is an effective barrier, representing a protective layer and an essential interface between the human body and the external environment. Based on its structure, it may affect the topical and transdermal bioavailability of various substances. Dermal absorption studies are routinely used to demonstrate benefits after topical application of cosmetics, pharmaceutical formulations containing active ingredients, transdermal patches, or medical devices, but also to predict risks from skin exposure to chemicals [126]. To receive reproducible data on percutaneous absorption, there is an increasing demand for reliable in vitro models, as the national legislation lays down that animal experiments should be avoided whenever scientifically feasible. In addition, the results of animal experiments do not always correlate with the results of human clinical studies due to differences in the structure of the skin [127]. Regarding human and animal models, the skin is associated with other organs, making it difficult to characterize skin diseases independently [128]. Furthermore, a standardized in vivo human or animal skin model is not yet available. Internationally accepted guidelines were created by the Organization for Economic Co-operation and Development (OECD), which give specifications for testing the in vitro percutaneous absorption of chemicals [129].

In recent years, several in vitro skin models have been developed using different cell cultures to assess the penetration and permeation profiles of active ingredients. The oldest but most used methods for constructing skin models are mainly the primary cells, for example, epidermal cells (keratinocytes and melanocytes) or dermal cells (fibroblasts and human dermal microvascular endothelial cells), and cell lines such as the immortalized human keratinocyte cell line (HaCaT), the human foreskin fibroblast cell line (HFF-1), and the murine NIH3T3 fibroblast cell line [130]. The biggest concern is that the primary cells and cell lines do not necessarily represent what happens in vivo, as the cell-cell and cell-matrix interactions, the diversity of the cells that make up the skin (e.g., melanocytes, Langerhans cells, and endothelial cells), and skin appendages (e.g., sweat glands and hair follicles) are missing. The cells do not grow on top of each other but are forced into a monolayer morphology, which is unnatural for most cell types. Despite these disadvantages, they are the most accurate methods of establishing scientific results for long-term research projects [131,132].

In vitro skin models, such as 2D monolayers of human skin cells created by tissue engineering, have shown the possibility of a more accurate, systematic characterization of the skin [128,130]. Establishing co-cultures (e.g., co-cultures of keratinocytes with immune cells and dermal fibroblasts) on Petri dishes or microtiter plates can increase natural intercellular contact and communication, but the 2D surface still inhibits the capacity for cells to form a multi-dimensional structure, which is limiting their accuracy in predicting the complicated effect of drug metabolism on the skin [133]. Therefore, cells grown in flat layers on plastic surfaces do not accurately model in vivo cells.

As a solution to the above-mentioned problems, many 3D models were developed in the form of reconstructed human epidermis (RHE) generated by seeding keratinocytes on a porous membrane. With the creation of these systems, the common goal was to bridge the gap between the use of animals and cellular monolayers [134].

Several RHEs are commercially available that exhibit actual similarities to the native human tissue in terms of morphology, biochemical markers, and lipid composition. These systems are appropriate devices for the testing of phototoxicity, corrosivity, and irritancy caused by different substances; moreover, transport studies can also be carried out. The EpiSkin™ (L'Oréal, Lyon, France), EpiDerm™ (MatTek Corporation, Ashland, MA, USA), SkinEthic™ (Lyon, France), and EpiCS® (CellSystems, Troisdorf, Germany) skin models are well documented in the literature [135,136]. EpiSkin™ and EpiDerm™ were the first 3D models developed and validated as predictive models for skin corrosion and skin irritation [137]. These two models contain human keratinocytes cultured on a collagen-based matrix, simulating the in vivo skin epidermis. Other models, such as SkinEthic® and the modified EpiDerm™ SIT, are used to test irritation on the skin [137–139].

Dreher et al. investigated the cutaneous bioavailability of formulations containing caffeine or alpha-tocopherol on RHEs (EpiDerm™ and EpiSkin™) and compared them with ex vivo studies conducted on human skin. They found that vehicles that contained alcohol showed more potent drug permeation rates in the case of EpiDerm™ and EpiSkin™ models compared to ex vivo results. This was attributed to the weaker barrier properties and the increased hydration of the outermost layer of the stratum corneum of the RHEs [140]. Similar studies were conducted by Schäfer-Korting et al. to evaluate the permeation of caffeine and testosterone across different RHE models (EpiDerm™, EpiSkin™, and SkinEthic™), human epidermis, and animal skin. The permeation coefficients of testosterone were in the following order: human epidermis, bovine udder skin, porcine skin < EpiDerm™, EpiSkin™ < SkinEthic™, while, for caffeine: bovine udder skin, EpiDerm™, porcine skin, human epidermis < SkinEthic™, EpiSkin™. Moreover, the investigated RHE models were validated by them, using nine different drugs with different physicochemical properties. The permeation rates of all substances were higher through the RHE models compared to the human epidermis and porcine skin; however, the ranking of drugs according to permeability was found to be similar on all membranes. They also found that the reproducibility of permeation parameters was very similar for RHEs and for excised skin [141].

Lotte et al. investigated the reproducibility of three RHEs (EpiDerm™, EpiSkin™, and SkinEthic™) regarding the permeation and skin absorption of topically applied compounds with different physicochemical properties (lauric acid, caffeine, and mannitol). They described that SkinEthic™ showed the worst reproducibility among these three models [142].

Jírová et al. examined the skin irritation of different chemicals with in vivo and in vitro methods using the 4-h human patch test (HPT). It was described that the concordance of human epidermis models with human data was 76% (EpiDerm™) and 70% (EpiSkin™). The sensitivity and accuracy of the irritant classification of the RHEs were higher than expected, and they showed better results compared with the tests conducted on rabbits [143].

These studies concluded that RHEs could be considered as alternatives to human, porcine, or rabbit skin for in vitro studies. However, despite the above-mentioned huge advancements, most of the 3D skin models still have some limitations such as weak barrier function, lack of vasculature and skin appendages, and thus, are not able to fully reproduce the complexity of human skin tissue [132,133,144].

In parallel with the development of RHE models, efforts have been made to add a living dermal compartment to produce models referred to as full-thickness (FT) skin models. These models make it possible to seed keratinocytes directly onto the surface of the formed dermal lattice layer, and thus, allowed the investigation of ultraviolet-A-induced aging [145], skin metabolism, genotoxicity [146], and the role of papillary and reticular fibroblast populations [147], as well as glycation in aging to be deciphered [148].

The development of an FT skin model is beginning with the generation of a mature dermis and with the expansion of melanocytes and keratinocytes on top of the dermis, followed by the development of the epidermis at the air–liquid interface [149].

The commercially available FT skin models such as PhenionFT™ (Henkel, Düsseldorf, Germany) and EpidermFT™ (T (MatTek, Ashland, MA) are widely used in the investigation of environmental and age-dependent effects [150], skin penetration, ultraviolet

(UV) irradiation effects, and skin disease mechanisms [151]. A novel FT skin model, T-Skin™, is an in vitro reconstructed skin that consists of a dermal equivalent with human fibroblasts overlaid by a stratified, well-differentiated epidermis derived from normal human keratinocytes cultured on an inert polycarbonate filter. Batallion et al. compared the structure and the layer-specific markers of the T-Skin™ (Episkin, Lyon, France)with normal human skin using histological and immunohistological staining. It was found that T-Skin™ exhibits a very similar structure and characteristics to the human skin, including a well-differentiated and organized epidermis and a functional dermis [152]. These results support the use of T-Skin™, as an alternative screening platform, to develop new cosmetics and to investigate dermatologically active ingredients.

Recently, given the increased interest in extending the experimental testing phase, a long-term FT skin model became commercially available (Phenion® Full-thickness LONG-LIFE skin model, (Henkel, Düsseldorf, Germany), which can be kept in culture for up to 50 days [149].

Significant progress for skin models may be achieved in the field of organ-on-chips, which can provide more physiological conditions with the combination of microsystem engineering and cell/tissue biology [132]. To develop a physiologically relevant in vitro skin model, human skin structures have been integrated into microfluidic systems to construct skin-on-chip models, which can mimic the complex in vivo situation [133]. Microfluidic technology makes it possible to develop an ideal skin-on-chip model by being able to create specific flow properties to ensure efficient chemical reactions, thus the cell-cell and cell-matrix interactions can work properly. Microfluidic-based organ-on-chip systems consist of microchannels, micropumps, valves, mixers, and integrated biosensors, with cell culture inserts used to develop in vitro functional models of healthy and diseased organs [128,153]. Using these devices, the skin tissue can be cultured under the control of several physical and biochemical parameters, such as flow, force, or chemical gradients [133,154].

The fabrication process, materials, and tissue maintenance of these in vitro models can vary greatly. There are two main groups to which the skin-on-chip models can be classified according to how the skin is generated in the chip: the first one is the direct transfer of a skin fragment from a biopsy or a human skin equivalent in the chip (transferred skin-on-a-chip), while the second one is based on the in situ generation of the tissue directly on the chip (in situ skin-on-a-chip) [154–156].

However, there would be some limitations in verifying the correct skin differentiation and structure. To overcome this problem, most of the researchers are using fluorescent-labeled cells or traditional immunocytochemistry for visual inspection, but in most cases, the detection process can be very complicated. This fact led to the development of biosensors which can be completely integrated into the chip to follow up the state of the skin in real time and to monitor the effects of the applied active agents [154].

Overall, skin-on-chip models could be the best platform to study intercellular interactions or even the immune response, as they can better reproduce the physiological environment of the tissue. Furthermore, they allow us to follow up several conditions at the same time under controlled parameters and measure drug efficiency rapidly.

4.3. Ex Vivo

The Franz diffusion cell is the most widely used ex vivo model for evaluating the release and skin permeation of API from topical and transdermal drug delivery systems. The main aim of these studies is to identify the main potential variables that may alter the in vivo bioavailability of the drug during formulation design [59]. The design and principle of operation of the test apparatus correspond to that described for the buccal ex vivo section. Several skin preparations were used, such as mouse [116], rat [157,158] porcine ear [159], newborn pig skin [160], or human skin [161]. Ears of porcine are used mostly because they are easily obtained and cheap; furthermore, the in vivo correlation is also good [120,162,163].

Evaluation of the penetration of active substances in the skin is essential for developing topical formulations, as the expected effect remains on the skin's surface. The concentration of the active ingredient in the skin layers (stratum corneum, epidermis, and dermis) can be determined by ex vivo and in vivo studies by skin retention tests [59]. After the Franz permeability test, the skin can be dried and separated into three main layers. Cellophane tapes can be used 25 times to remove the stratum corneum. The remaining epidermis and dermis can be divided into two parts by heating (60 °C) and mechanical. The API extractions can be carried out in methanol and using an ultrasonic bath at 40 °C for 15 min [164].

Information on the distribution of the active substance within the skin can be easily achieved using RAMAN spectroscopy. The Raman correlation map shows the incidence of the API in the different layers of the animal or human skin from the stratum corneum to the lower layer part of the epidermis. The Raman experiments give a good correlation with the Franz cell and skin PAMPA results, which, thus, closely approximate the in vivo results [7]. Techniques and methodologies used for the evaluation of transdermal bioavailability of drug formulation are summarized in Table 3 regarding their regulatory status.

Table 3. Regulatory opinions and acceptance of in vitro dissolution studies, permeability studies, cell culture models, and ex vivo models on the bioavailability of transdermal drugs/products.

Study Type	Regulatory Acceptance or Opinion
Dissolution *	• In vitro drug release test is defined only for patches by regulator's guidelines, the methods are described in Pharmacopeia (Ph. Eur., USP) [165,166]. • Official pharmacopoeia methods of in vitro drug release testing: Paddle over Disk (Apparatus 5), Cylinder (Apparatus 6), or Reciprocating Holder (Apparatus 7) [165]. • It is not correlated with in vivo, but it is necessary to be determined in the finished product release and shelf-life specification [166].
Permeability on artificial membrane	• In vitro release test (IVRT) is described as a permeability study for transdermal products involving artificial membranes. • The artificial membrane used must have adequate properties to separate the product from the receptor medium and must not interfere with the flow of the active substance or bind that. • In the case of receptor medium, sink conditions should be confirmed. The maximum concentration of the API in the receptor medium achieved during the experiment does not exceed 30% of its maximum solubility in the receptor medium [167].
Cell culture models	• Up to date, no guidelines enlist or describe permeability studies involving cell culture for transdermal products.
Ex vivo models	• Currently, FDA and EMA guidelines enlist permeation studies (IVPT) using excised human or animal skin tissues. • The most accepted is adult human skin, which does not contain tattoos, any diseases, and a hairy surface. • The use of aqueous buffers as a receptor/release medium is recommended, which does not damage the integrity of the tissue, otherwise, it is necessary to check it after the test. • During the test, 12 parallel experiments with samples taken from the same place from different donors are required to prove reproducibility, the test must be performed at 32 °C for 24 h. • Only tape stripping is accepted by the guidelines for testing the accumulation of the active substance in the tissue, RAMAN, and microdialysis methods can only provide additional information [167].

* To use for patches.

5. Ophthalmic

5.1. In Vitro

The unique anatomical structures of the eye represent multiple barriers, which modify drug absorption [168]. This and the different fluid dynamics make this organ an especially hard-to-simulate environment to develop in vitro, ex vivo, or cell culture techniques for bioavailability testing [169]. No true, validated method is available for the replacement of the in vivo Draize rabbit eye test, which is the gold standard for not only bioavailability but also toxicity testing due to its high similarity and ease to use compared to other mammalian models [170].

In the case of some APIs, FDA guidelines allow the use of bioequivalence testing according to 21 CFR part 320 with different in vitro methods for ophthalmic products instead of a human clinical end-point study in case of a special condition [171,172]. This is the qualitative (Q1) and quantitative (Q2) sameness of the test and the reference product, enabling a ±5% concentration difference in the case of inactive ingredients. Physicochemical characterization including measurement of pH, osmolality, viscosity, particle size distribution and charge (for emulsions and suspensions), phase distribution, specific gravity, and surface tension measurement is needed [173,174]. In vitro drug release tests can be carried out with the use of dialysis tubes and Franz diffusion cells [175]. These experiments are usually carried out in either artificial tear fluid or normal PBS solution with membranes and a dialysis bag made out of cellophane or some cellulose derivative with a molecular weight cut off around 10 kD [176–179].

5.2. Cell Culture

2D and 3D cell culture models vary in form and the utilized cell line. In general, they are cheap, easy to maintain, and reproducible ways to carry out drug transport experiments. Meanwhile, the modern but complicated in vitro 3D cell culture methods, such as the reconstructed human tissue assays SkinEthic™ Human Corneal Epithelium and EpiOcular Eye Irritation test, are rarely utilized by current researchers due to their high price, low repeatability, and limited transition towards in vivo results [169,180,181]. Apart from these, 2D cell cultures of immortalized cell lines such as ARPE-19 or TERT-RPE are mainly used to screen cytotoxicity before in vivo tests. Nevertheless, cell cultures can be useful tools to verify cellular uptake of the API before an animal experiment. Simple, 2D cultures ARPE-19 cells were successful in the study of Yang et al. in regards to the prediction of cellular retention of bovine serum albumin-loaded silk fibroin nanoparticles when compared to in vivo rabbit eye model [182]. In the case of atorvastatin-loaded solid nanoparticles, the same correlation can also be seen as the cells showed high levels of retention of the API [183]. Even the similarity of ocular PK values for melanin binding was found between ARPE-19 cells and rat eye model [184]. Human corneal epithelial cells in 2D cultures were also reported as good indicators of the resveratrol uptake [185]. Despite these positive examples in the study of Yousry et al., normal human primary corneal epithelial cell lines failed to predict the superior uptake of a terconazole SNES over simple suspension, which was later verified by animal experiments [186].

5.3. Ex Vivo

An upgraded version of the previously mentioned permeability test is when excised animal corneas are used as the "membrane" of a Franz diffusion cell, using artificial tear fluid as solvent [187–190]. Apart from corneas, even whole eyeballs can be used [191]. Overall, these methods are not officially validated, but the in vitro and ex vivo results are usually used to reduce the number of experimental formulations selected for the in vivo experiments. Thus, these methods usually act as a filter for the multiple original formulations with different excipients, as only those get a pass on to the animal model, which has the best pharmacokinetic/dissolution profiles.

Notably, apart from the traditional Draize test, the implantation of a microdialysis probe into the anterior segment of the eye gives the researchers the ability to test out multiple concentrations of an experimental formulation and gain additional dissolution profiles [190,192,193].

The regulatory acceptance and opinion are summarized in Table 4.

Table 4. Regulatory opinions and acceptance of in vitro dissolution studies, permeability studies, cell culture models, and ex vivo models on the bioavailability of ophthalmic drugs/products.

Study Type	Regulatory Acceptance or Opinion
Dissolution	• In vitro release studies can be performed in case of qualitative and quantitative sameness of the products. • The methodology used for in vitro drug release testing should be able to discriminate the effect of process and variability in the production of the test formulation [171,172]. • No concrete method is described; generally, Franz diffusion cell or dialysis tests are performed.
Permeability on artificial membrane	• To date, no guidelines enlist or describe permeability studies involving artificial membranes for ophthalmic products.
Cell culture models	• To date, no guidelines enlist or describe permeability studies involving cell culture for ophthalmic products.
Ex vivo models	• To date, no guidelines enlist or describe permeability studies involving ex vivo models for ophthalmic products.

6. Conclusions

Summarizing the methods and techniques to assess the drug availability during drug R&D or formulation development phases is essential for screening for optimal molecules and their dosage forms. When the bioavailability of drugs administered via oral, transdermal, intranasal/pulmonary, or ocular pathways is assessed, in vitro screening tests, due to their low cost and high throughput performance, are inevitable. Designing the in vitro tests, either for solubility assessment of the solid dispersion or the deposition of the fine particles, is all based on those physiological factors that are vital and responsible for effective drug therapy. Biopharmaceutical drug design also relies on the interaction among the drug, the carrier or dosage form, and the first biological barrier determining absorption. Cell culture models, either primary or immortalized cell lines, provide the first biorelevant permeability data, even with drawbacks such as different transporter or junctional protein expression. Dermal and ocular barriers are more complex compared to the intestinal, pulmonary, or nasal barriers. Modeling the complexity of such cellular barriers can be integrated into simplified 3D cell culture models. Due to their complexity, they are more biorelevant when drug permeability is investigated. In the case of RHE, a comparison of the drug with the standards could predict in vivo permeability rates. On the other hand, when passive diffusional pathways are considered in such cases, the actual in vivo data might not correlate with the data obtained in such models. The last step before investigating the drug or its formulation in vivo is to obtain data on human or animal tissues. Besides considering the ethical problems related to the origin and source, differences among the species are another issue researchers should not forget. Due to their limited lifetime, excised tissues or organs require experienced human resources and device setups. Expertise in these studies can be obtained in laboratories, where the surgical and analytical background is provided and validated. Considering the source of the excised tissues or organs, ethical questions almost immediately appear in our focus. All the efforts made to replace lab animals, reduce their number during preclinical studies, and refine study protocols and statistics in data analysis cannot completely predict the in vivo performance of the formulation. Regulatory authorities did not integrate artificial membrane studies into their guidelines when drug permeability is evaluated in vitro, except for transdermal dosage forms. Additionally, the Caco-2 cell culture model is only recommended by the FDA; thus, incomplete harmonization is present among the agencies. Still, a gap exists among the phases of drug development and characterization, starting from the in vitro evaluation through the cell culture laboratories and the absorption or distribution evaluation ex vivo.

Author Contributions: Conceptualization: Á.H. and G.V.; writing-original draft preparation: L.J., D.N., Á.P., D.K. and R.R.; writing—review and editing: I.B. and Á.H.; visualization: L.J. and G.V. All authors have read and agreed to the published version of the manuscript.

Funding: Supported by the ÚNKP-22-4-I New National Excellence Program of the Ministry for Innovation and Technology from the source of the National Research, Development, and Innovation Fund. Project no. TKP2021-EGA-19 has been implemented with the support provided by the National Research, Development, and Innovation Fund of Hungary, financed under the TKP2021-EGA funding scheme. The publication was supported by the GINOP-2.3.1-20-2020-00004 project. The project was co-financed by the European Union and the European Regional Development Fund.

Institutional Review Board Statement: Not applicable.

Informed Consent Statement: Not applicable.

Data Availability Statement: Not applicable.

Conflicts of Interest: The authors declare no conflict of interest.

References

1. Avila, A.M.; Bebenek, I.; Bonzo, J.A.; Bourcier, T.; Davis Bruno, K.L.; Carlson, D.B.; Dubinion, J.; Elayan, I.; Harrouk, W.; Lee, S.-L.; et al. An FDA/CDER Perspective on Nonclinical Testing Strategies: Classical Toxicology Approaches and New Approach Methodologies (NAMs). *Regul. Toxicol. Pharmacol.* **2020**, *114*, 104662. [CrossRef] [PubMed]
2. Jaroch, K.; Jaroch, A.; Bojko, B. Cell Cultures in Drug Discovery and Development: The Need of Reliable in vitro-in vivo Extrapolation for Pharmacodynamics and Pharmacokinetics Assessment. *J. Pharm. Biomed. Anal.* **2018**, *147*, 297–312. [CrossRef] [PubMed]
3. Castelo-Branco, D.d.S.C.M.; Amando, B.R.; Ocadaque, C.J.; Aguiar, L.d.; Paiva, D.D.d.Q.; Diógenes, E.M.; Guedes, G.M.d.M.; Costa, C.L.; Santos-Filho, A.S.P.; Andrade, A.R.C.d.; et al. Mini-Review: From in vitro to Ex Vivo Studies: An Overview of Alternative Methods for the Study of Medical Biofilms. *Biofouling* **2020**, *36*, 1129–1148. [CrossRef]
4. Kirk, R.G.W. Recovering the Principles of Humane Experimental Technique. *Sci. Technol. Hum. Values* **2018**, *43*, 622–648. [CrossRef]
5. Xu, Y.; Shrestha, N.; Préat, V.; Beloqui, A. An Overview of in vitro, Ex Vivo and in vivo Models for Studying the Transport of Drugs across Intestinal Barriers. *Adv. Drug Deliv. Rev.* **2021**, *175*, 113795. [CrossRef] [PubMed]
6. Meigs, L. Animal Testing and Its Alternatives—The Most Important Omics Is Economics. *ALTEX* **2018**, *35*, 275–305. [CrossRef] [PubMed]
7. Zsikó, S.; Csányi, E.; Kovács, A.; Budai-Szűcs, M.; Gácsi, A.; Berkó, S. Novel In Vitro Investigational Methods for Modeling Skin Permeation: Skin PAMPA, Raman Mapping. *Pharmaceutics* **2020**, *12*, 803. [CrossRef]
8. Peeters, E.; Nelis, H.J.; Coenye, T. Comparison of Multiple Methods for Quantification of Microbial Biofilms Grown in Microtiter Plates. *J. Microbiol. Methods* **2008**, *72*, 157–165. [CrossRef]
9. Roberts, A.E.L.; Kragh, K.N.; Bjarnsholt, T.; Diggle, S.P. The Limitations of In Vitro Experimentation in Understanding Biofilms and Chronic Infection. *J. Mol. Biol.* **2015**, *427*, 3646–3661. [CrossRef]
10. Pearce, S.C.; Coia, H.G.; Karl, J.P.; Pantoja-Feliciano, I.G.; Zachos, N.C.; Racicot, K. Intestinal in vitro and Ex Vivo Models to Study Host-Microbiome Interactions and Acute Stressors. *Front. Physiol.* **2018**, *9*, 1584. [CrossRef]
11. Štukelj, J.; Svanbäck, S.; Agopov, M.; Löbmann, K.; Strachan, C.J.; Rades, T.; Yliruusi, J. Direct Measurement of Amorphous Solubility. *Anal. Chem.* **2019**, *91*, 7411–7417. [CrossRef] [PubMed]
12. Wilson, V.; Lou, X.; Osterling, D.J.; Stolarik, D.F.; Jenkins, G.; Gao, W.; Zhang, G.G.Z.; Taylor, L.S. Relationship between Amorphous Solid Dispersion in vivo Absorption and in vitro Dissolution: Phase Behavior during Dissolution, Speciation, and Membrane Mass Transport. *J. Control. Release* **2018**, *292*, 172–182. [CrossRef] [PubMed]
13. Elkhabaz, A.; Moseson, D.E.; Brouwers, J.; Augustijns, P.; Taylor, L.S. Interplay of Supersaturation and Solubilization: Lack of Correlation between Concentration-Based Supersaturation Measurements and Membrane Transport Rates in Simulated and Aspirated Human Fluids. *Mol. Pharm.* **2019**, *16*, 5042–5053. [CrossRef] [PubMed]
14. Vertzoni, M.; Dressman, J.; Butler, J.; Hempenstall, J.; Reppas, C. Simulation of Fasting Gastric Conditions and Its Importance for the in vivo Dissolution of Lipophilic Compounds. *Eur. J. Pharm. Biopharm.* **2005**, *60*, 413–417. [CrossRef]
15. Jantratid, E.; Dressman, J. Biorelevant Dissolution Media Simulating the Proximal Human Gastrointestinal Tract: An Update. *Dissolution Technol.* **2009**, *16*, 21–25. [CrossRef]
16. Jantratid, E.; Janssen, N.; Chokshi, H.; Tang, K.; Dressman, J.B. Designing Biorelevant Dissolution Tests for Lipid Formulations: Case Example—Lipid Suspension of RZ-50. *Eur. J. Pharm. Biopharm.* **2008**, *69*, 776–785. [CrossRef]
17. Dressman, J.B.; Amidon, G.L.; Reppas, C.; Shah, V.P. Dissolution Testing as a Prognostic Tool for Oral Drug Absorption: Immediate Release Dosage Forms. *Pharm. Res.* **1998**, *15*, 11–22. [CrossRef]

18. Sorasitthiyanukarn, F.N.; Muangnoi, C.; Rojsitthisak, P.; Rojsitthisak, P. Chitosan Oligosaccharide/Alginate Nanoparticles as an Effective Carrier for Astaxanthin with Improving Stability, in vitro Oral Bioaccessibility, and Bioavailability. *Food Hydrocoll.* 2022, *124*, 107246. [CrossRef]
19. Dahan, A.; Hoffman, A. Use of a Dynamic in vitro Lipolysis Model to Rationalize Oral Formulation Development for Poor Water Soluble Drugs: Correlation with in vivo Data and the Relationship to Intra-Enterocyte Processes in Rats. *Pharm. Res.* 2006, *23*, 2165–2174. [CrossRef]
20. Caon, T.; Kratz, J.M.; Kuminek, G.; Heller, M.; Konig, R.A.; Micke, G.A.; Koester, L.S.; Simões, C.M.O. Oral Saquinavir Mesylate Solid Dispersions: In Vitro Dissolution, Caco-2 Cell Model Permeability and in vivo Absorption Studies. *Powder Technol.* 2015, *269*, 200–206. [CrossRef]
21. Zhao, Q.; Wang, Z.; Wang, X.; Yan, X.; Guo, Q.; Yue, Y.; Yue, T.; Yuan, Y. The Bioaccessibility, Bioavailability, Bioactivity, and Prebiotic Effects of Phenolic Compounds from Raw and Solid-Fermented Mulberry Leaves during in vitro Digestion and Colonic Fermentation. *Food Res. Int.* 2023, *165*, 112493. [CrossRef]
22. Feeney, O.M.; Crum, M.F.; McEvoy, C.L.; Trevaskis, N.L.; Williams, H.D.; Pouton, C.W.; Charman, W.N.; Bergström, C.A.S.; Porter, C.J.H. 50 Years of Oral Lipid-Based Formulations: Provenance, Progress and Future Perspectives. *Adv. Drug Deliv. Rev.* 2016, *101*, 167–194. [CrossRef]
23. Murshed, M.; Pham, A.; Vithani, K.; Salim, M.; Boyd, B.J. Controlling Drug Release by Introducing Lipase Inhibitor within a Lipid Formulation. *Int. J. Pharm.* 2022, *623*, 121958. [CrossRef] [PubMed]
24. Huang, Y.; Yu, Q.; Chen, Z.; Wu, W.; Zhu, Q.; Lu, Y. In vitro and in vivo Correlation for Lipid-Based Formulations: Current Status and Future Perspectives. *Acta Pharm. Sin. B* 2021, *11*, 2469–2487. [CrossRef]
25. Berlin, M.; Przyklenk, K.-H.; Richtberg, A.; Baumann, W.; Dressman, J.B. Prediction of Oral Absorption of Cinnarizine—A Highly Supersaturating Poorly Soluble Weak Base with Borderline Permeability. *Eur. J. Pharm. Biopharm.* 2014, *88*, 795–806. [CrossRef] [PubMed]
26. Pettarin, M.; Bolger, M.B.; Chronowska, M.; Kostewicz, E.S. A Combined in vitro In-Silico Approach to Predict the Oral Bioavailability of Borderline BCS Class II/IV Weak Base Albendazole and Its Main Metabolite Albendazole Sulfoxide. *Eur. J. Pharm. Sci.* 2020, *155*, 105552. [CrossRef] [PubMed]
27. Hate, S.S.; Mosquera-Giraldo, L.I.; Taylor, L.S. A Mechanistic Study of Drug Mass Transport from Supersaturated Solutions Across PAMPA Membranes. *J. Pharm. Sci.* 2022, *111*, 102–115. [CrossRef]
28. Đanić, M.; Pavlović, N.; Stanimirov, B.; Lazarević, S.; Vukmirović, S.; Al-Salami, H.; Mikov, M. PAMPA Model of Gliclazide Permeability: The Impact of Probiotic Bacteria and Bile Acids. *Eur. J. Pharm. Sci.* 2021, *158*, 105668. [CrossRef]
29. Borbás, E.; Nagy, Z.K.; Nagy, B.; Balogh, A.; Farkas, B.; Tsinman, O.; Tsinman, K.; Sinkó, B. The Effect of Formulation Additives on in vitro Dissolution-Absorption Profile and in vivo Bioavailability of Telmisartan from Brand and Generic Formulations. *Eur. J. Pharm. Sci.* 2018, *114*, 310–317. [CrossRef]
30. Li, J.; Tsinman, K.; Tsinman, O.; Wigman, L. Using PH Gradient Dissolution with In-Situ Flux Measurement to Evaluate Bioavailability and DDI for Formulated Poorly Soluble Drug Products. *AAPS PharmSciTech* 2018, *19*, 2898–2907. [CrossRef]
31. Patel, M.H.; Sawant, K.K. Self Microemulsifying Drug Delivery System of Lurasidone Hydrochloride for Enhanced Oral Bioavailability by Lymphatic Targeting: In vitro, Caco-2 Cell Line and in vivo Evaluation. *Eur. J. Pharm. Sci.* 2019, *138*, 105027. [CrossRef] [PubMed]
32. Jarc, T.; Novak, M.; Hevir, N.; Rižner, T.L.; Kreft, M.E.; Kristan, K. Demonstrating Suitability of the Caco-2 Cell Model for BCS-Based Biowaiver According to the Recent FDA and ICH Harmonised Guidelines. *J. Pharm. Pharmacol.* 2019, *71*, 1231–1242. [CrossRef] [PubMed]
33. Faralli, A.; Shekarforoush, E.; Ajalloueian, F.; Mendes, A.C.; Chronakis, I.S. In Vitro Permeability Enhancement of Curcumin across Caco-2 Cells Monolayers Using Electrospun Xanthan-Chitosan Nanofibers. *Carbohydr. Polym.* 2019, *206*, 38–47. [CrossRef] [PubMed]
34. Ferruzza, S.; Rossi, C.; Scarino, M.L.; Sambuy, Y. A Protocol for Differentiation of Human Intestinal Caco-2 Cells in Asymmetric Serum-Containing Medium. *Toxicol. Vitr.* 2012, *26*, 1252–1255. [CrossRef]
35. Fenyvesi, F.; Nguyen, T.L.P.; Haimhoffer, Á.; Rusznyák, Á.; Vasvári, G.; Bácskay, I.; Vecsernyés, M.; Ignat, S.-R.; Dinescu, S.; Costache, M.; et al. Cyclodextrin Complexation Improves the Solubility and Caco-2 Permeability of Chrysin. *Materials* 2020, *13*, 3618. [CrossRef]
36. Haimhoffer, Á.; Dossi, E.; Béresová, M.; Bácskay, I.; Váradi, J.; Afsar, A.; Rusznyák, Á.; Vasvári, G.; Fenyvesi, F. Preformulation Studies and Bioavailability Enhancement of Curcumin with a 'Two in One' PEG-β-Cyclodextrin Polymer. *Pharmaceutics* 2021, *13*, 1710. [CrossRef]
37. Gantzsch, S.P.; Kann, B.; Ofer-Glaessgen, M.; Loos, P.; Berchtold, H.; Balbach, S.; Eichinger, T.; Lehr, C.-M.; Schaefer, U.F.; Windbergs, M. Characterization and Evaluation of a Modified PVPA Barrier in Comparison to Caco-2 Cell Monolayers for Combined Dissolution and Permeation Testing. *J. Control. Release* 2014, *175*, 79–86. [CrossRef]
38. Remenyik, J.; Biró, A.; Klusóczki, Á.; Juhász, K.Z.; Szendi-Szatmári, T.; Kenesei, Á.; Szőllősi, E.; Vasvári, G.; Stündl, L.; Fenyvesi, F.; et al. Comparison of the Modulating Effect of Anthocyanin-Rich Sour Cherry Extract on Occludin and ZO-1 on Caco-2 and HUVEC Cultures. *Int. J. Mol. Sci.* 2022, *23*, 9036. [CrossRef]

39. Nguyen, T.L.P.; Fenyvesi, F.; Remenyik, J.; Homoki, J.R.; Gogolák, P.; Bácskay, I.; Fehér, P.; Ujhelyi, Z.; Vasvári, G.; Vecsernyés, M.; et al. Protective Effect of Pure Sour Cherry Anthocyanin Extract on Cytokine-Induced Inflammatory Caco-2 Monolayers. *Nutrients* **2018**, *10*, 861. [CrossRef]
40. Réti-Nagy, K.; Malanga, M.; Fenyvesi, É.; Szente, L.; Vámosi, G.; Váradi, J.; Bácskay, I.; Fehér, P.; Ujhelyi, Z.; Róka, E.; et al. Endocytosis of Fluorescent Cyclodextrins by Intestinal Caco-2 Cells and Its Role in Paclitaxel Drug Delivery. *Int. J. Pharm.* **2015**, *496*, 509–517. [CrossRef]
41. Rusznyák, Á.; Malanga, M.; Fenyvesi, É.; Szente, L.; Váradi, J.; Bácskay, I.; Vecsernyés, M.; Vasvári, G.; Haimhoffer, Á.; Fehér, P.; et al. Investigation of the Cellular Effects of Beta- Cyclodextrin Derivatives on Caco-2 Intestinal Epithelial Cells. *Pharmaceutics* **2021**, *13*, 157. [CrossRef]
42. Józsa, L.; Ujhelyi, Z.; Vasvári, G.; Sinka, D.; Nemes, D.; Fenyvesi, F.; Váradi, J.; Vecsernyés, M.; Szabó, J.; Kalló, G.; et al. Formulation of Creams Containing Spirulina Platensis Powder with Different Nonionic Surfactants for the Treatment of Acne Vulgaris. *Molecules* **2020**, *25*, 4856. [CrossRef] [PubMed]
43. Pamlényi, K.; Regdon, G.; Nemes, D.; Fenyvesi, F.; Bácskay, I.; Kristó, K. Stability, Permeability and Cytotoxicity of Buccal Films in Allergy Treatment. *Pharmaceutics* **2022**, *14*, 1633. [CrossRef] [PubMed]
44. Clarke, L.L. A Guide to Ussing Chamber Studies of Mouse Intestine. *Am. J. Physiol. Liver Physiol.* **2009**, *296*, G1151–G1166. [CrossRef] [PubMed]
45. Arnold, Y.E.; Kalia, Y.N. Using Ex Vivo Porcine Jejunum to Identify Membrane Transporter Substrates: A Screening Tool for Early—Stage Drug Development. *Biomedicines* **2020**, *8*, 340. [CrossRef]
46. Andlauer, W.; Kolb, J.; Fürst, P. Absorption and Metabolism of Genistin in the Isolated Rat Small Intestine. *FEBS Lett.* **2000**, *475*, 127–130. [CrossRef]
47. Luo, Z.; Liu, Y.; Zhao, B.; Tang, M.; Dong, H.; Zhang, L.; Lv, B.; Wei, L. Ex Vivo and in Situ Approaches Used to Study Intestinal Absorption. *J. Pharmacol. Toxicol. Methods* **2013**, *68*, 208–216. [CrossRef]
48. Jung, S.-M.; Kim, S. In Vitro Models of the Small Intestine for Studying Intestinal Diseases. *Front. Microbiol.* **2022**, *12*, 4102. [CrossRef]
49. Sjöberg, Å.; Lutz, M.; Tannergren, C.; Wingolf, C.; Borde, A.; Ungell, A.-L. Comprehensive Study on Regional Human Intestinal Permeability and Prediction of Fraction Absorbed of Drugs Using the Ussing Chamber Technique. *Eur. J. Pharm. Sci.* **2013**, *48*, 166–180. [CrossRef]
50. Miyake, M.; Koga, T.; Kondo, S.; Yoda, N.; Emoto, C.; Mukai, T.; Toguchi, H. Prediction of Drug Intestinal Absorption in Human Using the Ussing Chamber System: A Comparison of Intestinal Tissues from Animals and Humans. *Eur. J. Pharm. Sci.* **2017**, *96*, 373–380. [CrossRef]
51. Nunes, R.; Silva, C.; Chaves, L. Tissue-Based in vitro and Ex Vivo Models for Intestinal Permeability Studies. In *Concepts and Models for Drug Permeability Studies*; Elsevier: Amsterdam, The Netherlands, 2016; pp. 203–236. ISBN 9780081000946.
52. Streekstra, E.J.; Kiss, M.; van den Heuvel, J.; Nicolaï, J.; van den Broek, P.; Botden, S.M.B.I.; Stommel, M.W.J.; van Rijssel, L.; Ungell, A.; van de Steeg, E.; et al. A Proof of Concept Using the Ussing Chamber Methodology to Study Pediatric Intestinal Drug Transport and Age-dependent Differences in Absorption. *Clin. Transl. Sci.* **2022**, *15*, 2392–2402. [CrossRef] [PubMed]
53. Luo, L.-Y.; Fan, M.-X.; Zhao, H.-Y.; Li, M.-X.; Wu, X.; Gao, W.-Y. Pharmacokinetics and Bioavailability of the Isoflavones Formononetin and Ononin and Their in vitro Absorption in Ussing Chamber and Caco-2 Cell Models. *J. Agric. Food Chem.* **2018**, *66*, 2917–2924. [CrossRef]
54. Kalungwana, N.; Marshall, L.; Mackie, A.; Boesch, C. An Ex Vivo Intestinal Absorption Model Is More Effective than an in vitro Cell Model to Characterise Absorption of Dietary Carotenoids Following Simulated Gastrointestinal Digestion. *Food Res. Int.* **2023**, *166*, 112558. [CrossRef] [PubMed]
55. Li, Y.; Park, H.J.; Xiu, H.; Akoh, C.C.; Kong, F. Predicting Intestinal Effective Permeability of Different Transport Mechanisms: Comparing Ex Vivo Porcine and in vitro Dialysis Models. *J. Food Eng.* **2023**, *338*, 111256. [CrossRef]
56. Faiz, S.; Arshad, S.; Kamal, Y.; Imran, S.; Asim, M.H.; Mahmood, A.; Inam, S.; Irfan, H.M.; Riaz, H. Pioglitazone-Loaded Nanostructured Lipid Carriers: In-Vitro and in-Vivo Evaluation for Improved Bioavailability. *J. Drug Deliv. Sci. Technol.* **2023**, *79*, 104041. [CrossRef]
57. Wang, D.; Liu, R.; Zeng, J.; Li, C.; Xiang, W.; Zhong, G.; Xia, Z. Preliminary Screening of the Potential Active Ingredients in Traditional Chinese Medicines Using the Ussing Chamber Model Combined with HPLC-PDA-MS. *J. Chromatogr. B* **2022**, *1189*, 123090. [CrossRef] [PubMed]
58. Lennernas, H. Animal Data: The Contributions of the Ussing Chamber and Perfusion Systems to Predicting Human Oral Drug Delivery in vivo☆. *Adv. Drug Deliv. Rev.* **2007**, *59*, 1103–1120. [CrossRef]
59. Ruela, A.L.M.; Perissinato, A.G.; Lino, M.E.d.S.; Mudrik, P.S.; Pereira, G.R. Evaluation of Skin Absorption of Drugs from Topical and Transdermal Formulations. *Brazilian J. Pharm. Sci.* **2016**, *52*, 527–544. [CrossRef]
60. Castro, P.; Madureira, R.; Sarmento, B.; Pintado, M. Tissue-Based in vitro and Ex Vivo Models for Buccal Permeability Studies. In *Concepts and Models for Drug Permeability Studies*; Elsevier: Amsterdam, The Netherlands, 2016; pp. 189–202.
61. Wang, S.; Zuo, A.; Guo, J. Types and Evaluation of in vitro Penetration Models for Buccal Mucosal Delivery. *J. Drug Deliv. Sci. Technol.* **2021**, *61*, 102122. [CrossRef]
62. Sa, G.; Xiong, X.; Wu, T.; Yang, J.; He, S.; Zhao, Y. Histological Features of Oral Epithelium in Seven Animal Species: As a Reference for Selecting Animal Models. *Eur. J. Pharm. Sci.* **2016**, *81*, 10–17. [CrossRef]

63. Obradovic, T.; Hidalgo, I.J. In Vitro Models for Investigations of Buccal Drug Permeation and Metabolism. In *Drug Absorption Studies*; Springer: Boston, MA, USA; pp. 167–181.
64. Meng-Lund, E.; Marxen, E.; Pedersen, A.M.L.; Müllertz, A.; Hyrup, B.; Holm, R.; Jacobsen, J. Ex Vivo Correlation of the Permeability of Metoprolol across Human and Porcine Buccal Mucosa. *J. Pharm. Sci.* **2014**, *103*, 2053–2061. [CrossRef] [PubMed]
65. van Eyk, A.D.; van der Bijl, P. Comparative Permeability of Various Chemical Markers through Human Vaginal and Buccal Mucosa as Well as Porcine Buccal and Mouth Floor Mucosa. *Arch. Oral Biol.* **2004**, *49*, 387–392. [CrossRef] [PubMed]
66. Pinto, S.; Pintado, M.E.; Sarmento, B. In Vivo, Ex Vivo and in vitro Assessment of Buccal Permeation of Drugs from Delivery Systems. *Expert Opin. Drug Deliv.* **2020**, *17*, 33–48. [CrossRef] [PubMed]
67. Wilson, T.H.; Wiseman, G. The Use of Sacs of Everted Small Intestine for the Study of the Transference of Substances from the Mucosal to the Serosal Surface. *J. Physiol.* **1954**, *123*, 116–125. [CrossRef] [PubMed]
68. Cotter, P.; López-Expósito, I.; Kleiveland, C.; Lea, T.; Mackie, A.; Requena, T.; Swiatecka, D.; Harry, W. *The Impact of Food Bioactives on Health*; Verhoeckx, K., Cotter, P., López-Expósito, I., Kleiveland, C., Lea, T., Mackie, A., Requena, T., Swiatecka, D., Wichers, H., Eds.; Springer International Publishing: Cham, Switzerland, 2015; ISBN 978-3-319-15791-7.
69. Dixit, P.; Jain, D.K.; Dumbwani, J. Standardization of an Ex Vivo Method for Determination of Intestinal Permeability of Drugs Using Everted Rat Intestine Apparatus. *J. Pharmacol. Toxicol. Methods* **2012**, *65*, 13–17. [CrossRef]
70. Gandia, P.; Lacombe, O.; Woodley, J.; Houin, G. The Perfused Everted Intestinal Segment of Rat. *Arzneimittelforschung* **2011**, *54*, 467–473. [CrossRef]
71. Gagliardi, M.; Clemente, N.; Monzani, R.; Fusaro, L.; Ferrari, E.; Saverio, V.; Grieco, G.; Pańczyszyn, E.; Carton, F.; Santoro, C.; et al. Gut-Ex-Vivo System as a Model to Study Gluten Response in Celiac Disease. *Cell Death Discov.* **2021**, *7*, 45. [CrossRef]
72. Committee for Medicinal Products for Human Use (CHMP). *Guideline on the Investigation of Bioequivalence*; Committee for Medicinal Products for Human Use (CHMP): London, UK, 2010.
73. Committee for Medicinal Products for Human Use (CHMP). *ICH M9 on Biopharmaceutics Classification System Based Biowaivers—Scientific Guideline*; Committee for Medicinal Products for Human Use (CHMP): Amsterdam, The Netherlands, 2020.
74. United States. Department of Health and Human Services; United States. Food and Drug Administration; Center for Drug Evaluation and Research (U.S.). *Waiver of In Vivo Bioavailability and Bioequivalence Studies for Immediate-Release Solid Oral Dosage Forms Based on a Biopharmaceutics Classification System*; Guidance for Industry; Center for Drug Evaluation and Research: Silver Spring, MD, USA, 2017.
75. Committee for Medicinal Products for Human Use (CHMP). *Guideline on Quality of Oral Modified Release Products*; Committee for Medicinal Products for Human Use (CHMP): London, UK, 2014.
76. Committee for Medicinal Products for Human Use (CHMP). *Guideline on the Pharmacokinetic and Clinical Evaluation of Modified Release Dosage Forms*; Committee for Medicinal Products for Human Use (CHMP): London, UK, 2014.
77. Pu, Y.; Goodey, A.P.; Fang, X.; Jacob, K. A Comparison of the Deposition Patterns of Different Nasal Spray Formulations Using a Nasal Cast. *Aerosol Sci. Technol.* **2014**, *48*, 930–938. [CrossRef]
78. Le Guellec, S.; Ehrmann, S.; Vecellio, L. In Vitro—In Vivo Correlation of Intranasal Drug Deposition. *Adv. Drug Deliv. Rev.* **2021**, *170*, 340–352. [CrossRef]
79. Williams, G.; Suman, J.D. In Vitro Anatomical Models for Nasal Drug Delivery. *Pharmaceutics* **2022**, *14*, 1353. [CrossRef]
80. Hilton, C.; Wiedmann, T.; Martin, M.S.; Humphrey, B.; Schleiffarth, R.; Rimell, F. Differential Deposition of Aerosols in the Maxillary Sinus of Human Cadavers by Particle Size. *Am. J. Rhinol.* **2008**, *22*, 395–398. [CrossRef] [PubMed]
81. Okuda, T.; Tang, P.; Yu, J.; Finlay, W.H.; Chan, H.-K. Powder Aerosol Delivery through Nasal High-Flow System: In Vitro Feasibility and Influence of Process Conditions. *Int. J. Pharm.* **2017**, *533*, 187–197. [CrossRef] [PubMed]
82. Spence, C.J.T.; Buchmann, N.A.; Jermy, M.C.; Moore, S.M. Stereoscopic PIV Measurements of Flow in the Nasal Cavity with High Flow Therapy. *Exp. Fluids* **2011**, *50*, 1005–1017. [CrossRef]
83. Le Guellec, S.; Le Pennec, D.; Gatier, S.; Leclerc, L.; Cabrera, M.; Pourchez, J.; Diot, P.; Reychler, G.; Pitance, L.; Durand, M.; et al. Validation of Anatomical Models to Study Aerosol Deposition in Human Nasal Cavities. *Pharm. Res.* **2014**, *31*, 228–237. [CrossRef] [PubMed]
84. Shah, S.A.; Dickens, C.J.; Ward, D.J.; Banaszek, A.A.; George, C.; Horodnik, W. Design of Experiments to Optimize an In Vitro Cast to Predict Human Nasal Drug Deposition. *J. Aerosol Med. Pulm. Drug Deliv.* **2014**, *27*, 21–29. [CrossRef] [PubMed]
85. Hartigan, D.R.; Adelfio, M.; Shutt, M.E.; Jones, S.M.; Patel, S.; Marchand, J.T.; McGuinness, P.D.; Buchholz, B.O.; Ghezzi, C.E. In Vitro Nasal Tissue Model for the Validation of Nasopharyngeal and Midturbinate Swabs for SARS-CoV-2 Testing. *ACS Omega* **2022**, *7*, 12193–12201. [CrossRef] [PubMed]
86. Salade, L.; Wauthoz, N.; Goole, J.; Amighi, K. How to Characterize a Nasal Product. The State of the Art of in vitro and Ex Vivo Specific Methods. *Int. J. Pharm.* **2019**, *561*, 47–65. [CrossRef] [PubMed]
87. McFadden, E.R.; Pichurko, B.M.; Bowman, H.F.; Ingenito, E.; Burns, S.; Dowling, N.; Solway, J. Thermal Mapping of the Airways in Humans. *J. Appl. Physiol.* **1985**, *58*, 564–570. [CrossRef]
88. Radivojev, S.; Zellnitz, S.; Paudel, A.; Fröhlich, E. Searching for Physiologically Relevant in vitro Dissolution Techniques for Orally Inhaled Drugs. *Int. J. Pharm.* **2019**, *556*, 45–56. [CrossRef]
89. Steimer, A.; Haltner, E.; Lehr, C.-M. Cell Culture Models of the Respiratory Tract Relevant to Pulmonary Drug Delivery. *J. Aerosol Med.* **2005**, *18*, 137–182. [CrossRef]

90. Geraghty, R.J.; Stacey, G.N.; Masters, J.R.W.; Lovell-Badge, R.; Vias, M.; Davis, J.M.; Downward, J.; Thraves, P.; Knezevic, I.; Capes-Davis, A.; et al. Guidelines for the Use of Cell Lines in Biomedical Research. *Br. J. Cancer* **2015**, *111*, 1976–1977. [CrossRef]
91. Fulcher, M.L.; Randell, S.H. Human Nasal and Tracheo-Bronchial Respiratory Epithelial Cell Culture. In *Epithelial Cell Culture Protocols: Second Edition*; Springer: Berlin/Heidelberg, Germany, 2012; Volume 945, pp. 109–121. ISBN 9781627031257.
92. Mercier, C.; Perek, N.; Delavenne, X. Is RPMI 2650 a Suitable In Vitro Nasal Model for Drug Transport Studies? *Eur. J. Drug Metab. Pharmacokinet.* **2018**, *43*, 13–24. [CrossRef] [PubMed]
93. Sibinovska, N.; Žakelj, S.; Trontelj, J.; Kristan, K. Applicability of RPMI 2650 and Calu-3 Cell Models for Evaluation of Nasal Formulations. *Pharmaceutics* **2022**, *14*, 369. [CrossRef] [PubMed]
94. Sibinovska, N.; Žakelj, S.; Kristan, K. Suitability of RPMI 2650 Cell Models for Nasal Drug Permeability Prediction. *Eur. J. Pharm. Biopharm.* **2019**, *145*, 85–95. [CrossRef]
95. Callaghan, P.J.; Ferrick, B.; Rybakovsky, E.; Thomas, S.; Mullin, J.M. Epithelial Barrier Function Properties of the 16HBE14o- Human Bronchial Epithelial Cell Culture Model. *Biosci. Rep.* **2020**, *40*, BSR20201532. [CrossRef]
96. Forbes, B.; Shah, A.; Martin, G.P.; Lansley, A.B. The Human Bronchial Epithelial Cell Line 16HBE14o- as a Model System of the Airways for Studying Drug Transport. *Int. J. Pharm.* **2003**, *257*, 161–167. [CrossRef] [PubMed]
97. Lin, H.-L.; Chiu, Y.-W.; Wang, C.-C.; Tung, C.-W. Computational Prediction of Calu-3-Based in vitro Pulmonary Permeability of Chemicals. *Regul. Toxicol. Pharmacol.* **2022**, *135*, 105265. [CrossRef]
98. Ji, X.; Sheng, Y.; Guan, Y.; Li, Y.; Xu, Y.; Tang, L. Evaluation of Calu-3 Cell Lines as an in vitro Model to Study the Inhalation Toxicity of Flavoring Extracts. *Toxicol. Mech. Methods* **2022**, *32*, 171–179. [CrossRef]
99. Selo, M.A.; Sake, J.A.; Kim, K.-J.; Ehrhardt, C. In Vitro and Ex Vivo Models in Inhalation Biopharmaceutical Research—Advances, Challenges and Future Perspectives. *Adv. Drug Deliv. Rev.* **2021**, *177*, 113862. [CrossRef]
100. Andreasson, A.S.I.; Dark, J.H.; Fisher, A.J. Ex Vivo Lung Perfusion in Clinical Lung Transplantation–State of the Art. *Eur. J. Cardio-Thoracic Surg.* **2014**, *46*, 779–788. [CrossRef]
101. Paranjpe, M.; Neuhaus, V.; Finke, J.H.; Richter, C.; Gothsch, T.; Kwade, A.; Büttgenbach, S.; Braun, A.; Müller-Goymann, C.C. In Vitro and Ex Vivo Toxicological Testing of Sildenafil-Loaded Solid Lipid Nanoparticles. *Inhal. Toxicol.* **2013**, *25*, 536–543. [CrossRef] [PubMed]
102. Hansen, N.U.B.; Karsdal, M.A.; Brockbank, S.; Cruwys, S.; Rønnow, S.; Leeming, D.J. Tissue Turnover of Collagen Type I, III and Elastin Is Elevated in the PCLS Model of IPF and Can Be Restored Back to Vehicle Levels Using a Phosphodiesterase Inhibitor. *Respir. Res.* **2016**, *17*, 76. [CrossRef] [PubMed]
103. Liu, G.; Betts, C.; Cunoosamy, D.M.; Åberg, P.M.; Hornberg, J.J.; Sivars, K.B.; Cohen, T.S. Use of Precision Cut Lung Slices as a Translational Model for the Study of Lung Biology. *Respir. Res.* **2019**, *20*, 162. [CrossRef]
104. Cidem, A.; Bradbury, P.; Traini, D.; Ong, H.X. Modifying and Integrating in vitro and Ex Vivo Respiratory Models for Inhalation Drug Screening. *Front. Bioeng. Biotechnol.* **2020**, *8*, 1–15. [CrossRef] [PubMed]
105. U.S. Department of Health and Human Services Food and Drug Administration. *Guidance for Industry Bioavailability and Bioequivalence Studies for Nasal Aerosols and Nasal Sprays for Local Action*; U.S. Department of Health and Human Services Food and Drug Administration: Silver Spring, MD, USA, 2003.
106. Committee for Medicinal Products for Human Use(Chmp). *Guideline on the Pharmaceutical Quality of Inhalation and Nasal Products*; Committee for Medicinal Products for Human Use(Chmp): London, UK, 2004.
107. El-Nabarawi, M.A.; Bendas, E.R.; El Rehem, R.T.A.; Abary, M.Y.S. Transdermal Drug Delivery of Paroxetine through Lipid-Vesicular Formulation to Augment Its Bioavailability. *Int. J. Pharm.* **2013**, *443*, 307–317. [CrossRef]
108. Abdel Azim, A.M.; El-Ashmoony, M.; Swealem, A.M.; Shoukry, R.A. Transdermal Films Containing Tizanidine: In Vitro and in vivo Evaluation. *J. Drug Deliv. Sci. Technol.* **2014**, *24*, 92–99. [CrossRef]
109. Akhtar, B.; Muhammad, F.; Aslam, B.; Saleemi, M.K.; Sharif, A. Biodegradable Nanoparticle Based Transdermal Patches for Gentamicin Delivery: Formulation, Characterization and Pharmacokinetics in Rabbits. *J. Drug Deliv. Sci. Technol.* **2020**, *57*, 101680. [CrossRef]
110. Abouhussein, D.M.N. Enhanced Transdermal Permeation of BCS Class IV Aprepitant Using Binary Ethosome: Optimization, Characterization and Ex Vivo Permeation. *J. Drug Deliv. Sci. Technol.* **2021**, *61*, 102185. [CrossRef]
111. Kumar, A.; Singh, S.; Gautam, H. An Official Publication of Association of Pharmacy Professionals Theoretical aspects of transdermal drug. *Bull. Pharm. Res.* **2013**, *1*, 18–30.
112. Selzer, D.; Abdel-Mottaleb, M.M.A.; Hahn, T.; Schaefer, U.F.; Neumann, D. Finite and Infinite Dosing: Difficulties in Measurements, Evaluations and Predictions. *Adv. Drug Deliv. Rev.* **2013**, *65*, 278–294. [CrossRef]
113. Tsai, M.; Lu, I.; Fu, Y.; Fang, Y.; Huang, Y.; Wu, P. Colloids and Surfaces B: Biointerfaces Nanocarriers Enhance the Transdermal Bioavailability of Resveratrol: In-Vitro and in-Vivo Study. *Colloids Surf. B Biointerfaces* **2016**, *148*, 650–656. [CrossRef] [PubMed]
114. Krishnaiah, Y.S.R.; Yang, Y.; Hunt, R.L.; Khan, M.A. Cold Fl Ow of Estradiol Transdermal Systems: In Fl Uence of Drug Loss on the in vitro Fl Ux and Drug Transfer across Human Epidermis. *Int. J. Pharm.* **2014**, *477*, 73–80. [CrossRef] [PubMed]
115. Chien, Y.W.; Liu, J.C. Transdermal Drug Delivery Systems. *J. Biomater. Appl.* **1986**, *1*, 183–206. [CrossRef] [PubMed]
116. Jung, E.; Young, E.; Choi, H.; Ban, S.; Choi, S.; Sun, J.; Yoon, I.; Kim, D. Development of Drug-in-Adhesive Patch Formulations for Transdermal Delivery of Fl Uoxetine: In Vitro and in vivo Evaluations. *Int. J. Pharm.* **2015**, *487*, 49–55. [CrossRef]
117. Mohamed, L.A.; Kamal, N.; Elfakhri, K.H.; Ibrahim, S.; Ashraf, M.; Zidan, A.S. Application of Synthetic Membranes in Establishing Bio-Predictive IVPT for Testosterone Transdermal Gel. *Int. J. Pharm.* **2020**, *586*, 119572. [CrossRef] [PubMed]

118. Kuznetsova, D.A.; Vasileva, L.A.; Gaynanova, G.A.; Vasilieva, E.A.; Lenina, O.A.; Nizameev, I.R.; Kadirov, M.K.; Petrov, K.A.; Zakharova, L.Y.; Sinyashin, O.G. Cationic Liposomes Mediated Transdermal Delivery of Meloxicam and Ketoprofen: Optimization of the Composition, in vitro and in vivo Assessment of Efficiency. *Int. J. Pharm.* **2021**, *605*, 120803. [CrossRef]
119. Yang, Y.; Manda, P.; Pavurala, N.; Khan, M.A.; Krishnaiah, Y.S.R. Development and Validation of in vitro-in vivo Correlation (IVIVC) for Estradiol Transdermal Drug Delivery Systems. *J. Control. Release* **2015**, *210*, 58–66. [CrossRef]
120. Boscariol, R.; Oliveira Junior, J.M.; Baldo, D.A.; Balcão, V.M.; Vila, M.M.D.C. Transdermal Permeation of Curcumin Promoted by Choline Geranate Ionic Liquid: Potential for the Treatment of Skin Diseases. *Saudi Pharm. J.* **2022**, *30*, 382–397. [CrossRef]
121. Patel, N.; Jain, S.; Lin, S. Transdermal Iontophoretic Delivery of Tacrine Hydrochloride: Correlation between in vitro Permeation and in vivo Performance in Rats. *Int. J. Pharm.* **2016**, *513*, 393–403. [CrossRef]
122. Puri, A.; Frempong, D.; Mishra, D.; Dogra, P. Microneedle-Mediated Transdermal Delivery of Naloxone Hydrochloride for Treatment of Opioid Overdose. *Int. J. Pharm.* **2021**, *604*, 120739. [CrossRef]
123. Ottaviani, G.; Martel, S.; Carrupt, P.-A. Parallel Artificial Membrane Permeability Assay: A New Membrane for the Fast Prediction of Passive Human Skin Permeability. *J. Med. Chem.* **2006**, *49*, 3948–3954. [CrossRef] [PubMed]
124. Sinkó, B.; Garrigues, T.M.; Balogh, G.T.; Nagy, Z.K.; Tsinman, O.; Avdeef, A.; Takács-Novák, K. Skin–PAMPA: A New Method for Fast Prediction of Skin Penetration. *Eur. J. Pharm. Sci.* **2012**, *45*, 698–707. [CrossRef] [PubMed]
125. Sinkó, B.; Kökösi, J.; Avdeef, A.; Takács-Novák, K. A PAMPA Study of the Permeability-Enhancing Effect of New Ceramide Analogues. *Chem. Biodivers.* **2009**, *6*, 1867–1874. [CrossRef] [PubMed]
126. Pulsoni, I.; Lubda, M.; Aiello, M.; Fedi, A.; Marzagalli, M.; von Hagen, J.; Scaglione, S. Comparison Between Franz Diffusion Cell and a Novel Micro-Physiological System for In Vitro Penetration Assay Using Different Skin Models. *SLAS Technol.* **2022**, *27*, 161–171. [CrossRef]
127. Van De Sandt, J.J.M.; Van Burgsteden, J.A.; Cage, S.; Carmichael, P.L.; Dick, I.; Kenyon, S.; Korinth, G.; Larese, F.; Limasset, J.C.; Maas, W.J.M.; et al. In Vitro Predictions of Skin Absorption of Caffeine, Testosterone, and Benzoic Acid: A Multi-Centre Comparison Study. *Regul. Toxicol. Pharmacol.* **2004**, *39*, 271–281. [CrossRef]
128. Mohammadi, M.H.; Heidary Araghi, B.; Beydaghi, V.; Geraili, A.; Moradi, F.; Jafari, P.; Janmaleki, M.; Valente, K.P.; Akbari, M.; Sanati-Nezhad, A. Skin Diseases Modeling Using Combined Tissue Engineering and Microfluidic Technologies. *Adv. Healthc. Mater.* **2016**, *5*, 2459–2480. [CrossRef]
129. Hopf, N.B.; Champmartin, C.; Schenk, L.; Berthet, A.; Chedik, L.; Du Plessis, J.L.; Franken, A.; Frasch, F.; Gaskin, S.; Johanson, G.; et al. Reflections on the OECD Guidelines for in vitro Skin Absorption Studies. *Regul. Toxicol. Pharmacol.* **2020**, *117*, 104752. [CrossRef]
130. Yousuf, Y.; Amini-Nik, S.; Jeschke, M.G. Overall Perspective on the Clinical Importance of Skin Models. In *Skin Tissue Models for Regenerative Medicine*; Elsevier: Amsterdam, The Netherlands, 2018; pp. 39–54.
131. Edmondson, R.; Broglie, J.J.; Adcock, A.F.; Yang, L. Three-Dimensional Cell Culture Systems and Their Applications in Drug Discovery and Cell-Based Biosensors. *Assay Drug Dev. Technol.* **2014**, *12*, 207–218. [CrossRef]
132. van den Broek, L.J.; Bergers, L.I.J.C.; Reijnders, C.M.A.; Gibbs, S. Progress and Future Prospectives in Skin-on-Chip Development with Emphasis on the Use of Different Cell Types and Technical Challenges. *Stem Cell Rev. Reports* **2017**, *13*, 418–429. [CrossRef]
133. Zhang, Q.; Sito, L.; Mao, M.; He, J.; Zhang, Y.S.; Zhao, X. Current Advances in Skin-on-a-Chip Models for Drug Testing. *Microphysiological Syst.* **2018**, *2*, 4. [CrossRef]
134. Antoni, D.; Burckel, H.; Josset, E.; Noel, G. Three-Dimensional Cell Culture: A Breakthrough in vivo. *Int. J. Mol. Sci.* **2015**, *16*, 5517–5527. [CrossRef] [PubMed]
135. Netzlaff, F.; Lehr, C.-M.; Wertz, P.W.; Schaefer, U.F. The Human Epidermis Models EpiSkin®, SkinEthic® and EpiDerm®: An Evaluation of Morphology and Their Suitability for Testing Phototoxicity, Irritancy, Corrosivity, and Substance Transport. *Eur. J. Pharm. Biopharm.* **2005**, *60*, 167–178. [CrossRef] [PubMed]
136. Neupane, R.; Boddu, S.H.S.; Renukuntla, J.; Babu, R.J.; Tiwari, A.K. Alternatives to Biological Skin in Permeation Studies: Current Trends and Possibilities. *Pharmaceutics* **2020**, *12*, 152. [CrossRef] [PubMed]
137. Alépée, N.; Grandidier, M.-H.; Cotovio, J. Usefulness of the EpiSkin™ Reconstructed Human Epidermis Model within Integrated Approaches on Testing and Assessment (IATA) for Skin Corrosion and Irritation. *Toxicol. Vitr.* **2019**, *54*, 147–167. [CrossRef]
138. Kandárová, H.; Hayden, P.; Klausner, M.; Kubilus, J.; Kearney, P.; Sheasgreen, J. In Vitro Skin Irritation Testing: Improving the Sensitivity of the EpiDerm Skin Irritation Test Protocol. *Altern. to Lab. Anim.* **2009**, *37*, 671–689. [CrossRef]
139. Pellevoisin, C.; Videau, C.; Briotet, D.; Grégoire, C.; Tornier, C.; Alonso, A.; Rigaudeau, A.S.; Bouez, C.; Seyler, N. SkinEthic™ RHE for in vitro Evaluation of Skin Irritation of Medical Device Extracts. *Toxicol. Vitr.* **2018**, *50*, 418–425. [CrossRef]
140. Dreher, F.; Fouchard, F.; Patouillet, C.; Andrian, M.; Simonnet, J.-T.; Benech-Kieffer, F. Comparison of Cutaneous Bioavailability of Cosmetic Preparations Containing Caffeine or α-Tocopherol Applied on Human Skin Models or Human Skin Ex Vivo at Finite Doses. *Skin Pharmacol. Physiol.* **2002**, *15*, 40–58. [CrossRef]
141. Schäfer-Korting, M.; Bock, U.; Diembeck, W.; Düsing, H.-J.; Gamer, A.; Haltner-Ukomadu, E.; Hoffmann, C.; Kaca, M.; Kamp, H.; Kersen, S.; et al. The Use of Reconstructed Human Epidermis for Skin Absorption Testing: Results of the Validation Study. *Altern. to Lab. Anim.* **2008**, *36*, 161–187. [CrossRef]
142. Lotte, C.; Patouillet, C.; Zanini, M.; Messager, A.; Roguet, R. Permeation and Skin Absorption: Reproducibility of Various Industrial Reconstructed Human Skin Models. *Skin Pharmacol. Physiol.* **2002**, *15*, 18–30. [CrossRef]

143. Jírová, D.; Basketter, D.; Liebsch, M.; Bendová, H.; Kejlová, K.; Marriott, M.; Kandárová, H. Comparison of Human Skin Irritation Patch Test Data with in vitro Skin Irritation Assays and Animal Data. *Contact Dermat.* **2010**, *62*, 109–116. [CrossRef]
144. Van Gele, M.; Geusens, B.; Brochez, L.; Speeckaert, R.; Lambert, J. Three-Dimensional Skin Models as Tools for Transdermal Drug Delivery: Challenges and Limitations. *Expert Opin. Drug Deliv.* **2011**, *8*, 705–720. [CrossRef] [PubMed]
145. Bernerd, F.; Asselineau, D. An Organotypic Model of Skin to Study Photodamage and Photoprotection in vitro. *J. Am. Acad. Dermatol.* **2008**, *58*, S155–S159. [CrossRef] [PubMed]
146. Reisinger, K.; Blatz, V.; Brinkmann, J.; Downs, T.R.; Fischer, A.; Henkler, F.; Hoffmann, S.; Krul, C.; Liebsch, M.; Luch, A.; et al. Validation of the 3D Skin Comet Assay Using Full Thickness Skin Models: Transferability and Reproducibility. *Mutat. Res. Toxicol. Environ. Mutagen.* **2018**, *827*, 27–41. [CrossRef] [PubMed]
147. Pageon, H.; Zucchi, H.; Asselineau, D. Distinct and Complementary Roles of Papillary and Reticular Fibroblasts in Skin Morphogenesis and Homeostasis. *Eur. J. Dermatology* **2012**, *22*, 324–332. [CrossRef] [PubMed]
148. Markiewicz, E.; Jerome, J.; Mammone, T.; Idowu, O.C. Anti-Glycation and Anti-Aging Properties of Resveratrol Derivatives in the in-Vitro 3D Models of Human Skin. *Clin. Cosmet. Investig. Dermatol.* **2022**, *15*, 911–927. [CrossRef] [PubMed]
149. Zoio, P.; Ventura, S.; Leite, M.; Oliva, A. Pigmented Full-Thickness Human Skin Model Based on a Fibroblast-Derived Matrix for Long-Term Studies. *Tissue Eng. Part C Methods* **2021**, *27*, 433–443. [CrossRef] [PubMed]
150. Hamada, H.; Shimoda, K.; Horio, Y.; Ono, T.; Hosoda, R.; Nakayama, N.; Urano, K. Pterostilbene and Its Glucoside Induce Type XVII Collagen Expression. *Nat. Prod. Commun.* **2017**, *12*, 1934578X1701200. [CrossRef]
151. Ackermann, K.; Lombardi Borgia, S.; Korting, H.C.; Mewes, K.R.; Schäfer-Korting, M. The Phenion® Full-Thickness Skin Model for Percutaneous Absorption Testing. *Skin Pharmacol. Physiol.* **2010**, *23*, 105–112. [CrossRef]
152. Bataillon, M.; Lelièvre, D.; Chapuis, A.; Thillou, F.; Autourde, J.B.; Durand, S.; Boyera, N.; Rigaudeau, A.-S.; Besné, I.; Pellevoisin, C. Characterization of a New Reconstructed Full Thickness Skin Model, T-Skin™, and Its Application for Investigations of Anti-Aging Compounds. *Int. J. Mol. Sci.* **2019**, *20*, 2240. [CrossRef]
153. Li, Z.; Hui, J.; Yang, P.; Mao, H. Microfluidic Organ-on-a-Chip System for Disease Modeling and Drug Development. *Biosensors* **2022**, *12*, 370. [CrossRef]
154. Risueño, I.; Valencia, L.; Jorcano, J.L.; Velasco, D. Skin-on-a-Chip Models: General Overview and Future Perspectives. *APL Bioeng.* **2021**, *5*, 030901. [CrossRef] [PubMed]
155. Abaci, H.E.; Gledhill, K.; Guo, Z.; Christiano, A.M.; Shuler, M.L. Pumpless Microfluidic Platform for Drug Testing on Human Skin Equivalents. *Lab Chip* **2015**, *15*, 882–888. [CrossRef] [PubMed]
156. Song, H.J.; Lim, H.Y.; Chun, W.; Choi, K.C.; Sung, J.H.; Sung, G.Y. Fabrication of a Pumpless, Microfluidic Skin Chip from Different Collagen Sources. *J. Ind. Eng. Chem.* **2017**, *56*, 375–381. [CrossRef]
157. Mo, L.; Lu, G.; Ou, X.; Ouyang, D. Saudi Journal of Biological Sciences Formulation and Development of Novel Control Release Transdermal Patches of Carvedilol to Improve Bioavailability for the Treatment of Heart Failure. *Saudi J. Biol. Sci.* **2022**, *29*, 266–272. [CrossRef] [PubMed]
158. Morsi, N.M.; Aboelwafa, A.A.; Dawoud, M.H.S. Improved Bioavailability of Timolol Maleate via Transdermal Transfersomal Gel: Statistical Optimization, Characterization, and Pharmacokinetic Assessment. *J. Adv. Res.* **2016**, *7*, 691–701. [CrossRef]
159. Kalaria, D.R.; Singhal, M.; Patravale, V.; Merino, V. European Journal of Pharmaceutics and Biopharmaceutics Simultaneous Controlled Iontophoretic Delivery of Pramipexole and Rasagiline in vitro and in vivo: Transdermal Polypharmacy to Treat Parkinson ' s Disease. *Eur. J. Pharm. Biopharm.* **2018**, *127*, 204–212. [CrossRef]
160. Domínguez-robles, J.; Tekko, I.A.; Larra, E.; Ramadon, D.; Donnelly, R.F. Versatility of Hydrogel-Forming Microneedles in in vitro Transdermal Delivery of Tuberculosis Drugs. *Eur. J. Pharm. Biopharm.* **2021**, *158*, 294–312. [CrossRef]
161. Calatayud-pascual, M.A.; Balaguer-fernández, C.; Serna-jiménez, C.E.; Rio-sancho, S. Del Effect of Iontophoresis on in vitro Transdermal Absorption of Almotriptan. *Int. J. Pharm.* **2011**, *416*, 189–194. [CrossRef]
162. Herkenne, C.; Naik, A.; Kalia, Y.N.; Hadgraft, J.; Guy, R.H. Ibuprofen Transport into and through Skin from Topical Formulations: In vitro-in vivo Comparison. *J. Invest. Dermatol.* **2007**, *127*, 135–142. [CrossRef]
163. Godin, B.; Touitou, E. Transdermal Skin Delivery: Predictions for Humans from in vivo, Ex vivo and Animal Models☆. *Adv. Drug Deliv. Rev.* **2007**, *59*, 1152–1161. [CrossRef]
164. Argenziano, M.; Haimhoffer, A.; Bastiancich, C.; Jicsinszky, L.; Caldera, F.; Trotta, F.; Scutera, S.; Alotto, D.; Fumagalli, M.; Musso, T.; et al. In Vitro Enhanced Skin Permeation and Retention of Imiquimod Loaded in β-Cyclodextrin Nanosponge Hydrogel. *Pharmaceutics* **2019**, *11*, 138. [CrossRef]
165. U.S. Department of Health and Human Services Food and DrugAdministration. *Transdermal and Topical Delivery Systems—Product Development and Quality Considerations*; U.S. Department of Health and Human Services Food and Drug Administration: Silver Spring, MD, USA, 2019.
166. Committee for Medicinal Products for Human Use (CHMP). *Guideline on Quality of Transdermal Patches*; Committee for Medicinal Products for Human Use (CHMP): London, UK, 2014.
167. Committee for Medicinal Products for Human Use (CHMP). *Guideline on Quality and Equivalence of Topical Products*; Committee for Medicinal Products for Human Use (CHMP): London, UK, 2018.
168. Alvarez-Trabado, J.; Diebold, Y.; Sanchez, A. Designing Lipid Nanoparticles for Topical Ocular Drug Delivery. *Int. J. Pharm.* **2017**, *532*, 204–217. [CrossRef] [PubMed]

169. Lieto, K.; Skopek, R.; Lewicka, A.; Stelmasiak, M.; Klimaszewska, E.; Zelent, A.; Szymański, Ł.; Lewicki, S. Looking into the Eyes—In Vitro Models for Ocular Research. *Int. J. Mol. Sci.* **2022**, *23*, 9158. [CrossRef] [PubMed]
170. Draize, J.H.; Woodard, G.; Calvery, H.O. Methods for the Study of Irritation and Toxicity of Substances Applied Topically to the Skin and Mucous Membranes. *J. Pharmacol. Exp. Ther.* **1944**, *82*, 377–390.
171. Food and Drug Administration. *Draft Guidance on Nepafenac*; Food and Drug Administration: Silver Spring, MD, USA, 2016.
172. Food and Drug Administration. *Draft Guidance on Cyclosporine*; Food and Drug Administration: Silver Spring, MD, USA, 2022.
173. Le Merdy, M.; Fan, J.; Bolger, M.B.; Lukacova, V.; Spires, J.; Tsakalozou, E.; Patel, V.; Xu, L.; Stewart, S.; Chockalingam, A.; et al. Application of Mechanistic Ocular Absorption Modeling and Simulation to Understand the Impact of Formulation Properties on Ophthalmic Bioavailability in Rabbits: A Case Study Using Dexamethasone Suspension. *AAPS J.* **2019**, *21*, 65. [CrossRef] [PubMed]
174. Choi, S.H.; Lionberger, R.A. Clinical, Pharmacokinetic, and In Vitro Studies to Support Bioequivalence of Ophthalmic Drug Products. *AAPS J.* **2016**, *18*, 1032–1038. [CrossRef]
175. Rahman, Z.; Xu, X.; Katragadda, U.; Krishnaiah, Y.S.R.; Yu, L.; Khan, M.A. Quality by Design Approach for Understanding the Critical Quality Attributes of Cyclosporine Ophthalmic Emulsion. *Mol. Pharm.* **2014**, *11*, 787–799. [CrossRef]
176. Soliman, O.A.E.-A.; Mohamed, E.A.; Khatera, N.A.A. Enhanced Ocular Bioavailability of Fluconazole from Niosomal Gels and Microemulsions: Formulation, Optimization, and in vitro–in vivo Evaluation. *Pharm. Dev. Technol.* **2019**, *24*, 48–62. [CrossRef]
177. Verma, P.; Gupta, R.N.; Jha, A.K.; Pandey, R. Development, in vitro and in vivo Characterization of Eudragit RL 100 Nanoparticles for Improved Ocular Bioavailability of Acetazolamide. *Drug Deliv.* **2013**, *20*, 269–276. [CrossRef]
178. Luo, Q.; Yang, J.; Xu, H.; Shi, J.; Liang, Z.; Zhang, R.; Lu, P.; Pu, G.; Zhao, N.; Zhang, J. Sorafenib-Loaded Nanostructured Lipid Carriers for Topical Ocular Therapy of Corneal Neovascularization: Development, in-Vitro and in vivo Study. *Drug Deliv.* **2022**, *29*, 837–855. [CrossRef]
179. Ashraf, O.; Nasr, M.; Nebsen, M.; Said, A.M.A.; Sammour, O. In Vitro Stabilization and in vivo Improvement of Ocular Pharmacokinetics of the Multi-Therapeutic Agent Baicalin: Delineating the Most Suitable Vesicular Systems. *Int. J. Pharm.* **2018**, *539*, 83–94. [CrossRef] [PubMed]
180. Kaluzhny, Y.; Klausner, M. In Vitro Reconstructed 3D Corneal Tissue Models for Ocular Toxicology and Ophthalmic Drug Development. *Vitr. Cell. Dev. Biol.-Anim.* **2021**, *57*, 207–237. [CrossRef] [PubMed]
181. Agarwal, P.; Rupenthal, I.D. In Vitro and Ex Vivo Corneal Penetration and Absorption Models. *Drug Deliv. Transl. Res.* **2016**, *6*, 634–647. [CrossRef]
182. Yang, P.; Dong, Y.; Huang, D.; Zhu, C.; Liu, H.; Pan, X.; Wu, C. Silk Fibroin Nanoparticles for Enhanced Bio-Macromolecule Delivery to the Retina. *Pharm. Dev. Technol.* **2019**, *24*, 575–583. [CrossRef]
183. Yadav, M.; Schiavone, N.; Guzman-Aranguez, A.; Giansanti, F.; Papucci, L.; Perez de Lara, M.J.; Singh, M.; Kaur, I.P. Atorvastatin-Loaded Solid Lipid Nanoparticles as Eye Drops: Proposed Treatment Option for Age-Related Macular Degeneration (AMD). *Drug Deliv. Transl. Res.* **2020**, *10*, 919–944. [CrossRef]
184. Jakubiak, P.; Cantrill, C.; Urtti, A.; Alvarez-Sánchez, R. Establishment of an In Vitro–In Vivo Correlation for Melanin Binding and the Extension of the Ocular Half-Life of Small-Molecule Drugs. *Mol. Pharm.* **2019**, *16*, 4890–4901. [CrossRef] [PubMed]
185. Li, M.; Zhang, L.; Li, R.; Yan, M. New Resveratrol Micelle Formulation for Ocular Delivery: Characterization and in vitro/in vivo Evaluation. *Drug Dev. Ind. Pharm.* **2020**, *46*, 1960–1970. [CrossRef] [PubMed]
186. Yousry, C.; Zikry, P.M.; Salem, H.M.; Basalious, E.B.; El-Gazayerly, O.N. Integrated Nanovesicular/Self-Nanoemulsifying System (INV/SNES) for Enhanced Dual Ocular Drug Delivery: Statistical Optimization, in vitro and in vivo Evaluation. *Drug Deliv. Transl. Res.* **2020**, *10*, 801–814. [CrossRef]
187. Okur, N.Ü.; Yozgatlı, V.; Okur, M.E. In vitro–in vivo Evaluation of Tetrahydrozoline-loaded Ocular in Situ Gels on Rabbits for Allergic Conjunctivitis Management. *Drug Dev. Res.* **2020**, *81*, 716–727. [CrossRef]
188. Mohamed, H.B.; Attia Shafie, M.A.; Mekkawy, A.I. Chitosan Nanoparticles for Meloxicam Ocular Delivery: Development, In Vitro Characterization, and In Vivo Evaluation in a Rabbit Eye Model. *Pharmaceutics* **2022**, *14*, 893. [CrossRef]
189. Liang, Z.; Zhang, Z.; Yang, J.; Lu, P.; Zhou, T.; Li, J.; Zhang, J. Assessment to the Antifungal Effects in vitro and the Ocular Pharmacokinetics of Solid-Lipid Nanoparticle in Rabbits. *Int. J. Nanomed.* **2021**, *16*, 7847–7857. [CrossRef]
190. Li, X.; Nie, S.; Kong, J.; Li, N.; Ju, C.; Pan, W. A Controlled-Release Ocular Delivery System for Ibuprofen Based on Nanostructured Lipid Carriers. *Int. J. Pharm.* **2008**, *363*, 177–182. [CrossRef] [PubMed]
191. Rathod, L.V.; Kapadia, R.; Sawant, K.K. A Novel Nanoparticles Impregnated Ocular Insert for Enhanced Bioavailability to Posterior Segment of Eye: In vitro, in vivo and Stability Studies. *Mater. Sci. Eng. C* **2017**, *71*, 529–540. [CrossRef] [PubMed]
192. Gai, X.; Cheng, L.; Li, T.; Liu, D.; Wang, Y.; Wang, T.; Pan, W.; Yang, X. In Vitro and In Vivo Studies on a Novel Bioadhesive Colloidal System: Cationic Liposomes of Ibuprofen. *AAPS PharmSciTech* **2018**, *19*, 700–709. [CrossRef] [PubMed]
193. Lai, S.; Wei, Y.; Wu, Q.; Zhou, K.; Liu, T.; Zhang, Y.; Jiang, N.; Xiao, W.; Chen, J.; Liu, Q.; et al. Liposomes for Effective Drug Delivery to the Ocular Posterior Chamber. *J. Nanobiotechnol.* **2019**, *17*, 64. [CrossRef] [PubMed]

Disclaimer/Publisher's Note: The statements, opinions and data contained in all publications are solely those of the individual author(s) and contributor(s) and not of MDPI and/or the editor(s). MDPI and/or the editor(s) disclaim responsibility for any injury to people or property resulting from any ideas, methods, instructions or products referred to in the content.

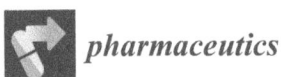

Article

Development of Robust Tablet Formulations with Enhanced Drug Dissolution Profiles from Centrifugally-Spun Micro-Fibrous Solid Dispersions of Itraconazole, a BCS Class II Drug

Stefania Marano [1,†], Manish Ghimire [2], Shahrzad Missaghi [2], Ali Rajabi-Siahboomi [2], Duncan Q. M. Craig [1] and Susan A. Barker [1,*,‡]

[1] School of Pharmacy, University College London (UCL), 29-39 Brunswick Square, London WC1N 1AX, UK
[2] Colorcon Inc., Global Headquarters, 275 Ruth Road, Harleysville, PA 19438, USA
[*] Correspondence: s.barker@greenwich.ac.uk
[†] Present address: Dipartimento di Scienze e Ingegneria della Materia dell'Ambiente ed Urbanistica, Università Politecnica delle Marche, Via Brecce Bianche, 60131 Ancona, Italy.
[‡] Present address: Medway School of Pharmacy, Universities of Greenwich and Kent, Anson Building, Chatham Maritime, Kent ME4 4TB, UK.

Citation: Marano, S.; Ghimire, M.; Missaghi, S.; Rajabi-Siahboomi, A.; Craig, D.Q.M.; Barker, S.A. Development of Robust Tablet Formulations with Enhanced Drug Dissolution Profiles from Centrifugally-Spun Micro-Fibrous Solid Dispersions of Itraconazole, a BCS Class II Drug. *Pharmaceutics* 2023, 15, 802. https://doi.org/10.3390/pharmaceutics15030802

Academic Editors: Gábor Vasvári and Ádám Haimhoffer

Received: 7 February 2023
Revised: 16 February 2023
Accepted: 22 February 2023
Published: 1 March 2023

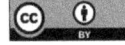

Copyright: © 2023 by the authors. Licensee MDPI, Basel, Switzerland. This article is an open access article distributed under the terms and conditions of the Creative Commons Attribution (CC BY) license (https://creativecommons.org/licenses/by/4.0/).

Abstract: Fibre-based oral drug delivery systems are an attractive approach to addressing low drug solubility, although clear strategies for incorporating such systems into viable dosage forms have not yet been demonstrated. The present study extends our previous work on drug-loaded sucrose microfibres produced by centrifugal melt spinning to examine systems with high drug loading and investigates their incorporation into realistic tablet formulations. Itraconazole, a model BCS Class II hydrophobic drug, was incorporated into sucrose microfibres at 10, 20, 30, and 50% w/w. Microfibres were exposed to high relative humidity conditions (25 °C/75% RH) for 30 days to deliberately induce sucrose recrystallisation and collapse of the fibrous structure into powdery particles. The collapsed particles were successfully processed into pharmaceutically acceptable tablets using a dry mixing and direct compression approach. The dissolution advantage of the fresh microfibres was maintained and even enhanced after humidity treatment for drug loadings up to 30% w/w and, importantly, retained after compression into tablets. Variations in excipient content and compression force allowed manipulation of the disintegration rate and drug content of the tablets. This then permitted control of the rate of supersaturation generation, allowing the optimisation of the formulation in terms of its dissolution profile. In conclusion, the microfibre-tablet approach has been shown to be a viable method for formulating poorly soluble BCS Class II drugs with improved dissolution performance.

Keywords: centrifugal spinning; microfibre; amorphous solid dispersion; sucrose; poorly water-soluble drug; itraconazole; dissolution enhancement; supersaturation; tabletting; oral formulation

1. Introduction

Appropriate formulation of Biopharmaceutics Classification System (BCS) Class II drugs, characterised by low solubility and high permeability, is essential to maximising their oral bioavailability and thereby minimising waste. Many formulation approaches have been investigated in an attempt to increase the rate and extent of dissolution of BCS Class II drugs, with solid dispersion technology being especially well studied. Over the last decade, advanced fabrication technologies such as electrospinning and centrifugal spinning (melt and solution) have been used to prepare solid dispersions in the form of polymer- or sugar-based nano- and micro-fibres [1–6]. Typically, the formulation design is for the drug to be molecularly dispersed within the fibres, leading to enhanced in vitro dissolution and in vivo bioavailability. Several excellent reviews on this area of pharmaceutical formulation science have recently been published, providing an in-depth analysis of the current understanding of the subject [7–11].

Despite the potential dissolution and oral bioavailability advantages of fibre-based formulations, they require further processing into a patient-friendly format before use. However, due to the particular morphological features of nano- or micro-fibres (high surface area to volume ratio, high porosity, and low density), the incorporation of these systems into a conventional oral dosage form capable of being manufactured reproducibly on a large scale may be challenging. In particular, content (dose) uniformity in the final product is critical and will be dependent on adequate mixing of the fibres and the additional formulation excipients, potentially requiring a milling stage with concomitant risks of both chemical and physical instability of the drug. Tabletting (compression) of "fluffy" material such as fibre mats to obtain a robust product may be mechanically difficult, carries a risk of inducing recrystallisation of an amorphous material, and may result in a decrease in the dissolution rate compared with the native uncompressed fibres due to effective surface area changes. Finally, if the dissolution and oral bioavailability advantages of the original fibres are dependent on the drug being present in the amorphous state, the risks of recrystallisation on storage, leading to deleterious changes in the dissolution profile over time, need to be evaluated and mitigated by judicious choice of packaging and storage conditions.

There have been relatively few studies on the downstream processing of electrospun fibres. Electrospun drug-loaded fibre mats have been manually folded and placed in gelatine capsule shells [12], although this was more of a processing aid for dissolution studies than an attempt to develop a viable pharmaceutical product. Some studies [13–16] have shown that electrospun drug-loaded fibre mats can be manually compressed after direct loading of the fibre mat into the tablet die. Other authors have ground the fibre mats to effect size reduction and mixed them with large quantities of conventional tabletting excipients prior to compression, reflecting a more conventional oral tablet formulation [17–22]. Two recent studies have focussed on the mixing step in the conversion of electrospun drug-loaded fibre mats into tablets. Fülöp et al. [23] showed that it is possible to prepare low-dose tablets with acceptable content uniformity from electrospun drug-loaded fibre mats after high-shear dry mixing with conventional tabletting excipients on a reasonable development lab scale (500 g) and compression on a rotary tablet press. Szabó et al. [24] successfully applied continuous manufacturing processing techniques (mixing, compression) with inline analysis to prepare tablets from electrospun drug-loaded microfibre mats; in this case, the milled fibres were treated as a starting material. A detailed study on the mechanical and compression behaviour of electrospun drug-loaded nanofibre mats has recently been published [25]. The presence of the drug, at 10% w/w loading, was shown to affect the mechanical properties of the nanofibre mat, in that the drug-loaded samples exhibited greater stiffness and lower ductility than the placebos. Interestingly, only the drug-loaded nanofibrous tablets showed clear fracture behaviour during diametral compression testing after preparation, with the placebo nanofibrous tablets and the tablets prepared from equivalent physical mixtures all showing continuous yielding and tablet shape change instead. The study by Démuth et al. [26] illustrated the need for judicious choice of excipients in developing tablet formulations from amorphous solid dispersions. They studied electrospun nanofibres containing itraconazole, a poorly water-soluble drug. A total drug release of only 80% of the theoretical amount was observed from tablets containing the water-insoluble lubricant magnesium stearate, which was attributed to the amorphous itraconazole in the nanofibres crystallising on the magnesium stearate during the dissolution test. When a more water-soluble lubricant (sodium stearyl fumarate) was used instead, dissolution was both faster and more extensive, with drug release values of >95% of the theoretical value being achieved.

Much less attention has been paid to the technique of centrifugal spinning (sometimes described as rotary spinning), either in the solution mode or the melt mode, as a means of preparing micro- and nanofibres that can be further processed for pharmaceutical use. Two studies [27,28] used centrifugal solution spinning of aqueous solutions of drug and polymer to generate drug-loaded nanofibre mats, which were then micronised, mixed with standard tabletting excipients, and compressed into tablets. Centrifugal melt spinning was used in two studies [29,30] to prepare nanofibre mats of drug and sucrose/polyvinylpyrrolidone (PVP), which were then directly compressed into tablets with no further processing. In both cases, dissolution from the tablets was slightly slower than from the nanofibre mats, and in one case [29], the tablets were observed to be sticky, indicating that, although the nanofibre mats could be compacted, further work is required to convert the nanofibres into a useable formulation.

In our previous work [3,4], we have used centrifugal melt spinning to successfully manufacture sucrose-based microfibres containing three clinically significant BCS Class II drugs (itraconazole, olanzapine, and piroxicam) at 10% w/w drug loading. Upon manufacture, both the drug and the carrier (sucrose) were observed to exist in an amorphous state in the microfibres, although small amounts of crystalline drug were detected in the piroxicam-loaded microfibres. Under both sink and non-sink conditions, all the fresh drug-loaded microfibres showed significantly superior dissolution behaviour to the raw drugs and to simple physical mixtures of equivalent formulation, with supersaturation being observed in the non-sink testing protocol. The amorphous nature of both the drug and the microfibre matrix, the solubilizing capability of sucrose, and the high surface area to volume ratio of the microfibres all contributed to these effects. Surprisingly, all three drug-loaded microfibres retained their dissolution and supersaturation advantages after exposure to 75% relative humidity (RH) at 25 °C for short periods (around 1 day), which resulted in the crystallisation of the sucrose carrier leading to the collapse of the microfibres to powder. No change in the dissolution profile was observed after 8 months of further exposure to 25 °C/75% RH. Interestingly, while olanzapine and piroxicam recrystallised along with the sucrose, itraconazole appeared to be present in an amorphous state in the humidity-treated samples. These results show that there is considerable potential for the use of centrifugally melt-spun microfibres in enhancing the dissolution profiles of poorly water-soluble drugs. Additionally, these studies indicate that the relationship between the physical form of the system and the drug dissolution behaviour may be more complex than anticipated, with recrystallisation on exposure to high humidity conditions not necessarily leading to the decrease in dissolution rate that may be commonly expected.

This then raises the question of whether it is possible to deliberately recrystallise freshly prepared drug-loaded microfibres by exposure to an environment with controlled high humidity, causing the collapse of the microfibres into powder, and use this powder as the drug source for further processing into conventional tablets for ease of administration to patients. Such an approach should have the dual advantages of retaining the dissolution benefit of the microfibres while using a source material (powder) that is more easily processed into tablets than the freshly prepared microfibres themselves. It is this question that is explored in the current study. Here we have investigated the feasibility of preparing tablet formulations using standard pharmaceutical excipients and processing methods that contain drug-loaded microfibres produced by centrifugal melt spinning and exposed to high humidity conditions. Our aim is to develop a tablet product with a fast dissolution profile that is both scalable and economically viable. Itraconazole was chosen as the model drug for this study, as there is a particular need for an improved oral formulation of itraconazole, given its relatively low oral bioavailability (55%), and the variability in plasma levels reported following oral administration under different feeding regimes [31,32]. However, as a low level of drug loading in the microfibres (10% w/w in our previous studies) will inevitably lead to a low drug content in the final tablets, the effects of increasing the itraconazole content of the microfibres have also been investigated. The flow properties of the drug-loaded microfibres, alone and in formulation mixtures, were studied, along with their mixing and segregation potentials. Selected formulations were compressed, and their pharmaceutical performance was assessed in terms of compliance with standard mandatory pharmacopoeial tests and their disintegration and dissolution profiles.

2. Materials and Methods

2.1. Materials

Itraconazole (ITZ) (molecular weight 705.64 g/mol, melting point 166 °C, glass transition temperature 60 °C) was purchased from Watson Noke Scientific Ltd. (Suzhou, China), and sucrose was obtained from Sigma-Aldrich Co. (St Louis, MO, USA). All buffer salts used for the dissolution media, as well as acetic acid ($\geq$99.85%), acetonitrile ($\geq$99.93%), and sodium n-dodecyl sulphate ($\geq$99%), were purchased from Sigma-Aldrich (Taufkirchen, Germany). Avicel PH102® was purchased from FMC (Cork, Ireland). StarTab® was obtained from Colorcon (Harleysville, PA, USA). Compressol SM® (SPI-Pharma, Wilmington, DE, USA), Kollidon CL-F® (BASF, Ludwigshafen, Germany), and Compritol 888 ATO® (Gattefossé UK Ltd., Ascot, UK) were obtained as gift samples. All other chemical reagents were of analytical grade.

2.2. Methods

2.2.1. Preparation of Fresh Microfibres by Centrifugal Melt Spinning

Sucrose-based itraconazole-loaded microfibres with varying itraconazole content (20, 30, and 50% w/w) and pure drug microfibres (100% w/w) were prepared using the previously described centrifugal melt spinning process [3,4]. For samples containing up to 50% w/w drug loading, microfibres were prepared by spinning the appropriate physical mixture of sucrose and itraconazole at a fixed rotational speed of 2400 rpm and operating temperature of 197 °C. Pure crystalline itraconazole was directly spun in the absence of sucrose at a fixed rotational speed of 2400 rpm and a range of operating temperatures to produce 100% w/w pure itraconazole microfibres.

For comparison purposes, equivalent quench-cooled solid dispersion samples were prepared in situ in a DSC pan by heating sucrose-itraconazole physical mixes and pure itraconazole at a rate of 10 °C/minute to a final temperature 3 °C above the melting temperature of the mix (previously determined), holding isothermally for 1 minute, then cooling at a rate of 20 °C/minute to −20 °C. These samples were analysed immediately using the same modulated temperature differential scanning calorimetry (MTDSC) protocol as the microfibre samples [3,4].

2.2.2. High-Humidity Treatment of Fresh Microfibres

All freshly prepared samples were stored at 25 °C/75% RH in open glass vials, as previously described (4), to induce recrystallisation and microfibre collapse. The samples were stored in a sealed desiccator containing a saturated salt solution of sodium chloride to generate the 75% RH condition. The desiccator was stored in a 25 °C chamber to maintain the temperature.

2.2.3. Physical and Chemical Characterisation of Fresh and Aged Microfibres

The methods used here to characterise the drug-loaded sucrose microfibres have been described in detail in our previous work [3,4], so only brief details are given here.

Drug content of the microfibres was assessed immediately after preparation and after 30 days exposure to 25 °C/75% RH. Itraconazole was extracted using 50:50 acetonitrile:pH 6.8 phosphate buffer, then measured using reversed-phase HPLC (Synergi 4 µm Polar-RP 80 Å, 50 × 3 mm column (Phenomenex, Macclesfield, UK)) with a mobile phase of 50:50 acetontrile: water-acetic acid (0.1% v/v) and UV detection at 264 nm.

The physical state of itraconazole and sucrose within the microfibre samples was measured immediately after preparation and then monitored on a daily basis by MTDSC and X-ray Powder Diffraction (XRPD). For the MTDSC studies, a fully calibrated Q2000 (TA Instruments Q2000, New Castle, DE, USA) with a refrigerated cooling system and a dry nitrogen sample purge was used. All samples were tested in PerkinElmer 40 µL aluminium pans with pinholed lids, with an underlying heating rate of 2 °C/minute and a ±0.212 °C modulation amplitude over a 60 second period. For the XRPD studies, a MiniFlex diffractometer (RigaKu, Tokyo, Japan) was used. XRPD patterns were recorded using diffraction angles (2θ) from 5° to 50° (step size 0.05°; time per step 0.2 s).

Scanning Electron Microscopy (SEM) was used to assess the morphology of microfibre samples on preparation and after humidity treatment. Samples were gold-coated (20 nm) under vacuum using a Quorum Q150T Turbo-Pumped Sputter Coater (Quorum Technologies, Laughton, UK) and then imaged with a Quanta 200F instrument (FEI, Hillsborough, OR, USA).

Non-sink dissolution testing was performed on the fresh and aged microfibre samples, each sample containing the equivalent of 10 mg of drug. The dissolution medium was 50 mL of phosphate buffer (pH: 6.8) containing 0.1% w/v of sodium dodecyl sulfate (SDS), maintained at 37 ± 0.2 °C in a shaking incubator. One (1) mL samples were withdrawn at pre-determined time intervals and filtered through a 0.22 µm Millipore Millex® GT filter. The drawn volume was replaced with the same amount of blank dissolution medium at 37 ± 0.2 °C. Drug concentration was measured using the HPLC-UV system after appropriate dilution.

2.2.4. Preparation of Powder Blends

Powder blends of aged microfibres and relevant excipients were prepared by initial mixing by geometric dilution with a mortar and pestle. Powder blends were then transferred into plastic containers and further mixed for 10 min using a Turbula T2G blender (Willy A. Bachofen AG, Muttenz, Switzerland). The powder blends were analysed for their flow properties and segregation potential, as described below.

2.2.5. Powder Flow Analysis

Powder flow was assessed via analysis of bulk and tapped densities, according to the method described in the United States Pharmacopeia (USP) Chapter <616>, "Bulk Density and Tapped Density of Powders." A Sotax TD2 tap density tester (Hopkinton, MA, USA) was used with a 100 mL glass measuring cylinder and 25 g of sample. Initial (V_0) and final (V_F) volumes were measured after 1 tap and 1250 taps, respectively. The Carr index was calculated as in Equation (1) below.

$$Carr\ index\ (\%) = 100 \times (V_0 - V_F)/V_0 \qquad (1)$$

2.2.6. Powder Segregation Analysis

A novel approach to segregation testing, based on the bulk and tapped density analytical method, was used here to assess the segregation tendency of microfibres in excipient mixtures. The Sotax TD2 tap density tester (Hopkinton, MA, USA) was used, but the conventional single measuring cylinder was replaced with a 100 mL outer plastic cylinder with a removable base and a set of seven stacking inner plastic cylinders to enable sampling at specific heights in the powder bed. Powder mixes (25 g) were tapped 100 times, and then samples weighing 300 mg (corresponding to the target tablet weight used in later studies) were taken at the evenly-spaced sampling points.

Drug content in the segregation test samples was measured by dissolving samples containing a theoretical load of 3 mg itraconazole in 100 mL of methanol, followed by appropriate dilution for UV detection at 260 nm. Solutions were sonicated for at least 30 min to ensure complete drug dissolution prior to the analysis. No interference from the excipients or methanol was observed at the detection wavelength.

2.2.7. Preparation of Tablets

The formulation of the initial eleven batches of tablets is shown in Table 1. For each batch, 25 g of powder mix was prepared. The powder blends were first prepared as described above in the absence of lubricant, then the lubricant was added and the mixture blended for another minute. Tablets with a target weight of 300 mg were prepared by compression using an instrumented eccentric tablet press (Atlas Auto T8, Specac, Kent, UK) equipped with 10 mm round, flat-faced punches. Tablets were produced at compression forces of 10, 16, 20, and 26 kN. Further batches of tablets based on the analysis of these batches were produced in an analogous fashion.

Table 1. Tablet compositions for the 11 different batches (F1-F11) based on the 10% itraconazole-loaded microfibres (Fibres$_{10\%ITZ}$). Values are rounded to one decimal place, so they may not sum to exactly 100%.

Ingredient	Composition (% w/w)										
	Group 1			Group 2			Group 3			Group 4	
	F1	F2	F3	F4	F5	F6	F7	F8	F9	F10	F11
StarTab®	27.8	41.7	50.1	21.1	31.7	38.1	14.5	21.7	26.1	-	-
Avicel PH102®	27.8	20.9	16.7	21.1	15.9	12.7	14.5	10.8	8.7	-	-
Compressol SM®	27.8	20.9	16.7	21.1	15.9	12.7	14.5	10.8	8.7	-	-
Kollidon CL-F®	5.0	5.0	5.0	5.0	5.0	5.0	5.0	5.0	5.0	5.0	5.0
Glyceryl dibehenate	1.5	1.5	1.5	1.5	1.5	1.5	1.5	1.5	1.5	1.5	1.5
Fibres$_{10\%ITZ}$	10.0	10.0	10.0	30.0	30.0	30.0	50.0	50.0	50.0	93.5	-
Raw itraconazole	-	-	-	-	-	-	-	-	-	-	9.3
Raw sucrose	-	-	-	-	-	-	-	-	-	-	84.2

2.2.8. Physical and Analytical Characterisation of Tablets

Tablet dimensions were measured using a digital caliper (Manchester, UK). Tablet crushing strength was measured using an 8M hardness tester (Thun, Switzerland) on 10 randomly selected tablets according to USP chapter <1217> "Tablet Breaking Force." Subsequently, the tablet tensile strength T (MPa) was calculated as in Equation (2) below, where F (N) is the tablet crushing strength, d (mm) is the tablet diameter, and h (mm) is the tablet thickness (Fell and Newton, 1970).

$$T = 2F/\pi dh \tag{2}$$

Tablet friability was measured according to USP chapter <1216> "Tablet Friability Test." A unit of ten pre-weighed tablets was rotated at 25 rpm for 4 min using a TAR 20 Friability tester (Erweka, Germany). Tablets were then dusted off and reweighed, and the percentage weight loss was calculated.

The disintegration times of six random tablets from each batch were measured at 37 ± 2 °C in 900 mL of distilled water on a ZT54 dissolution tester (Erweka, Milford, CT, USA) according to USP Chapter <701> "Disintegration."

Selected batches of tablets were assessed for drug content uniformity as per the requirements of USP Chapter <905> "Uniformity of Dosage Units." Ten tablets of each batch were crushed individually, and itraconazole extracted and analysed as described above for the segregation test samples.

Non-sink dissolution testing was performed on selected tablets in the same manner as for the microfibres. However, in this case, the tablets were tested intact, and the itraconazole content varied from 3 mg to 45 mg.

Solid-State ^{13}C NMR Spectroscopy was used to assess the physical state of the itraconazole in the tablets, using the procedures described in our previous work [4]. High-resolution spectra were recorded using cross-polarisation (CP), MAS, high-power proton decoupling, and total suppression of sidebands (TOSS). The tablets were crushed prior to testing in order to facilitate the experiment.

2.2.9. Statistical Analysis

All results are expressed as mean ± SD. For the dissolution studies, the maximum drug concentration in solution (C_{max}) and the time of its occurrence (T_{max}) were obtained from the drug concentration–time profiles. The supersaturation profiles between formulations were compared by measuring the area under the curve (AUC). Data from different formulations were compared for statistical significance by one-way analysis of variance (ANOVA). Differences were considered statistically significant at $p < 0.05$.

3. Results and Discussion

3.1. Preparation of Microfibres with Increasing Drug Loading and Characterisation of the Fresh Microfibres

Microfibres were successfully prepared by centrifugal melt spinning of physical mixtures of sucrose and itraconazole as described above. The calculated percentage yields (% of theoretical, mean ± SD, n = 6) were 94.6 ± 1.5, 93.4 ± 1.7, and 94.1 ± 1.4, respectively, for the 20, 30, and 50% w/w drug-loaded microfibres, similar to the value of 95.4 ± 2.1 observed for the 10% w/w sample [4]. Drug content uniformity values (% of theoretical, mean ± SD, n = 6) of 98.6 ± 1.5 and 99.4 ± 1.3 for the 20 and 30% w/w samples, respectively, were again similar to that seen for the 10% w/w sample, 99.5 ± 1.1 [4], indicating full incorporation and homogeneous distribution of the drug in the microfibre product. However, at 50% w/w itraconazole loading, a higher mean value and greater variation were observed, i.e., 117.1 ± 9.8, suggesting that the drug may not be homogeneously distributed within the sucrose matrix at high drug incorporation, possibly due to the limited loading capacity of the sucrose carrier. This is discussed in more detail below. Surprisingly, itraconazole was able to form microfibres alone, with no sucrose carrier. The optimum temperature for spinning pure itraconazole was found to be 183 °C, with a yield of 65.7 ± 4.3% of theoretical. At lower temperatures, no microfibres were formed even though the drug was molten, whereas at higher temperatures, the yields were lower as some of the drug stuck to the spinneret. The lower spinning temperature for pure itraconazole compared with the mixed itraconazole-sucrose systems is a consequence of itraconazole's lower melting point of 166 °C [33] compared with that of sucrose (186 °C) [34]. We believe this is the first report of pure itraconazole microfibres being formed using any production technique.

As shown in Figure 1, under SEM, all freshly prepared itraconazole-loaded sucrose microfibres showed smooth surface morphology with no defects or evidence of surface or bulk drug crystallisation.

The mean microfibre diameter was independent of itraconazole content, with values of circa 7 μm being observed for all samples, as detailed in Table 2. However, visual inspection of the 50% w/w itraconazole-loaded samples and closer analysis of their SEM images showed the presence of thin (1 to 5 μm diameter), grey-coloured microfibres with a visibly different texture from the bulk of the microfibres. These thinner microfibres were similar in appearance and diameter to the pure itraconazole microfibres (3.22 ± 2.54 μm, mean ± SD), suggesting that some of the thinner microfibres in the 50% w/w itraconazole-loaded sample were in fact pure itraconazole microfibres.

XRPD diffractograms of all fresh drug-loaded sucrose microfibres (20, 30, and 50% w/w) and the pure drug microfibres showed the typical broad halo pattern of an amorphous material, as shown in Figure 2, as had previously been observed for the freshly prepared drug-free and 10% w/w drug-loaded sucrose systems.

Figure 3 shows the MTDSC reversing heat flow traces of the spun microfibres and the equivalent quench-cooled samples.

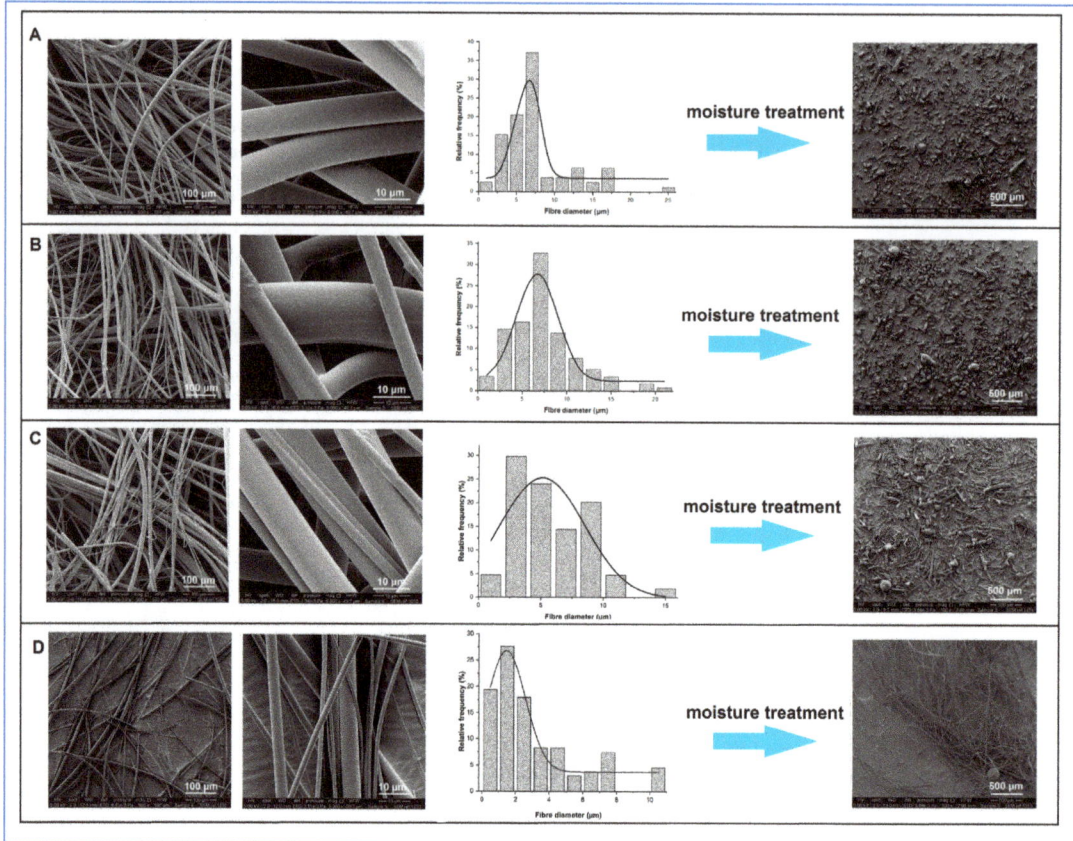

Figure 1. From left to right: SEM micrographs of freshly prepared itraconazole-loaded sucrose microfibres (500× and 6000× magnification), microfibre diameter frequency diagrams, SEM images of the corresponding samples (100× magnification) after 30 days exposure to 25 °C/75%RH. (**A**) 20% w/w, (**B**) 30% w/w, (**C**) 50% w/w itraconazole-loaded sucrose microfibres, and (**D**) 100% w/w itraconazole microfibres.

Table 2. Average microfibre diameter of freshly prepared samples and particle size (short and long diameter lengths) of the corresponding aged samples after 24 h storage (for microfibres containing 0 and 10% w/w itraconazole) and 30 days storage (for microfibres containing 20, 30, 50, and 100% w/w itraconazole) at 25 °C/75% RH.

Itraconazole Loading (% w/w)	Freshly Prepared Sample	Moisture-Treated Sample	
	Fibre diameter (mean ± SD) (μm)	Long axis diameter (mean ± SD) (μm)	Short axis diameter (mean ± SD) (μm)
0	9.77 ± 3.10	426.29 ± 88.67	301.27 ± 76.11
10 [a]	6.23 ± 3.88	67.33 ± 29.23	27.48 ± 6.18
20	7.12 ± 2.45	80.13 ± 31.65	26.52 ± 6.78
30	7.49 ± 3.12	83.44 ± 37.23	30.18 ± 6.67
50	6.67 ± 3.89	242.87 ± 45.19	21.52 ± 9.36
100	3.22 ± 2.54	No fibre collapse observed. Fibre diameter (mean ± SD) = 3.13 ± 2.50 μm	

[a] The data for the pure sucrose and the 10% w/w itraconazole-loaded samples are reported in [4].

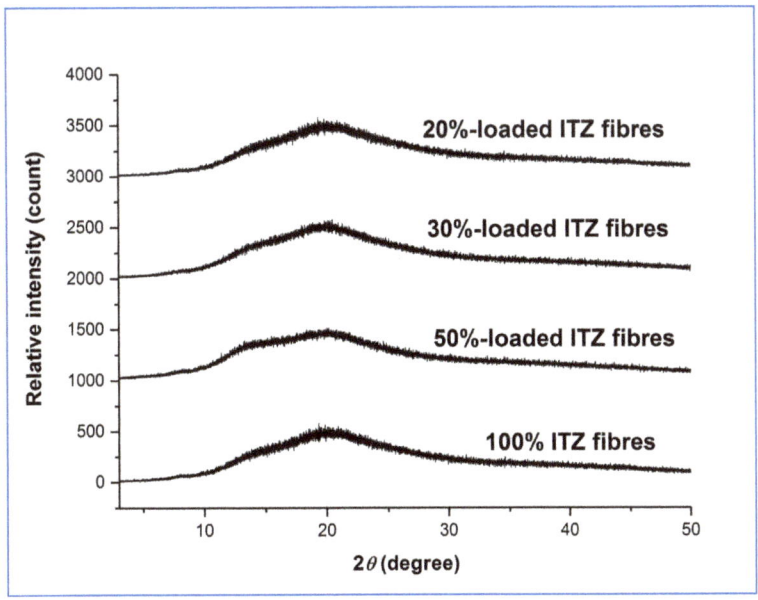

Figure 2. XRPD diffractograms of freshly prepared itraconazole-loaded sucrose microfibres (containing 20, 30, and 50% w/w itraconazole) and pure itraconazole microfibres. (ITZ = itraconazole).

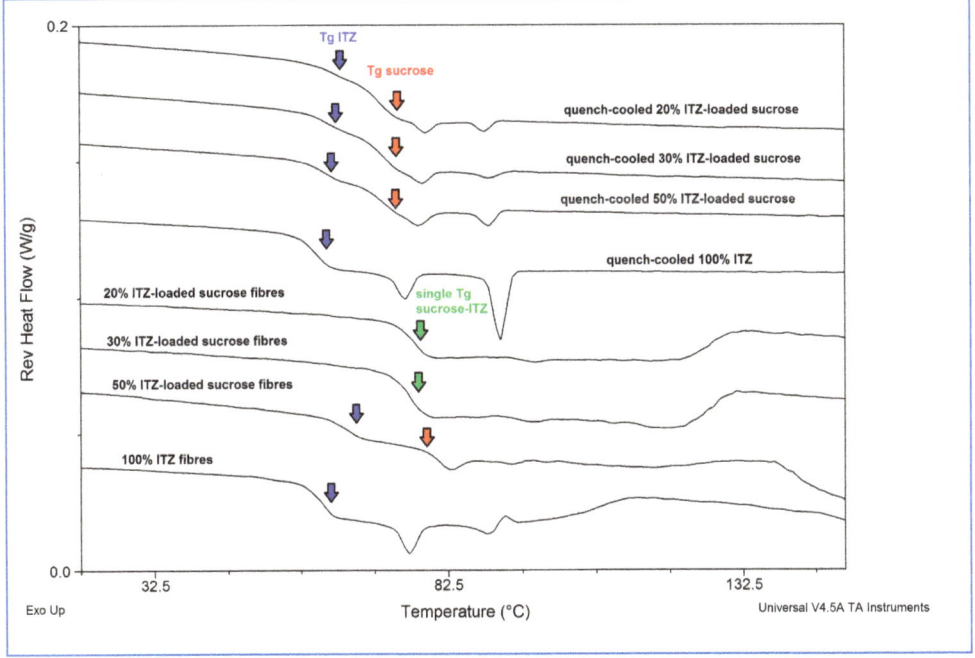

Figure 3. Reversing heat flow traces of freshly prepared itraconazole-loaded sucrose microfibres (containing 20, 30, and 50% w/w itraconazole), pure itraconazole microfibres, and solid dispersions with equivalent compositions prepared by quench-cooling from the melt. (ITZ = itraconazole).

All samples showed glass transitional behaviour, indicating the generation of amorphous dispersions. Interestingly, the quench-cooled sucrose-itraconazole samples all showed two separate glass transitions assigned to the individual components, with that of sucrose occurring at 68 ± 4.3 °C, indicated with a red arrow, and that of itraconazole occurring at 60 ± 0.2 °C, indicated with a blue arrow. These data indicate phase separation, i.e., lack of miscibility, of the two components, as discussed previously [35] for other systems. Further evidence of phase separation is offered by the presence of the two endothermic events occurring at around 74 and 90 °C, ascribed to the formation of a chiral nematic mesophase of pure itraconazole (90 °C) and rotational restriction of the molecules (74 °C) upon cooling from the melt, which are reversible upon re-heating, leading to the observed endotherms [36]. Both of these endothermic transitions and the glass transition are clearly visible for the quench-cooled pure itraconazole sample here. Microfibres containing 20 and 30% w/w itraconazole showed a single mixed-phase glass transition, indicated with a green arrow, at 74.7 ± 1.1 °C and 73.2 ± 1.3 °C, respectively, similar to that observed for the 10% w/w drug-loaded sample at 74.1 ± 1.9 °C [4]. Conversely, the thermal behaviour of the 50% w/w itraconazole-loaded microfibres was more similar to that of the corresponding quench-cooled sample, with both individual substance glass transitions and both itraconazole endothermic events being observed. It is interesting to note that the endothermic transitions are less pronounced for the microfibres, possibly indicating a lower degree of phase separation compared with the equivalent quench-cooled sample. The pure itraconazole microfibres showed the expected glass transition and endothermic transitions.

Taken together, these initial characterisation data suggest that the melt centrifugal process may increase the degree of mixing and miscibility of the drug (itraconazole) in the carrier (sucrose) compared with the simple melt quenching method, possibly due to the application of high centrifugal forces, with the true limit of miscibility being between 30 and 50% w/w of itraconazole. In the 50% w/w itraconazole-loaded samples, at least some of the excess drug appears to be ejected as pure drug microfibres rather than solidifying as conventional drug particles. This observation also provides an explanation for the more variable content uniformity data seen for the 50% w/w-loaded samples than those with lower drug content: each sample taken for analysis is likely to contain a different proportion of the various populations of microfibres, leading to greater variability in the results.

3.2. High Humidity Treatment of Fresh Microfibres

All high-drug-loaded microfibres showed sucrose recrystallisation after storage at 25 °C/75% RH in open containers, as demonstrated by the appearance of sucrose Bragg peaks in the XRPD diffractograms and collapse of the microfibre structure, as described previously for the 10% w/w system [4]. Interestingly, the time required for the microfibres to collapse increases as a function of the itraconazole content. The 10% w/w sample was observed to collapse within 24 h, whereas microfibres containing higher amounts of itraconazole required significantly longer times to do so. Specifically, systems containing 20, 30, and 50% w/w itraconazole were seen to collapse in 4.2 ± 1.3, 7.4 ± 1.9, and 19.7 ± 2.4 days, respectively (n = 3 for each formulation). This is likely due to differences in the water uptake tendency of the microfibres with the higher concentrations of this highly lipophilic drug. Our previous studies [4] on centrifugally spun sucrose microfibres containing 10% w/w of olanzapine (log P = 2.2), piroxicam (log P = 3.06), or itraconazole (log P = 5.66) showed that the more hydrophobic the drug, the lower the moisture uptake as determined by dynamic vapour sorption, and the slower the sucrose recrystallisation and microfibre collapse. This was attributed to the increased hydrophobicity of the microfibre surface in the presence of the drug. It is logical, therefore, to expect that increasing the quantity of itraconazole in the microfibres would further retard the diffusion of water through the hydrophilic sucrose matrix, slowing down the sucrose recrystallisation and the collapse of fibrous structure.

For all subsequent studies, all microfibre formulations were held at 25 °C/75% RH in open containers for 30 days in order to ensure that the sucrose had fully recrystallised in all samples and comparisons between formulations were valid.

3.3. Characterisation of the 30-Day Humidity-Treated Microfibres

After exposure of freshly prepared samples to high humidity conditions, microfibres with 20 and 30% w/w itraconazole collapsed into powders with similar average particle size and morphology to those observed for the previously investigated system containing 10% w/w itraconazole [4]. At 50% w/w drug loading, there are more particles with a more elongated morphology compared with all other systems. However, in all cases, the moisture-treated itraconazole-sucrose systems collapsed into significantly smaller particles than the drug-free sucrose sample. Figure 1 shows the SEM micrographs of the fresh microfibres with their corresponding diameter frequency diagrams and the SEM images of the collapsed powder after humidity treatment. Table 2 summarises the size data for the samples studied here and the 10% w/w drug-loaded and pure sucrose samples for comparison. The pure itraconazole microfibres showed no change in appearance after exposure to the high humidity conditions for 30 days, with the measured diameter of 3.13 ± 2.50 µm (mean $\pm$ SD) showing no significant difference to that of the fresh samples ($p > 0.05$). The different collapse behaviour of the microfibres (total collapse for the pure sucrose and 10, 20, and 30% w/w itraconazole-loaded microfibres; partial collapse of the 50% w/w itraconazole-loaded microfibres; no observable collapse for the pure itraconazole microfibres) suggest that the dominant factor in the collapse process is the sucrose. For the 50% w/w itraconazole-loaded samples, those microfibres containing sucrose will collapse after humidity treatment, whereas microfibres containing pure or almost pure drug will not, leading to the observation of a mixed population of particles and microfibres after treatment.

Figure 4 shows the XRPD diffractograms for the high humidity-treated microfibre formulations.

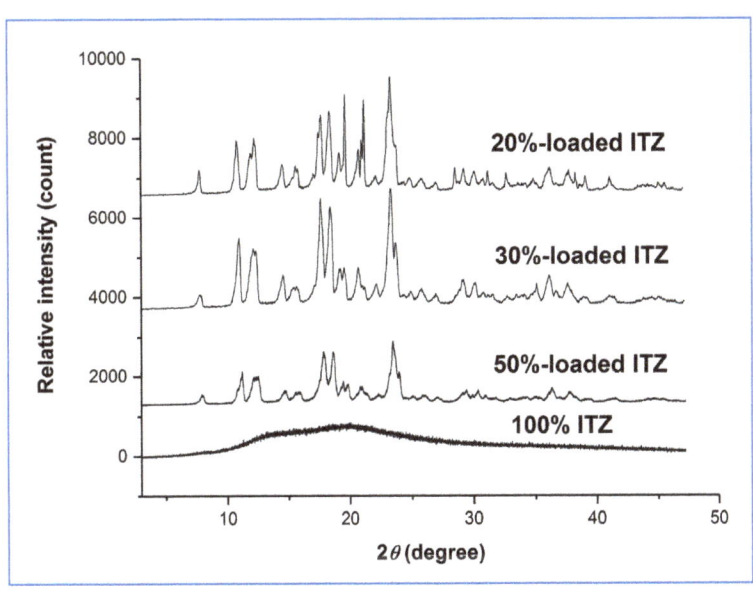

Figure 4. XRPD diffractograms of itraconazole-loaded sucrose microfibres (containing 20, 30, and 50% w/w itraconazole) and pure itraconazole microfibres after 30 days exposure to 25 °C/75% RH. (ITZ = itraconazole).

The presence of the characteristic Bragg peaks for crystalline sucrose and the absence of peaks corresponding to crystalline itraconazole confirmed that the sucrose had largely or fully recrystallised from all the aged sucrose-itraconazole systems, whereas it is inferred that the itraconazole remained in the amorphous state. We had previously observed this behaviour for the itraconazole-sucrose system containing 10% w/w drug [4]. However, no recrystallisation of the pure itraconazole microfibre system was observed after 30 days, as indicated by the presence of a broad halo pattern and the absence of any Bragg peaks for crystalline itraconazole. The MTDSC reversing heat flow traces of the high humidity-treated microfibre formulations are shown in Figure 5.

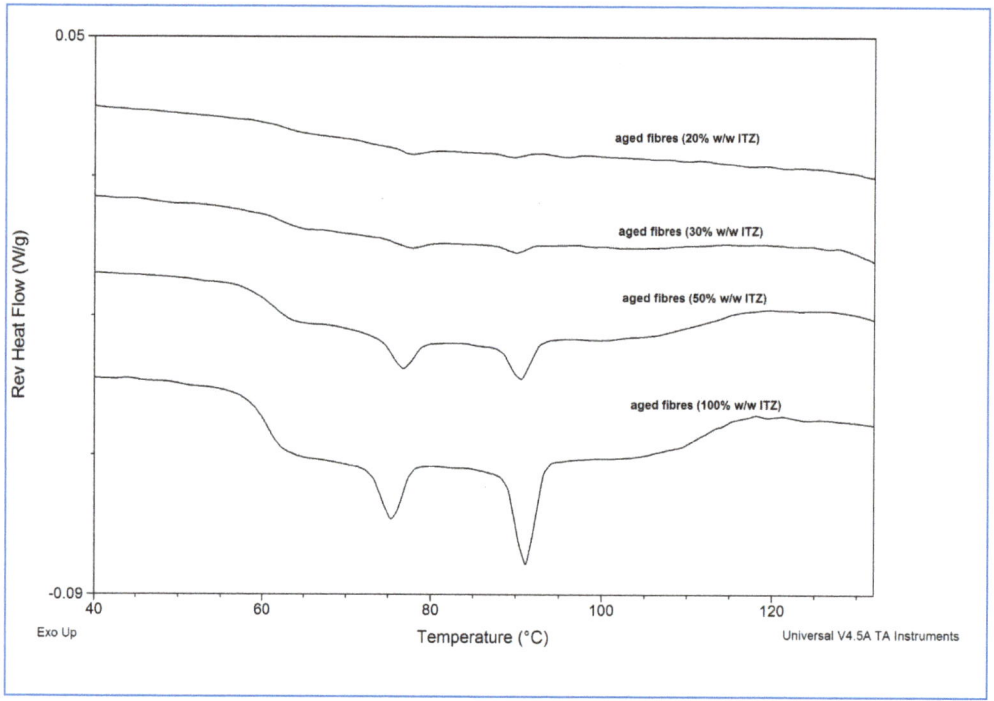

Figure 5. Reversing heat flow traces of itraconazole-loaded sucrose microfibres (containing 20, 30, and 50% w/w itraconazole) and pure itraconazole microfibres after 30 days exposure to 25 °C/75% RH. (ITZ = itraconazole).

The absence of the glass transition associated with sucrose (circa 68 °C) and the presence of the glass transition corresponding to itraconazole (circa 60 °C), followed by the two endothermic transitions associated with amorphous itraconazole (circa 74 °C and 90 °C) confirmed that sucrose fully recrystallised from all the itraconazole-sucrose systems, whereas itraconazole remained in the amorphous state.

Drug content uniformity was measured for the moisture-treated samples, with values (% of theoretical, mean ± SD, n = 6) of 99.1 ± 1.2, 97.9 ± 1.7 and 106.3 ± 11.2 for the 20, 30, and 50% w/w samples, respectively. These are essentially unchanged from the fresh samples, suggesting that the microfibre collapse did not adversely affect the drug distribution in the samples.

Overall, physical and chemical analysis of the humidity-treated microfibres shows that the collapse is due to recrystallisation of the sucrose carrier and that the drug remains in the amorphous form, possibly explained by its high hydrophobicity, which reduces its interaction with water during storage.

3.4. Non-Sink Dissolution Testing of Fresh and Aged Microfibres

In our previous study [4], humidity-treated 10% w/w itraconazole-loaded sucrose microfibres exhibited an unexpected increase (circa 1.25-fold) in the solubility of itraconazole, observed under non-sink conditions, compared with the freshly prepared microfibres, which themselves showed very significant itraconazole solubility increases (circa 8-fold) compared with the pure crystalline drug or an equivalent physical mix. The solubility advantage of the treated samples was maintained even after 8 months of further exposure to high humidity conditions. Here, we have studied the dissolution and solubility behaviour of the samples with higher drug content, both fresh and aged for 30 days at 25 °C/75% RH, under the same non-sink test conditions and with the same total amount of drug in each experiment. The concentration–time profiles of the fresh and aged samples are shown in Figures 6 and 7, respectively.

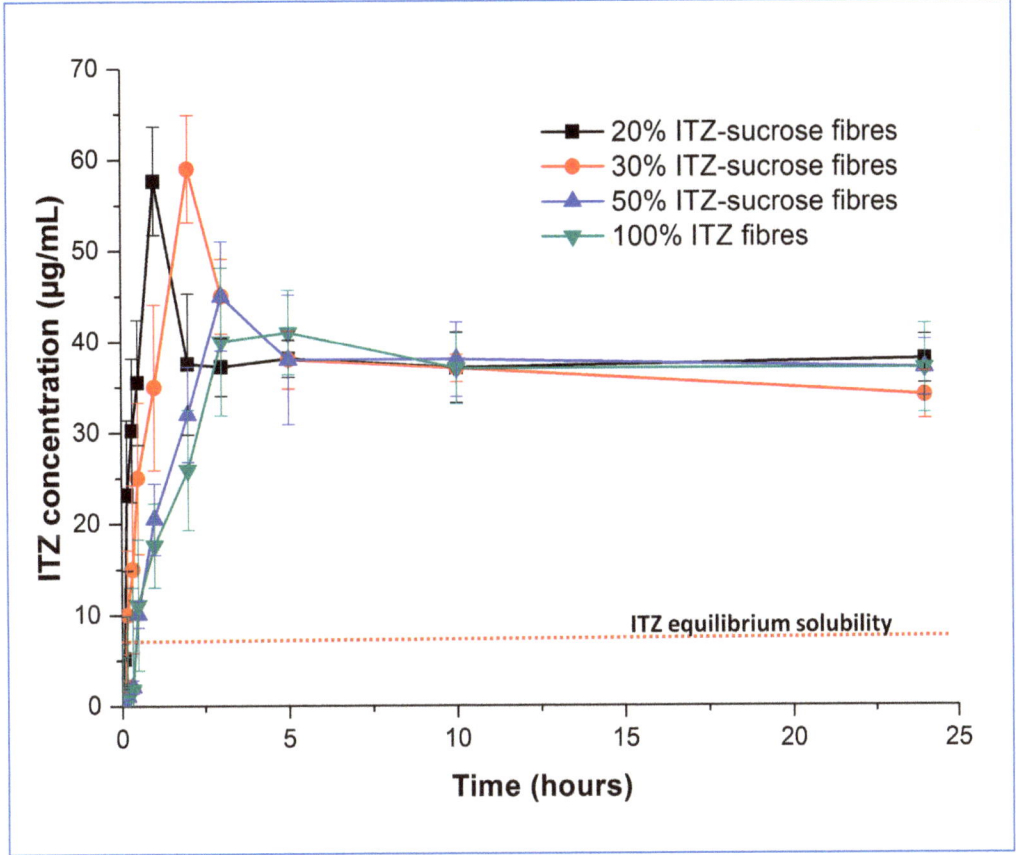

Figure 6. Dissolution–supersaturation profiles obtained under non-sink conditions for freshly prepared itraconazole-loaded sucrose microfibres (containing 20, 30, and 50% w/w itraconazole) and pure itraconazole microfibres. The red dotted line indicates the equilibrium solubility of crystalline itraconazole. (ITZ = itraconazole).

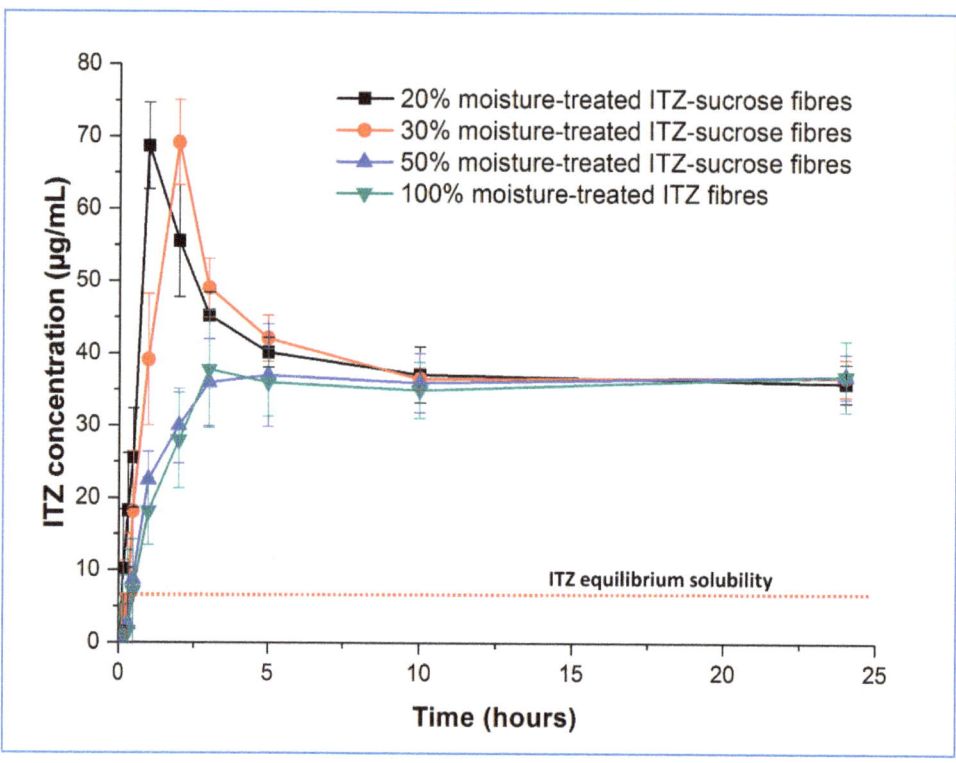

Figure 7. Dissolution–supersaturation profiles obtained under non-sink conditions for itraconazole-loaded sucrose microfibres (containing 20, 30, and 50% w/w itraconazole) and pure itraconazole microfibres after 30 days exposure to 25 °C/75% RH. The red dotted line indicates the equilibrium solubility of crystalline itraconazole. (ITZ = itraconazole).

Examining the fresh samples first, in all cases, the initial drug dissolution process was relatively rapid, forming supersaturated solutions with itraconazole concentrations far exceeding the measured crystalline itraconazole equilibrium solubility (approximately 7 µg/mL). It is interesting to note the behaviour of the pure amorphous itraconazole microfibres, as this gives an indication of the amorphous itraconazole equilibrium solubility (approximately 40 µg/mL) as well as allowing interrogation of the role of sucrose in the dissolution and supersaturation processes.

Both the rate of supersaturation generation and the peak concentration of the itraconazole in solution are affected by the drug-carrier ratio. The time required (T_{max}) to reach the maximum level of drug supersaturation (C_{max}) increases with increasing drug loading, with T_{max} values being approximately 1, 2, and 3 h for the 20, 30, and 50% w/w itraconazole-loaded microfibres, respectively. Samples containing 20 and 30% w/w of itraconazole reached an equivalent maximum level of supersaturation ($p > 0.05$) (C_{max} = 57.7 ± 5.9 and 59.2 ± 4.7 µg/mL, respectively), following which drug precipitation occurred, with the final observed dissolved concentrations stabilising at the level of the equilibrium solubility of amorphous itraconazole. In contrast, at 50% w/w drug loading, the C_{max} was significantly lower ($p < 0.05$), reaching only 44.9 ± 3.9 µg/mL and rapidly decreasing down to the pure amorphous itraconazole solubility. The 10% w/w drug-loaded sample showed the same trend as the 20 and 30% w/w drug-loaded samples: T_{max} was shorter at approximately 30 min, and C_{max} was not significantly different ($p > 0.05$) at 56.78 ± 5.9 µg/mL [4].

This observed pattern of supersaturation behaviour can be explained by a combination of the effect of the dissolving hydrophilic sucrose and the solid-state characteristics of the microfibres. At 50% w/w drug loading, the sucrose-itraconazole system is at least partially phase-separated, and the actual amount of sucrose in the dissolving sample is low. It is reasonable to suggest that the rapid dissolution of this small amount of sucrose is able to affect only marginally the initial drug dissolution step, leaving the phase-separated amorphous drug to regulate the final dissolution step, hence the final drug concentration cannot substantially exceed the solubility of the equivalent pure amorphous drug. At higher sucrose ratios (lower drug content), where the drug and carrier are molecularly dispersed in the solid microfibres, the initial drug dissolution profiles are more controlled by the concomitant dissolution of the carrier and some of the amorphous drug. This will lead to a more consistent C_{max}, as this will ultimately be dependent on the extent of the interactions between the two components and the maximum increase in solubility of itraconazole that may be effected by the presence of sucrose. The shorter T_{max} with the lower drug contents is a reflection of the higher sucrose:drug ratio, leading to greater interaction between the two components initially and a faster rate of supersaturation generation. The decrease in measured drug concentration from the C_{max} down to the level of equilibrium amorphous drug solubility is likely caused by the complete dissolution of the carrier, leaving the remaining undissolved amorphous drug to control the rest of the process. Even though the very high levels of supersaturation are maintained for a relatively short period (up to about 2 h), this may be sufficient to allow enhanced oral absorption, as considered in more detail below.

Examining now the dissolution–supersaturation profiles for the humidity-treated samples, at first sight, the profiles of the aged samples are very similar to those of the fresh samples. As expected based on the physical analysis described above, there was no change in the behaviour of the pure amorphous itraconazole microfibres, and the dissolution profile of the 50% w/w itraconazole sample has decreased to match that of the pure itraconazole microfibres, losing the initial solubility benefit seen in the fresh sample. In contrast, the initial dissolution rate of the 20 and 30% w/w drug-loaded samples decreased compared with the fresh samples, but the T_{max} values remained the same and the supersaturation (C_{max}) levels were increased, to 68.15 ± 4.12 and 69.17 ± 7.45 µg/mL, respectively, a similar profile to the 10% w/w-loaded samples previously described [4]. The C_{max} values for the aged 20 and 30% w/w drug-loaded samples were not significantly different from each other but were significantly different ($p < 0.05$) from the corresponding fresh samples. This may be explained by the slower dissolution of crystalline sucrose in the aged samples compared with the amorphous sucrose in the fresh samples, leading to slower initial dissolution of the drug but preventing a too-rapid buildup of supersaturation, which would then lead to rapid precipitation back to the equilibrium amorphous itraconazole solubility levels. These observations are in agreement with the theoretical model proposed by Han and Lee [37], in which rapid supersaturation generation above a critical value is followed by rapid desaturation based on the decreasing energy barrier to nucleation and precipitation seen at high supersaturation levels.

The overall dissolution performance can be further evaluated by comparing the area under the curve (AUC) of the dissolution–supersaturation profiles for the same quantity of drug, displayed in Figure 8, for the full 24 h of study. The 10, 20, and 30% w/w itraconazole-loaded aged samples all showed a statistically significant increase in AUC compared with their fresh counterparts, although the effect was much greater for the 10% w/w drug-loaded sample. Importantly, the aged 10% w/w drug-loaded samples showed a statistically significant better AUC performance than all other aged samples. Overall, the dissolution advantage of the microfibre generation and humidity treatment seems to be greater for the lower drug loading samples, but this must be balanced against the downstream formulation constraints and product size issues, as will be discussed in the next section.

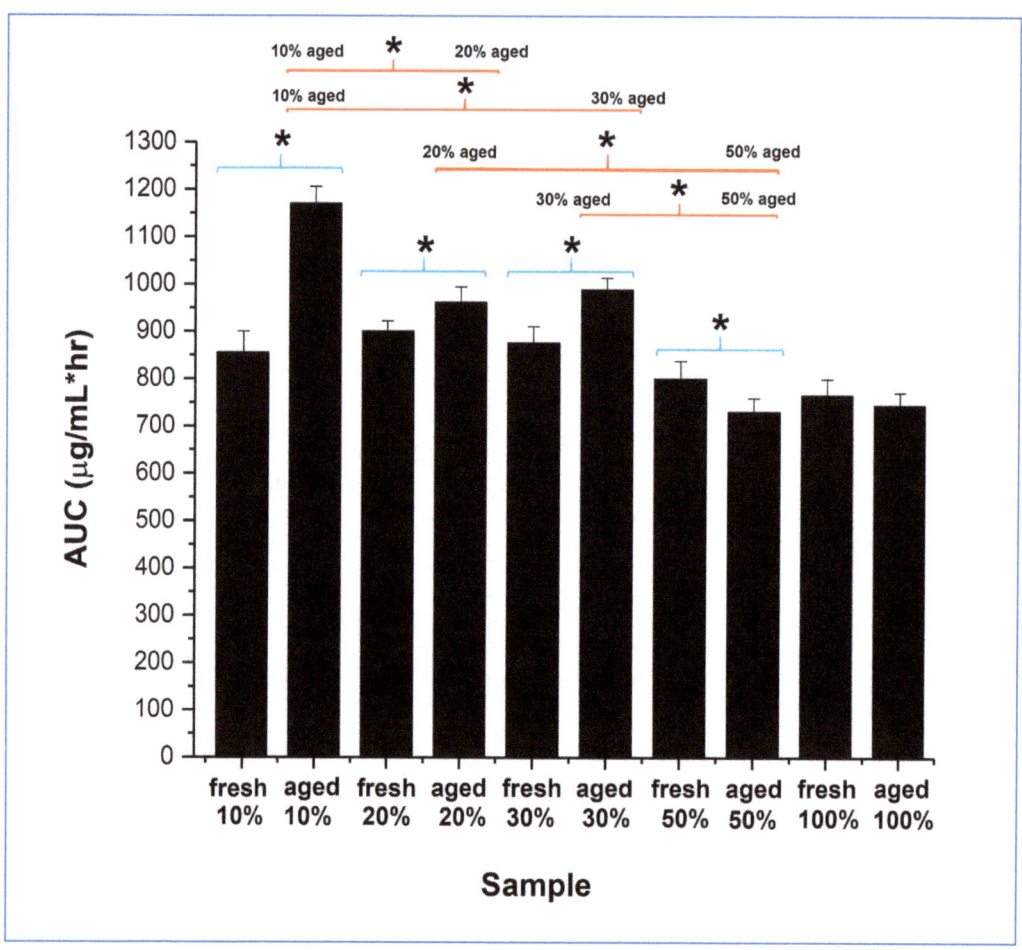

Figure 8. Overall (24 h) AUC of the dissolution–supersaturation profiles obtained under non-sink conditions for itraconazole-loaded sucrose microfibres (containing 20, 30, and 50% w/w itraconazole) and pure itraconazole microfibres, both freshly prepared and after 30 days exposure to 25 °C/75% RH (aged). * with blue brackets indicates a significant difference ($p < 0.05$) between fresh and aged samples of the same formulation. * with red brackets indicates a significant difference ($p < 0.05$) between different aged formulations.

3.5. Tablet Development—Powder Characterisation

Tablet development focussed on the 10 and 30% w/w drug-loaded aged microfibres, as these respectively showed the greatest dissolution/supersaturation advantage and the likely benefits of size reduction of the final product due to greater drug incorporation. Wet granulation was not considered to be a desirable method of tablet production here due to the risk of damage to the microfibres because of the presence of water (or other granulation solvents) and heat; a direct compression method was therefore selected. However, this approach requires careful consideration of the mixing and flow properties of the individual components and the formulation as a whole; hence, the collapsed microfibres were studied without further processing.

Both the aged microfibre samples showed poor flow characteristics, as would be expected given their morphologies, with Carr indices of > 30%. Binary mixtures of the aged microfibre samples with Compressol SM® or StarTab® showed significant improvements in flow behaviour: even at 60% w/w microfibre content, the Carr indices were < 20%, indicating good to fair flow. Conversely, binary mixtures with Avicel PH102® showed no improvement in flow properties compared with the microfibre samples alone, except at the lowest microfibre incorporation (10% w/w). The segregation potential of the binary mixtures was assessed using a novel segregation cell based on a tapped density apparatus. Here, the arrangement of an outer plastic cylinder with a removable base and a set of stacking inner plastic cylinders, rather than the normal single measuring cylinder, allows for ease of sampling at specific heights in the powder bed, after tapping to simulate the vibration and particle movement expected in the tabletting processes.

The mixing and segregation profiles of the aged microfibres were assessed using the 10% w/w itraconazole-loaded system. No segregation was seen with binary mixtures based on StarTab® containing 10 to 60%w/w microfibres, with drug content values of all individual unit-sized samples (300 mg total weight) comfortably within the range of 95 to 105% of theoretical, significantly better than the pharmacopoeial content uniformity specification of 85 to 115% of theoretical. Binary mixtures based on Avicel PH102® or Compressol SM® showed inappropriate segregation behaviour at low microfibre loadings (10% w/w), with content uniformity data outside the pharmacopoeial limits, but this improved as the microfibre loadings increased, such that at 60% w/w microfibre loading, the content uniformity values were within the range of 95 to 105% of theoretical. The lack of segregation seen with StarTab® is attributable to its morphology, with the high specific surface area and porosity providing greater opportunity for mechanical interlocking of the microfibres and the carrier particles. Subsequent experiments showed that a pre-mixing step of microfibres, equivalent to 10% w/w loading in the final mix, with StarTab® prior to dilution with either Avicel PH102®, Compressol SM®, or a 1:1 mix of these two excipients, led to non-segregating powders, with all measured drug content values being in the range of 95 to 105% of theoretical. These results suggest that, as long as the processed microfibres are initially mixed with StarTab®, other components with alternative functionalities may be added to generate a fully functional tablet formulation.

3.6. Tablet Development—Physical Characterisation

Using the aged 10% w/w itraconazole-loaded microfibres, nine different tablet formulations, labelled F1 to F9 and shown in Table 1, were produced via a direct compression process, i.e., pre-mixing of the microfibres with StarTab® to prevent segregation, dry mixing with other ingredients, lubrication, and compression. In all formulations, the level of the disintegrant (crospovidone (Kollidon CL-F®)) was kept constant at 5% w/w, and the level of the lubricant (glyceryl dibehenate (Compritol 888 ATO®)) was maintained at 1.5% w/w. The formulations are divided into three groups (Groups 1, 2, and 3) based on the content of the drug-loaded microfibres (10, 30, and 50% w/w, respectively). Within each group, the amount of StarTab® relative to Avicel PH102® and Compressol SM® was increased in the ratios of 1:1:1 (formulations F1, F4, and F7), 2:1:1 (formulations F2, F5, and F8), and 3:1:1 (formulations F3, F6, and F9). Finally, for comparative purposes, Group 4 included the highest possible loading of the microfibres (93.5% w/w) with just the disintegrant and lubricant in formulation F10 and the raw, unprocessed ingredients in the same ratios in formulation F11. All formulations were compressed at four compression forces: 10, 16, 20, and 26 kN.

Figure 9A–D shows the tensile strength–compression force and disintegration time–compression force curves for tablets from all 11 formulations.

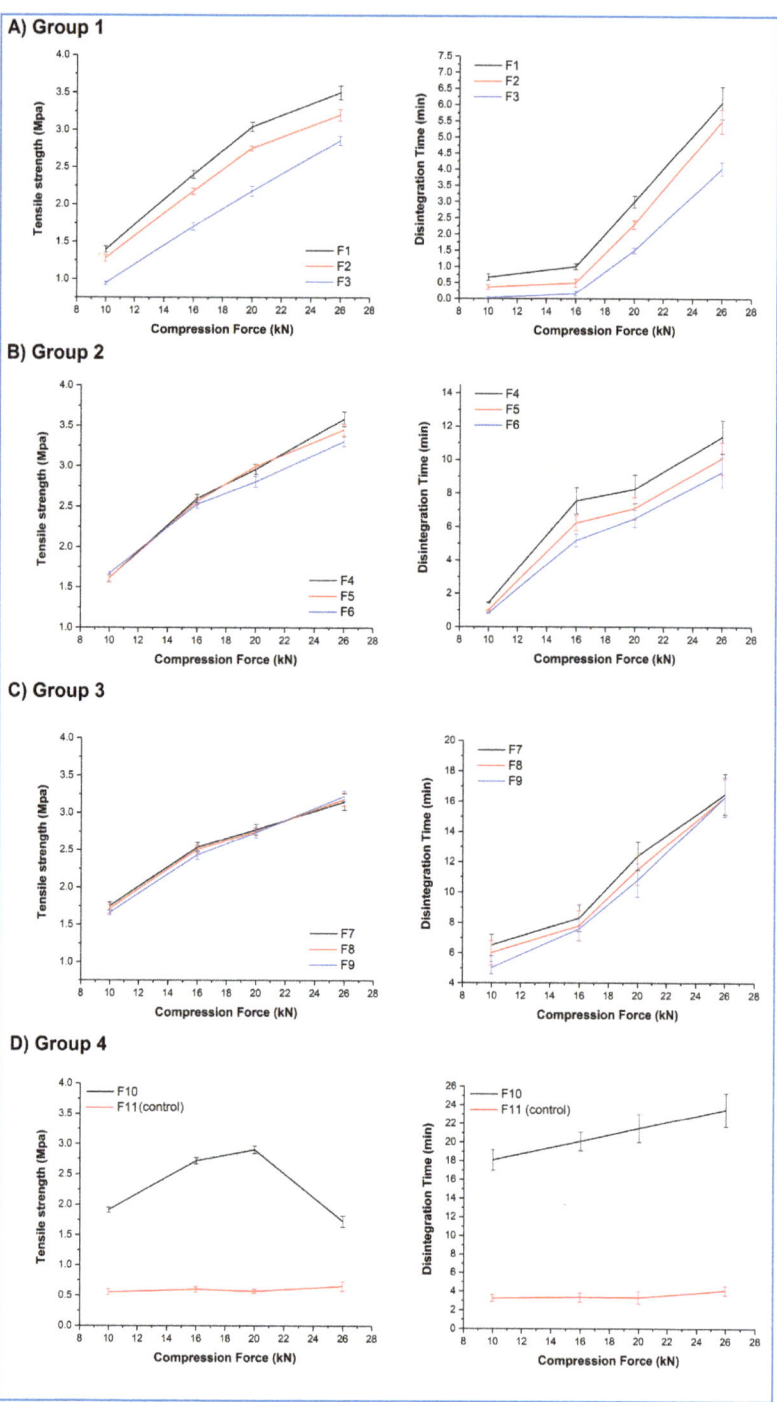

Figure 9. Tensile strength and disintegration time profiles as a function of compression force applied for tablets belonging to (**A**) Group 1, (**B**) Group 2, (**C**) Group 3, and (**D**) Group 4.

Both F10 and F11 mixtures stuck to the tablet punches during compression, illustrating the adhesive nature of their major constituents. F11 tablets showed low tensile strengths (circa 0.6 MPa) and correspondingly short disintegration times (circa 3.5 min) at all compression forces, along with lamination during the tensile strength testing. In contrast, F10 tablets showed an increase in tensile strength as a function of compression force up to 20 kN (ranging from 1.9 to 2.9 MPa), then a decrease at 26 kN, along with lamination during testing at this compression force. No significant differences ($p > 0.05$) in the disintegration time were observed for F10 tablets, with all tablets disintegrating in 20 to 23 min. All F11 tablet batches and the F10 tablet batch showing lamination failed the pharmacopoeial friability test; all other F10 tablet batches passed this test.

Within Groups 1, 2, and 3, a roughly linear increase in tablet tensile strength with increasing compression force was observed, with a concomitant increase in disintegration time. A closer inspection of the data highlights that both the percentage of aged microfibres and the ratio of the excipients affected the behaviour of the tablets. Within each group, tablets with the lowest relative content of StarTab® (F1, F4, F7) generally showed numerically greater values of tensile strength than the formulations with the middle (F2, F5, F8) and highest (F3, F6, F9) relative content of this excipient, although the differences were statistically significant ($p < 0.05$) only for Group 1 formulations at all compression forces and Group 2 formulations at the highest compression forces. A similar pattern was observed with the disintegration times. Comparing between groups, increasing the aged microfibre content from 10% w/w to 30% w/w resulted in an increase in tensile strength and disintegration time for formulations compressed at the same force and with the same excipient ratio. For example, F2 (Group 1) tablets compressed at 16 kN showed mean values of 2.1 MPa and 30 s, respectively, whereas the mean values for F5 (Group 2) tablets were significantly higher ($p < 0.05$) at 2.6 MPa and 6.2 min. However, as the microfibre content increases still further to 50% w/w, the differences become less significant. For example, F4 (Group 2) tablets compressed at 20 kN show statistically ($p > 0.05$) similar mean tensile strength and disintegration time values (2.9 MPa and 8.2 min, respectively) compared with the equivalent F7 (Group 3) tablets (2.8 MPa and 10.2 min, respectively). No sticking or lamination was observed for any of these formulations (F1 to F9), and all batches passed the pharmacopoeial friability test.

These results suggest that, although it is possible to directly compress the aged microfibres into tablets, a more considered formulation approach is required to produce robust tablets. A complex relationship exists between the formulation components in terms of the effect on the tensile strength and dissolution time of the resultant tablets, but the dominant formulation factor appears to be the content of the aged microfibres, with the excipient ratio playing a smaller role, most obviously observed at lower microfibre contents when the excipient content is correspondingly greater. The effect of increasing the compression force is predictable in that increasing compression force leads to increased tensile strength and disintegration time. However, these findings also demonstrate that it is possible to fine-tune the tensile strength and disintegration time of the tablets by varying the microfibre content, excipient ratios, and compression forces, potentially allowing the development of tablets for different purposes.

3.7. Tablet Development—Non-Sink Dissolution Testing

Formulations F3 and F9 were chosen for the non-sink dissolution study, representing the extremes of microfibre content, tensile strength, and disintegration time and having the same excipient ratio. Replicate formulations, labelled as F3* and F9*, containing the aged 30% w/w itraconazole-loaded microfibres were also studied. This sample selection allows investigation of the effects of both drug content and rate of supersaturation generation on the overall dissolution performance of the tablets. Table 3 shows the characterisation data of all these batches.

Table 3. Tablet characterisation data for tablet batches F3 and F9 [containing 10% w/w itraconazole-loaded microfibres (fibres$_{10\%ITZ}$)] and F3* and F9* [containing 30% w/w itraconazole-loaded microfibres (fibres$_{30\%ITZ}$)]. (ITZ = itraconazole).

Formulation Code	Compression Force Applied (kN)	Disintegration Time (Seconds or Minutes)	Tensile Strength (MPa)	Weight (mg)	ITZ Content (% of Theoretical)
F3	10	2 ± 1 s	0.60 ± 0.03	299.5 ± 1.1	98.6 ± 1.5
(contains	16	10 ± 2 s	1.09 ± 0.04	301.2 ± 0.9	100.6 ± 1.8
fibres$_{10\%ITZ}$)	20	92 ± 11 s	1.35 ± 0.03	298.9 ± 1.2	98.9 ± 2.0
	26	241 ± 24 s	1.71 ± 0.06	300.7 ± 0.7	101.1 ± 1.9
F3*	10	5 ± 2 s	0.66 ± 0.02	299.8 ± 0.9	98.8 ± 0.7
(contains	16	13 ± 2 s	1.13 ± 0.03	300.1 ± 0.8	99.6 ± 1.1
fibres$_{30\%ITZ}$)	20	126 ± 21 s	1.28 ± 0.05	299.5 ± 0.8	97.9 ± 1.9
	26	307 ± 39 s	1.77 ± 0.07	300.6 ± 0.9	100.2 ± 2.1
F9	10	5.0 ± 0.4 min	1.06 ± 0.02	298.6 ± 1.3	100.9 ± 2.5
(contains fibres$_{10\%ITZ}$)	26	16.3 ± 1.3 min	1.84 ± 0.03	301.2 ± 0.8	101.5 ± 1.9
F9*	10	5.5 ± 0.7 min	1.09 ± 0.04	299.7 ± 0.7	100.9 ± 2.1
(contains fibres$_{30\%ITZ}$)	26	16.5 ± 0.9 min	1.73 ± 0.06	298.8 ± 1.4	102.3 ± 1.8

Drug content uniformity and weight uniformity data were excellent, with all tablet batches clearly passing the relevant pharmacopoeial specifications. No significant differences ($p > 0.05$) were observed in any test between equivalent batches varying only in the drug content, i.e., F3/F3* and F9/F9*. This is a significant result, as it demonstrates that the microfibres show the same mechanical and formulation behaviour irrespective of drug content in the range of 10 to 30% w/w.

Concentration–time profiles, generated under the same non-sink conditions as used earlier for the microfibres, of the tablets and the corresponding uncompressed blends and pure crystalline itraconazole are shown in Figure 10 (F3 and F3*) and Figure 11 (F9 and F9*), respectively.

Examining the fast-disintegrating F3 formulations first, the uncompressed microfibres and the tablets compressed at 10, 16, and 20 kN showed broadly equivalent dissolution performance, achieving and maintaining supersaturation (C_{max}) at levels of approximately 20 µg/mL, i.e., approximately 2.8-fold higher than the pure crystalline drug solubility, although there was a trend towards slightly lower rates of drug dissolution from the tablets as the compression force increased. Tablets compressed at the highest compression force (26 kN) did not show supersaturation, and the corresponding dissolution profiles were similar to those of the pure crystalline drug. F3* microfibres and tablets showed similar dissolution behaviour to the equivalent F3 microfibres and tablets in relation to the effects of compression force and supersaturation generation. However, for F3* tablets compressed at forces up to and including 20 kN, some drug precipitation occurred shortly after the initial high values of C_{max} (in the range of 58 to 68 µg/mL) were attained, leading to the maintenance supersaturation levels being approximately 50 µg/mL, i.e., approximately 7.1-fold higher than the pure crystalline drug solubility and approximately 25% higher than the solubility of amorphous itraconazole established earlier. There was a trend toward lower peak C_{max} levels and lower maintenance supersaturation levels with increasing compression force. The plateau supersaturation levels obtained for the F3* tablets, which contain 9 mg itraconazole, were approximately 2.5-fold higher than those for the F3* tablets, which contain 3 mg itraconazole, demonstrating that the dissolution advantage of the microfibres is preserved at the higher drug loading, even if there is not a completely linear relationship between drug loading and plateau drug concentrations.

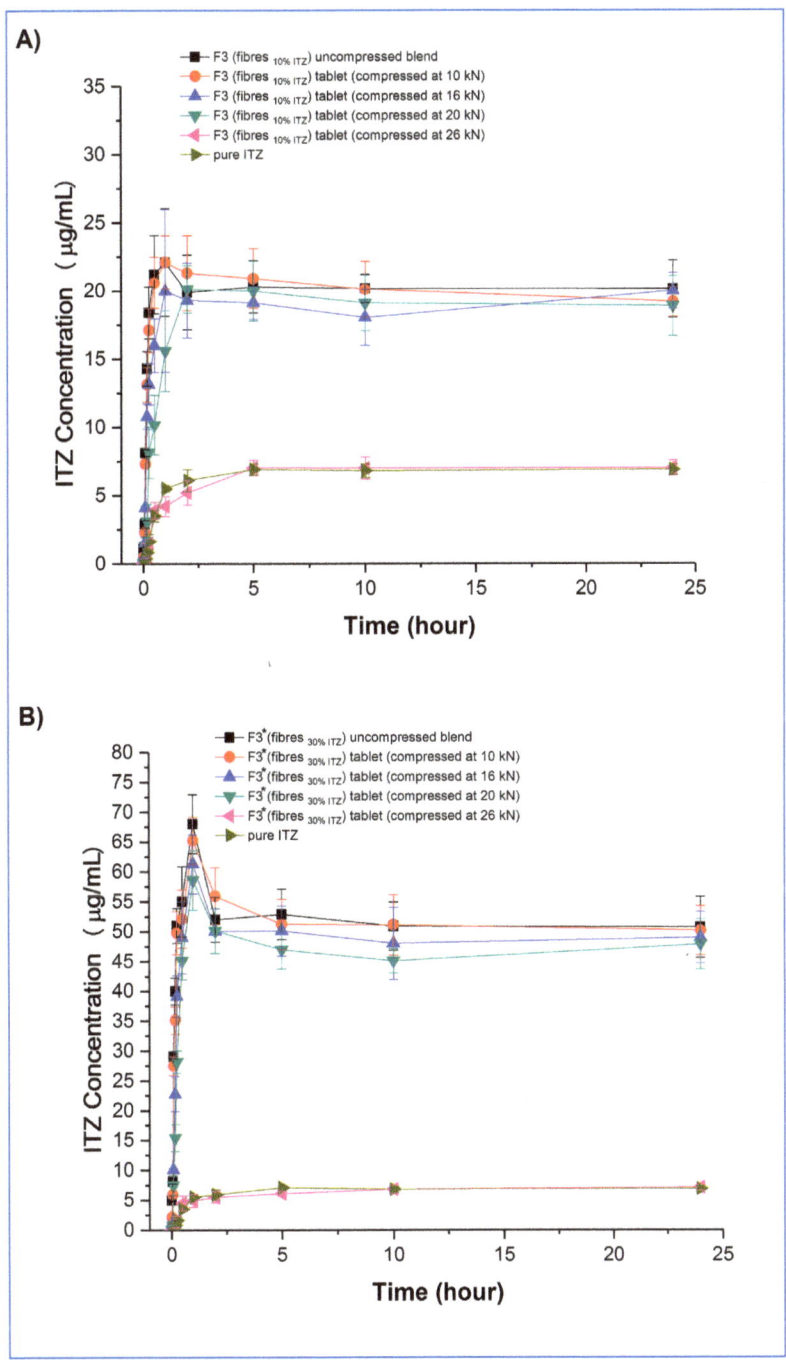

Figure 10. Dissolution–supersaturation profiles obtained under non-sink conditions for tablets, the corresponding uncompressed blends, and pure crystalline itraconazole. (**A**) F3 tablets, and (**B**) F3* tablets. (ITZ = itraconazole).

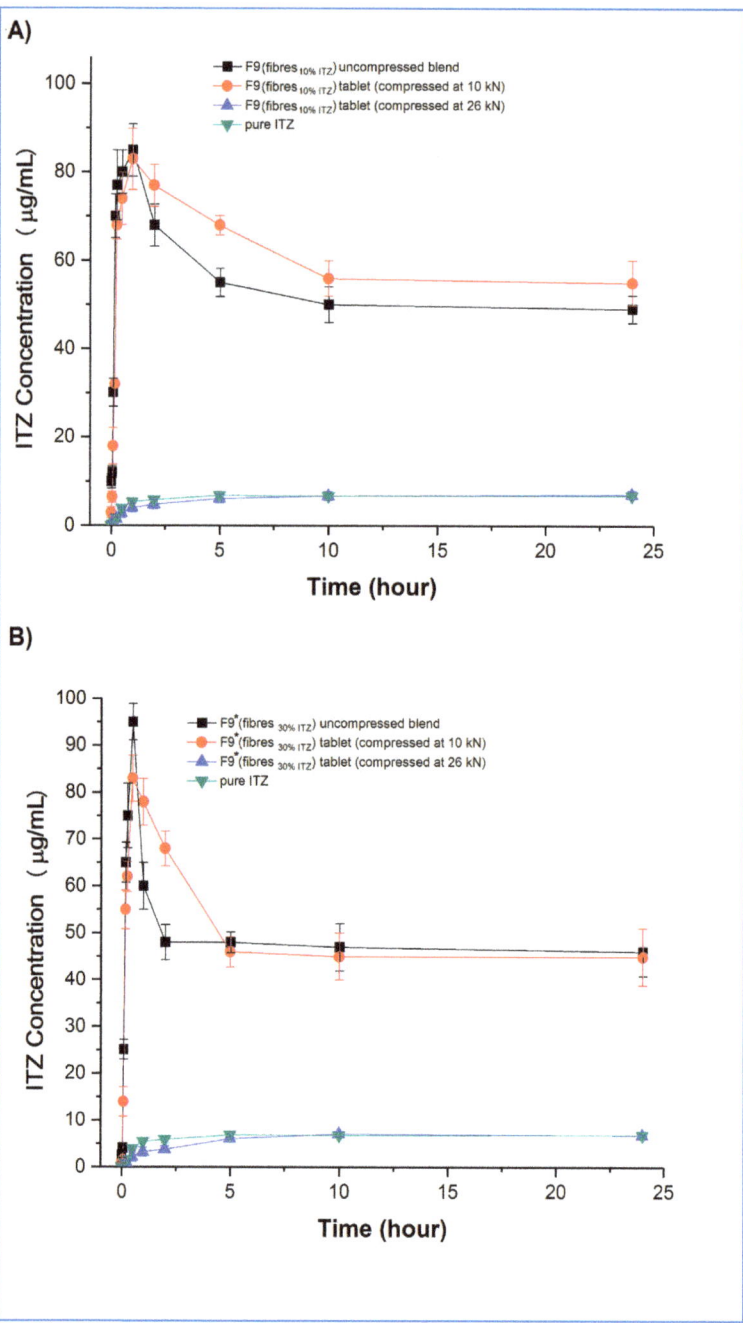

Figure 11. Dissolution–supersaturation profiles obtained under non-sink conditions for tablets, the corresponding uncompressed blends, and pure crystalline itraconazole. (**A**) F9 tablets, and (**B**) F9* tablets. (ITZ = itraconazole).

Both F9 and F9* tablets compressed at 26 kN force showed dissolution profiles indistinguishable from the raw crystalline drug. F9 uncompressed microfibres and tablets compressed at 10 kN both showed an initial fast dissolution and high C_{max} (approximately 85 and 83 µg/mL, respectively), with subsequent precipitation and stabilisation of supersaturation levels at approximately 50 and 56 µg/mL, respectively. The higher drug-loaded F9* formulation showed similar behaviour. In this case, the C_{max} values were approximately 83 and 95 µg/mL, respectively, for the uncompressed microfibres and tablets compressed at 10 kN, with the supersaturation concentration plateauing for both products at approximately 48 µg/mL. Closer inspection of the data reveals that, for both F9 and F9*, the tablets compressed at 10 kN showed significantly ($p < 0.05$) lower dissolution at the very early stages of the experiment, up to 15 min for F9 and 30 min for F9*, than the corresponding powder blend, which may be attributable to the 5 min disintegration time for these tablets reducing the initial rate of dissolution. This slower buildup of supersaturation is then responsible for the retention of the higher supersaturation concentrations in the tablets compared with the powder blends, following the model of Han and Lee [37].

Taken together, these results indicate that the rate and extent of supersaturation can be controlled by varying the drug content of the formulation and the disintegration time of the tablets, which will then affect the total amount of drug available for absorption in the intestine. The overall effect of this may be quantified by calculating the 24 h AUC values of the dissolution–supersaturation profiles: values (mean ± sd) of 480 ± 14, 1223 ± 18, 1448 ± 44 and 1178 ± 36 µg/mL.h were observed for F3, F3*, F9, and F9* tablets compressed at 10 kN, respectively, with the equivalent value for crystalline itraconazole being 158 ± 4 µg/mL.h. The 3-fold increase in overall drug content between F3 and F3*, achieved via an increase in the drug loading of the microfibres (10 and 30% w/w), led to a 2.5-fold increase in both final sustained concentration and AUC. However, a similarly derived 3-fold itraconazole content increase between F9 and F9* did not result in a similar dissolution advantage, and indeed, a lower AUC was observed for the F9* tablets, indicating that, above a certain limit, increasing the drug content has no effect on the final dissolution profile. The 5-fold increase in overall drug content between F3 and F9, achieved via an increase in the microfibre content of the tablets (10 and 50% w/w), led to an almost 3-fold increase in both final sustained concentration and AUC. Conversely, the similarly derived 5-fold itraconazole content increase between F3* and F9* tablets resulted in a slight decrease in overall AUC, again suggesting that there is a maximal effect of increasing the content of the drug. This dose effect is attributable to the initial supersaturated concentrations exceeding the critical value whereby the energy barrier to recrystallisation is sufficiently low to allow precipitation to occur. From these data, F9 would appear to be the most beneficial formulation. However, the absorption site for itraconazole is the small intestine, which has a commonly accepted transit time of 3 to 5 h. Therefore, considering only the first five hours of the dissolution experiment to simulate the likely absorption window, the corresponding AUC (mean ± SD) values for F3, F3*, F9, F9* tablets, and crystalline drug are 103 ± 5, 272 ± 9, 361 ± 14, 307 ± 12, and 18 ± 2 µg/mL·h, confirming that F9 is the best of the current formulations.

3.8. Tablet Development—Physical State of the Drug in the Compressed Tablets

The non-sink dissolution study highlighted that all tablet batches compressed at 26 kN showed dissolution profiles indistinguishable from the raw crystalline itraconazole, suggesting that compression at this force had resulted in the recrystallisation of the amorphous itraconazole in the microfibres. This was confirmed by ^{13}C CP/MAS SSNMR analysis. Figure 12 shows the responses of F3 and F9* tablets, with the lowest (1% w/w) and highest (15% w/w) itraconazole content, respectively, compressed at 10 and 26 kN, and the peaks attributable to crystalline and amorphous drug [4] shown by arrows. All tablets compressed at 10, 16, and 20 kN showed the amorphous response, and all tablets compressed at 26 kN showed the crystalline response, indicating that the recrystallisation process is compression force dependent, with the critical force being between 20 and 26 kN. These results highlight the need to understand the effect of process variables on the physical structure and behaviour of the formulation and, by extension, the likely effect on the biological performance of the drug.

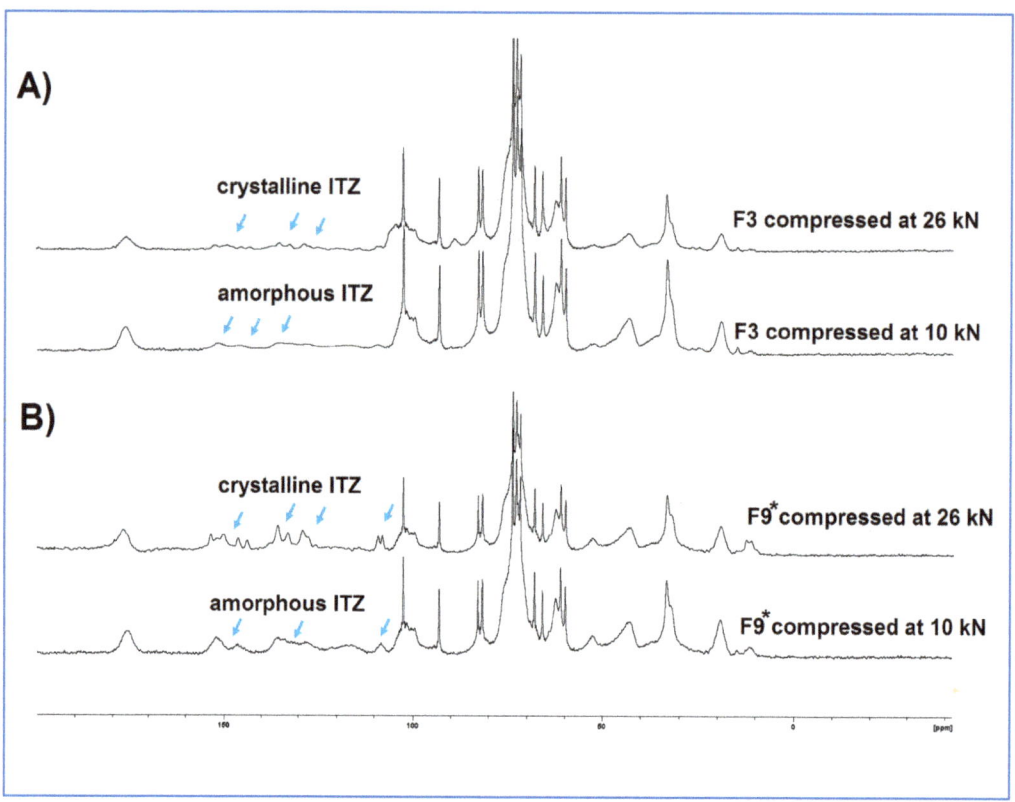

Figure 12. Comparison of ^{13}C CP/MAS NMR spectra of tablets compressed at 10 kN and 26 kN for (**A**) F3 tablets (with the lowest itraconazole content) and (**B**) F9* tablets (with the highest itraconazole content). (ITZ = itraconazole).

4. General Discussion and Future Perspectives

Building on our previous work [3,4], this study has shown that it is possible to prepare fully amorphous, one-phase itraconazole-loaded sucrose microfibres using melt centrifugal spinning, up to a drug content of 30% w/w. At 50% w/w drug loading, phase separation was seen, including the generation of pure itraconazole microfibres in the amorphous state. Fresh microfibres with up to 30% w/w itraconazole showed similar non-sink dissolution behaviour to that previously observed for the 10% w/w drug-loaded samples, i.e., a fast initial dissolution with high supersaturated concentrations being generated and subsequent partial drug precipitation with lower supersaturation concentrations being maintained for up to 24 h. Exposure for 30 days to 25 °C/75% RH resulted in the recrystallisation of the sucrose component of the microfibres, but the itraconazole remained in the amorphous state. The dissolution–supersaturation advantage seen in the fresh samples was maintained and even enhanced in the aged systems, ascribed to the slower initial dissolution of crystalline sucrose preventing a too-rapid rise in supersaturation and hence reducing the extent of precipitation thereafter.

An in-depth tablet formulation development study was carried out using aged itraconazole-loaded microfibres and commonly used direct compression tabletting excipients. To enhance mixing and prevent segregation, a pre-mixing step of the microfibres with StarTab®, a partially pregelatinised starch, was necessary prior to subsequent mixing with the remainder of the excipients, lubrication, and compression. The content of the aged microfibres was observed to have the greatest influence on the physical behaviour of the tablets, with the excipient mix playing a lesser role. Non-sink dissolution studies showed that the dissolution–supersaturation advantage of the itraconazole-loaded (10 and 30% w/w) aged microfibres was maintained in the tablet formulations containing 10% w/w microfibres and even enhanced for a microfibre content of 50% w/w in the final tablets when tablets were compressed at low and medium forces. However, compression at the highest force resulted in the recrystallisation of the amorphous drug, and the dissolution profiles became indistinguishable from those of the crystalline raw drug. All tablet batches tested for dissolution passed all relevant pharmacopoeial tests, with excellent drug content uniformity and weight uniformity being demonstrated. Tablet formulation F9, containing 50% w/w microfibres composed of 10% w/w itraconazole, showed the greatest AUC advantage when measured over 5 h to simulate intestinal transit and itraconazole's likely absorption window, or 24 h to simulate transit through the entire gastro-intestinal tract. This was attributed to a relatively slow rate of supersaturation generation and a subsequent slow precipitation rate, which led to a high maintenance supersaturation level. The lack of further increase in C_{max} or AUC seen with the microfibres and tablets with the highest drug loading (F9* compared with F9) demonstrates the overall limit of supersaturation that may be achieved with this approach and this drug. Additionally, it allows a rough estimation of the critical supersaturation concentration, above which drug precipitation occurs rapidly, as described by Han and Lee [37]. This value can be estimated here as being in the range of 90 to 100 µg/mL.

F9 and F9* tablets, which contain 50% w/w microfibres, showed longer disintegration times (around 5 min) compared with their equivalent formulations containing 10% w/w microfibres (a few seconds), which was thought to contribute to the slower onset of supersaturation. Extending this approach and developing a tablet with an even longer disintegration time may then lead to greater overall dissolution performance. In this case, the rate of supersaturation generation and hence the potential for drug precipitation would be expected to be reduced further while still maintaining the overall dissolution advantage of the amorphous state of the drug and the increase in solubility due to the presence of sucrose in the microfibres. This may be achieved by reducing the content of disintegrant in the tablet formulation. Increasing the compression force, which would also be expected to increase disintegration time and slow the initial dissolution rate, carries the risk of causing the in situ recrystallisation of the amorphous itraconazole, thus losing all benefit of this formulation approach.

From a commercial perspective, the potential scalability and speed of the centrifugal melt spinning process are important considerations. On a lab scale, 10 g of powder mix can be converted into microfibres in approximately 5 min once the equipment is at the correct temperature. The spinning process has the potential to be made into a (semi)-continuous process, as long as there is a balance between feeding of the starting materials (the powder mix) and collection of the product (the microfibres); hence, it is potentially scalable into a commercially viable process. However, as there is a need to humidity-treat the microfibres prior to formulation into tablets, the overall process will need to remain a batch process.

5. Conclusions

This study has demonstrated that fully amorphous sucrose microfibres can be prepared with high drug loading by a centrifugal melt-spinning process. Under non-sink conditions, fresh microfibres showed a significant dissolution and supersaturation advantage compared with the raw drug and physical mixtures of the drug and sucrose, which was maintained after humidity treatment (25 °C/75% RH for 30 days), which caused recrystallisation of the sucrose and collapse of the microfibres. It is possible to directly compress the aged microfibres to form tablets, although sticking to the punches was observed. A detailed tablet formulation study using aged microfibres as the drug source demonstrated that high-quality tablets can be prepared using a direct compression approach; these tablets easily passed all relevant pharmacopoeial specifications. A pre-mixing step with StarTab® was required to overcome the flow and segregation issues caused by the morphology of the collapsed microfibres. Importantly, the dissolution advantage of the microfibres was retained after compression into tablets. By varying the disintegration rate and drug content of the tablets, the rate of supersaturation generation and subsequent drug precipitation can be controlled, allowing the optimisation of the formulation in terms of dissolution profile. Overall, this investigation showed that the microfibre-tablet approach to formulating poorly soluble BCS Class II drugs leads to improved dissolution behaviour of the drug, which in turn should lead to enhanced oral bioavailability of the drug.

Author Contributions: Conceptualization: S.A.B., D.Q.M.C., S.M. (Stefania Marano), A.R.-S.; Data curation: S.M. (Stefania Marano); Formal Analysis: S.M. (Stefania Marano); Funding acquisition: D.Q.M.C., A.R.-S.; Investigation: M.G., S.M. (Stefania Marano); Methodology: M.G., S.M. (Stefania Marano), S.A.B., D.Q.M.C.; Supervision: S.A.B., D.Q.M.C.; Visualization: S.M. (Stefania Marano); Writing—original draft preparation: S.A.B.; Writing—review and editing: M.G., S.M. (Stefania Marano), S.M. (Shahrzad Missaghi), S.A.B., D.Q.M.C. All authors have read and agreed to the published version of the manuscript.

Funding: This work was funded by the Biotechnology and Biological Sciences Research Council (BBSRC) Industrial CASE studentship (BBSRC reference BB/K011731/1), formerly known as 'Collaborative Awards in Science and Engineering' and Colorcon Inc. The APC was funded by UCL.

Institutional Review Board Statement: Not applicable.

Informed Consent Statement: Not applicable.

Data Availability Statement: The data presented in this study are contained within this article.

Conflicts of Interest: The authors declare no conflict of interest.

References

1. Alshaya, H.A.; Alfahad, A.J.; Alsulaihem, F.M.; Aodah, A.H.; Alshehri, A.A.; Almughem, F.A.; Alfassam, H.A.; Aldossary, A.M.; Halwani, A.A.; Bukhary, H.A.; et al. Fast-Dissolving Nifedipine and Atorvastatin Calcium Electrospun Nanofibers as a Potential Buccal Delivery System. *Pharmaceutics* **2022**, *14*, 358. [CrossRef]
2. Becelaere, J.; Van Den Broeck, E.; Schoolaert, E.; Vanhoorne, V.; Van Guyse, J.F.R.; Vergaelen, M.; Borgmans, S.; Creemers, K.; Van Speybroeck, V.; Vervaet, C.; et al. Stable Amorphous Solid Dispersion of Flubendazole with High Loading via Electrospinning. *J. Control. Release* **2022**, *351*, 123–136. [CrossRef] [PubMed]
3. Marano, S.; Barker, S.A.; Raimi-Abraham, B.T.; Missaghi, S.; Rajabi-Siahboomi, A.; Craig, D.Q.M. Development of Micro-fibrous Solid Dispersions of Poorly Water-soluble Drugs in Sucrose Using Temperature-controlled Centrifugal Spinning. *Eur. J. Pharm. Biopharm.* **2016**, *103*, 84–94. [CrossRef]
4. Marano, S.; Barker, S.A.; Raimi-Abraham, B.T.; Missaghi, S.; Rajabi-Siahboomi, A.; Allev, A.E.; Craig, D.Q.M. Microfibrous Solid Dispersions of Poorly Water-Soluble Drugs Produced via Centrifugal Spinning: Unexpected Dissolution Behavior on Recrystallization. *Mol. Pharm.* **2017**, *14*, 1666–1680. [CrossRef] [PubMed]
5. Hussain, A.; Nasir, S.; Hussain, F.; Abbas, N.; Bukhari, N.I.; Arshad, M.S.; Mudassir, J.; Latif, S.; Ali, A. Improved Dissolution Rate of Oxcarbazepine by Centrifugal Spinning: In-Vitro and In-Vivo Implications. *Proceedings* **2021**, *78*, 7. [CrossRef]
6. Raimi-Abraham, B.T.; Mahalingam, S.; Davies, P.J.; Edirisinghe, M.; Craig, D.Q.M. Development and Characterization of Amorphous Nanofiber Drug Dispersions Prepared Using Pressurized Gyration. *Mol. Pharm.* **2015**, *12*, 3851–3861. [CrossRef]
7. Bhujbal, S.V.; Mitra, B.; Jain, U.; Gong, Y.; Agrawal, A.; Karki, S.; Taylor, L.S.; Kumar, S.; Zhou, Q. Pharmaceutical Amorphous Solid Dispersion: A Review of Manufacturing Strategies. *Acta Pharm. Sin. B* **2021**, *11*, 2505–2536. [CrossRef] [PubMed]
8. Mehta, P.; Rasekh, M.; Patel, M.; Onaiwu, E.; Nazari, K.; Kucuk, I.; Wilson, P.B.; Arshad, M.S.; Ahmad, Z.; Chang, M.W. Recent Applications of Electrical, Centrifugal, and Pressurised Emerging Technologies for Fibrous Structure Engineering in Drug Delivery, Regenerative Medicine and Theranostics. *Adv. Drug Delivery Rev.* **2021**, *175*, 113823. [CrossRef] [PubMed]
9. Ansari, M.J. An Overview of Techniques for Multifold Enhancement in Solubility of Poorly Soluble Drugs. *Curr. Issues Pharm. Med. Sci.* **2019**, *32*, 203–209. [CrossRef]
10. Nambiar, A.G.; Singh, M.; Mali, A.R.; Serrano, D.R.; Kumar, R.; Healy, A.M.; Agrawal, A.K.; Kumar, D. Continuous Manufacturing and Molecular Modeling of Pharmaceutical Amorphous Solid Dispersions. *AAPS PharmSciTech* **2022**, *23*, 249. [CrossRef] [PubMed]

11. Pattnaik, S.; Swain, K.; Ramakrishna, S. Optimal Delivery of Poorly Soluble Drugs using Electrospun Nanofiber Technology: Challenges, State of the Art, and Future Directions. *Wiley Interdisc. Rev. Nanomed. Nanobiotechnol.* **2022**, e1859. [CrossRef] [PubMed]
12. Illangakoon, U.E.; Nazir, T.; Williams, G.R.; Chatterton, N.P. Mebeverine-loaded Electrospun Nanofibers: Physicochemical Characterization and Dissolution Studies. *J. Pharm. Sci.* **2014**, *103*, 283–292. [CrossRef]
13. Brettmann, B.K.; Cheng, K.; Myerson, A.S.; Trout, B.L. Electrospun Formulations Containing Crystalline Active Pharmaceutical Ingredients. *Pharm. Res.* **2013**, *30*, 238–246. [CrossRef] [PubMed]
14. Hamori, M.; Nagano, K.; Kakimoto, S.; Naruhashi, K.; Kiriyama, A.; Nishimura, A.; Shibata, N. Preparation and Pharmaceutical Evaluation of Acetaminophen Nano-fiber Tablets: Application of a Solvent-based Electrospinning Method for Tableting. *Biomed. Pharmacother.* **2016**, *78*, 14–22. [CrossRef] [PubMed]
15. Poller, B.; Strachan, C.; Broadbent, R.; Walker, G.F. A Minitablet Formulation Made from Electrospun Nanofibers. *Eur. J. Pharm. Biopharm.* **2017**, *114*, 213–220. [CrossRef]
16. Vlachou, M.; Kikionis, S.; Siamidi, A.; Kyriakou, S.; Tsotinis, A.; Ioannou, E.; Roussis, V. Development and Characterization of Eudragit®-based Electrospun Nanofibrous Mats and Their Formulation into Nanofiber Tablets for the Modified Release of Furosemide. *Pharmaceutics* **2019**, *11*, 480. [CrossRef]
17. Démuth, B.; Farkas, A.; Szabó, B.; Balogh, A.; Nagy, B.; Vágó, E.; Vigh, T.; Tinke, A.P.; Kazsu, Z.; Demeter, Á.; et al. Development and Tableting of Directly Compressible Powder from Electrospun Nanofibrous Amorphous Solid Dispersion. *Adv. Powder Technol.* **2017**, *28*, 1554–1563. [CrossRef]
18. Vigh, T.; Démuth, B.; Balogh, A.; Galata, D.L.; Van Assche, I.; Mackie, C.; Vialpando, M.; Van Hove, B.; Psathas, P.; Borbás, E.; et al. Oral Bioavailability Enhancement of Flubendazole by Developing Nanofibrous Solid Dosage Forms. *Drug Dev. Ind. Pharm.* **2017**, *43*, 1126–1133. [CrossRef]
19. Casian, T.; Borbás, E.; Ilyés, K.; Démuth, B.; Farkas, A.; Rapi, Z.; Bogdan, C.; Iurian, S.; Toma, V.; Ştiufiuc, R.; et al. Electrospun Amorphous Solid Dispersions of Meloxicam: Influence of Polymer Type and Downstream Processing to Orodispersible Dosage Forms. *Int. J. Pharm.* **2019**, *569*, 118593. [CrossRef]
20. Vass, P.; Hirsch, E.; Kóczián, R.; Démuth, B.; Farkas, A.; Fehér, C.; Szabó, E.; Németh, Á.; Andersen, S.K.; Vigh, T.; et al. Scaled-up Production and Tableting of Grindable Electrospun Fibers Containing a Protein-type Drug. *Pharmaceutics* **2019**, *11*, 329. [CrossRef]
21. Pisani, S.; Friuli, V.; Conti, B.; Bruni, G.; Maggi, L. Tableted Hydrophilic Electrospun Nanofibers to Promote Meloxicam Dissolution Rate. *J. Drug Deliv. Sci. Technol.* **2021**, *66*, 102878. [CrossRef]
22. Friuli, V.; Pisani, S.; Conti, B.; Bruni, G.; Maggi, L. Tablet Formulations of Polymeric Electrospun Fibers for the Controlled Release of Drugs with pH-dependent Solubility. *Polymers* **2022**, *14*, 2127. [CrossRef]
23. Fülöp, G.; Balogh, A.; Farkas, B.; Farkas, A.; Szabó, B.; Démuth, B.; Borbás, E.; Nagy, Z.K.; Marosi, G. Homogenization of Amorphous Solid Dispersions Prepared by Electrospinning in Low-dose Tablet Formulation. *Pharmaceutics* **2018**, *10*, 114. [CrossRef] [PubMed]
24. Szabó, E.; Záhonyi, P.; Gyürkés, M.; Nagy, B.; Galata, D.L.; Madarász, L.; Hirsch, E.; Farkas, A.; Andersen, S.K.; Vígh, T.; et al. Continuous Downstream Processing of Milled Electrospun Fibers to Tablets Monitored by Near-Infrared and Raman Spectroscopy. *Eur. J. Pharm. Sci.* **2021**, *164*, 105907. [CrossRef] [PubMed]
25. Partheniadis, I.; Athanasiou, K.; Laidmäe, I.; Heinämäki, J.; Nikolakakis, I. Physicomechanical Characterization and Tablet Compression of Theophylline Nanofibrous Mats Prepared by Conventional and Ultrasound Enhanced Electrospinning. *Int. J. Pharm.* **2022**, *616*, 121448. [CrossRef] [PubMed]
26. Démuth, B.; Farkas, A.; Balogh, A.; Bartosiewicz, K.; Kállai-Szabó, B.; Bertels, J.; Vigh, T.; Mensch, J.; Verreck, G.; Van Assche, I.; et al. Lubricant-induced Crystallization of Itraconazole from Tablets Made of Electrospun Amorphous Solid Dispersion. *J. Pharm. Sci.* **2016**, *105*, 2982–2988. [CrossRef]
27. Sebe, I.; Bodai, Z.; Eke, Z.; Kállai-Szabó, B.; Szabó, P.; Zelkó, R. Comparison of Directly Compressed Vitamin B12 Tablets Prepared from Micronized Rotary-spun Microfibers and Cast Films. *Drug Dev. Ind. Pharm.* **2015**, *41*, 1438–1442. [CrossRef]
28. Szabó, P.; Sebe, I.; Stiedl, B.; Kállai-Szabó, B.; Zelkó, R. Tracking of Crystalline-Amorphous Transition of Carvedilol in Rotary Spun Microfibers and Their Formulation to Orodispersible Tablets for in vitro Dissolution Enhancement. *J. Pharm. Biomed. Anal.* **2015**, *115*, 359–367. [CrossRef]
29. Hussain, A.; Hussain, F.; Arshad, M.S.; Abbas, N.; Nasir, S.; Mudassir, J.; Mahmood, F.; Ali, E. Ibuprofen-loaded Centrifugally Spun Microfibers for Quick Relief of Inflammation in Rats. *Drug Dev. Ind. Pharm.* **2021**, *47*, 1786–1793. [CrossRef]
30. Nasir, S.; Hussain, A.; Abbas, N.; Bukhari, N.I.; Hussain, F.; Arshad, M.S. Improved Bioavailability of Oxcarbazepine, a BCS Class II Drug by Centrifugal Melt Spinning: In-vitro and in-vivo Implications. *Int. J. Pharm.* **2021**, *604*, 120775. [CrossRef]
31. Miller, D.A.; DiNunzio, J.C.; Yang, W.; McGinity, J.W.; Williams, R.O. Enhanced in vivo Absorption of Itraconazole via Stabilization of Supersaturation Following Acidic-to-Neutral pH Transition. *Drug Dev. Ind. Pharm.* **2008**, *34*, 890–902. [CrossRef] [PubMed]
32. Janssen-Cilag Ltd. Sporanox 100 mg Capsules SmPC. Available online: https://www.medicines.org.uk/emc/product/1513/smpc (accessed on 20 October 2022).
33. Fernández-Ronco, M.P.; Salvalaglio, M.; Kluge, J.; Mazzotti, M. Study of the Preparation of Amorphous Itraconazole Formulations. *Cryst. Growth Des.* **2015**, *15*, 2686–2694. [CrossRef]
34. Rowe, R.C.; Sheskey, P.J.; Quinn, M.E. *Handbook of Pharmaceutical Excipients*, 6th ed.; Pharmaceutical Press: London, UK, 2009.

35. Meng, F.; Dave, V.; Chauhan, H. Qualitative and Quantitative Methods to Determine Miscibility in Amorphous Drug-polymer Systems. *Eur. J. Pharm. Sci.* **2015**, *77*, 106–111. [CrossRef] [PubMed]
36. Six, K.; Verreck, G.; Peeters, J.; Binnemans, K.; Berghmans, H.; Augustijns, P.; Kinget, R.; Van den Mooter, G. Investigation of Thermal Properties of Glassy Itraconazole: Identification of a Monotropic Mesophase. *Thermochim. Acta* **2001**, *376*, 175–181. [CrossRef]
37. Han, Y.R.; Lee, P.I. Effect of Extent of Supersaturation on the Evolution of Kinetic Solubility Profiles. *Mol. Pharm.* **2017**, *14*, 206–220. [CrossRef] [PubMed]

Disclaimer/Publisher's Note: The statements, opinions and data contained in all publications are solely those of the individual author(s) and contributor(s) and not of MDPI and/or the editor(s). MDPI and/or the editor(s) disclaim responsibility for any injury to people or property resulting from any ideas, methods, instructions or products referred to in the content.

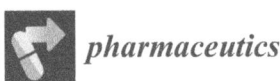

Article

The Pharmaceutical Formulation Plays a Pivotal Role in Hydroxytyrosol Pharmacokinetics

Laura Di Renzo [1], Antonella Smeriglio [2,*], Mariarosaria Ingegneri [2], Paola Gualtieri [1] and Domenico Trombetta [2]

[1] Section of Clinical Nutrition and Nutrigenomic, Department of Biomedicine and Prevention, University of Tor Vergata, Via Montpellier 1, 00133 Rome, Italy
[2] Department of Chemical, Biological, Pharmaceutical and Environmental Sciences, University of Messina, Viale Ferdinando Stagno d'Alcontres 31, 98166 Messina, Italy
* Correspondence: antonella.smeriglio@unime.it; Tel.: +39-0906765630

Abstract: Current evidence supports the use of extra virgin olive oil (EVOO) and its minor components such as hydroxytyrosol or 3,4-dihydroxyphenyl ethanol (DOPET), to improve cardiovascular and metabolic health. Nevertheless, more intervention studies in humans are needed because some gaps remain in its bioavailability and metabolism. The aim of this study was to investigate the DOPET pharmacokinetics on 20 healthy volunteers by administering a hard enteric-coated capsule containing 7.5 mg of bioactive compound conveyed in EVOO. The treatment was preceded by a washout period with a polyphenol and an alcohol-free diet. Blood and urine samples were collected at baseline and different time points, and free DOPET and metabolites, as well as sulfo- and glucuro-conjugates, were quantified by LC-DAD-ESI-MS/MS analysis. The plasma concentration versus time profiles of free DOPET was analyzed by a non-compartmental approach, and several pharmacokinetic parameters (C_{max}, T_{max}, $T_{1/2}$, $AUC_{0-440\ min}$, $AUC_{0-\infty}$, $AUC_{t-\infty}$, AUC_{extrap_pred}, C_{last} and K_{el}) were calculated. Results showed that DOPET C_{max} (5.5 ng/mL) was reached after 123 min (T_{max}), with a $T_{1/2}$ of 150.53 min. Comparing the data obtained with the literature, the bioavailability of this bioactive compound is about 2.5 times higher, confirming the hypothesis that the pharmaceutical formulation plays a pivotal role in the bioavailability and pharmacokinetics of hydroxytyrosol.

Keywords: hydroxytyrosol; pharmaceutical formulation; pharmacokinetics; bioavailability; DOPET; DOPAC; MOPET; HVA; human volunteers

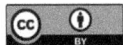

1. Introduction

The Mediterranean diet (MD) is considered a healthy and complete dietary model from a nutritional point of view [1]. Many of the beneficial effects for human health recognized and associated with this type of diet, such as longevity and the decreased incidence of chronic and inflammatory diseases [2], are due to reduced consumption of saturated fatty acids and animal proteins, a high intake of antioxidants, fibers, phytosterols, probiotics, monounsaturated fatty acids, and a correct balance of ω3/ω6 polyunsaturated fatty acids [1,3,4]. Extra virgin olive oil (EVOO), a cornerstone food of MD [5], plays a pivotal role in this dietary model thanks to its beneficial properties due to the high content of unsaturated fatty acids and phenolic compounds [6]. The main simple phenolic constituent within the EVOO is the 3,4-dihydroxy-phenylethanol (DOPET), namely also hydroxytyrosol [3,7]. Known to be the most potent antioxidant compound after gallic acid [8], hydroxytyrosol can be found in nature, mainly in olive leaves, olives, and olive oil [3]. DOPET originates from the hydrolysis of the phenolic secoiridoid oleuropein, which occurs naturally during olive ripening and olive oil production [9,10]. Indeed, the concentration of oleuropein, which is responsible for the olives' bitter taste, progressively decreases with the fruit ripening, first transforming into its non-glycosylated form by enzymatic hydrolysis, the oleuropein aglycone, and finally into elenoic acid (non-phenolic part), and hydroxytyrosol [5,11]. Due to its amphipathic features, hydroxytyrosol can be found in free form, as acetate, or as a derivative such as oleacein, oleuropein, and verbascoside, both in olive oil and in its by-products such as pomace and olive mill wastewater [3,10].

Another natural source of this phenol is wine, although concentrations are lower than those normally found in olive oil or olive leaf extracts [3,5]. In addition to exogenous sources, DOPET can form endogenously in humans starting from dopamine [12]. Several studies have shown an increase in hydroxytyrosol biosynthesis following ethanol intake [13]. De la Torre et al. [14] compared the short-term and postprandial effects of moderate doses of EVOO and wine and found that, despite the difference in the administered doses (1.7 mg and 0.35 mg for EVOO and wine, respectively), urinary recovery of DOPET was greater after wine-coadministration, thanks to the endogenous formation of this compound from dopamine in response to alcohol intake [12].

Hydroxytyrosol shows a wide range of biological activities useful for human health [6]. Its antioxidant properties have been widely demonstrated in several in vitro and in vivo models [6], as well as in clinical studies carried out both on healthy subjects and pediatric patients affected by non-alcoholic fatty liver disease (NAFLD). In the first case, it improved body composition parameters and modulated the antioxidant profile and the expression of inflammation and oxidative stress-related genes [15], whereas, in pediatric subjects, it improved the main oxidative stress parameters, insulin resistance, and steatosis [16] as well as systemic inflammation [17]. Moreover, it has been observed that combination treatment with hydroxytyrosol and vitamin E improves NAFLD-related fibrosis [18]. Hydroxytyrosol is a powerful free radical scavenger and metal chelator, and works mainly as a chain breaker by donating a hydrogen atom to peroxyl radicals [2]. In addition to this, this compound exhibits marked anti-inflammatory, antimicrobial, antiatherogenic, and antithrombotic activities [19–21]. Furthermore, it has beneficial effects on endothelial dysfunction, lipids, and hemostatic profiles and can therefore be considered an effective neuroprotective, cardioprotective, and chemo-preventive compound [21]. Moreover, recently, it has been demonstrated that hydroxytyrosol could play a pivotal role in counteract long-COVID syndrome by recovering SARS-CoV-2-PLpro-dependent impairment of interferon-related genes in the polarized human airway, intestinal and liver epithelial cells [22].

Considering this, interest in hydroxytyrosol has grown a lot in recent years [20]. By the way, it has been shown that hydroxytyrosol is safe even at high doses and that it does not exhibit any genotoxicity or mutagenicity in vitro [12]. This excellent safety profile makes hydroxytyrosol an excellent candidate for nutraceutical and food industry applications [21].

All these positive aspects, however, collide with a rather lacking literature on the best formulation of this bioactive compound. Indeed, experimental studies have shown that the intestinal absorption of hydroxytyrosol is strongly influenced by the food matrix in which it is incorporated. Making a comparison between different oily and aqueous vehicles, it has been shown that when this bioactive compound is conveyed in EVOO, its bioavailability increase [20]. However, it has been recently demonstrated that both the administered DOPET and the resulting DOPET from the hydrolysis of oleuropein and other secoiridoids, main bioactive compounds within the EVOO, suffer phase II metabolism also at the gastric level, with sulphation being the main conjugation process [23]. This observation is supported by the fact that the presence of the Sulfotransferase Family 1C Member 2 (SULT1C2) isoform was detected in the stomach [24]. This could modify, even conspicuously, the amount of free DOPET available for intestinal absorption. Furthermore, to date, there are no studies available on the pharmacokinetics of this molecule in an enteric-coated pharmaceutical formulation in which DOPET is delivered in EVOO.

Based on these considerations, the aim of the present study was to evaluate, for the first time, the DOPET pharmacokinetics by administration of a new nutraceutical product consisting of enteric-coated capsules containing 7.5 mg of DOPET conveyed in EVOO to healthy volunteers.

2. Materials and Methods

2.1. Chemicals

Ethylenediaminetetraacetic Acid (EDTA), citric acid, L-ascorbic acid, β-glucuronidase type H2 from *Helix pomatia*, LC-MS grade formic acid (HCOOH), methanol, HPLC-grade (purity ≥ 97%) DOPET, 3,4-dihydroxyphenylacetic acid (DOPAC), 4-hydroxy-3-methoxyphenethanol (MOPET) and homovanillic acid (HVA) were purchased from Merck KGaA (Darmstadt, Germany).

The pharmaceutical formulation FENÒLIA® enteric-coated capsules, kindly provided by P&P Farma (Turin, Italy), consists of extra virgin organic olive oil (*Olea Europaea* L., oleum ex fructibus), gelatin (shell component), coating agent: E1420, anti-caking agents: talc, silicon dioxide, dry olive extract (*Olea europaea* L., fructus) 15% titrated in DOPET, vitamin E (DL-alpha tocopheryl acetate), stabilizer: glycerol and pigment: E 171, E 141, E 161b.

2.2. Study Design

The study protocol, approved by the local ethics committee (Register Protocol No. 146 17/05/2018), was conducted on 20 healthy Caucasian volunteers, aged 25–60 years with BMI ranging from 19 and 25 kg/m^2, enrolled at the University hospital facility of the Clinical Research Unit of the Department of Biomedicine and Prevention, University of Tor Vergata (Rome, Italy). Two enteric-coated capsules, each containing 7.5 mg of DOPET, were administered orally. All subjects fulfilled the following eligibility criteria: non-smokers, non-alcoholics, healthy diet, and no drugs during the experimental procedure. The administration was preceded by a 4-day washout with polyphenols and an alcoholic-free diet to avoid any interference, and by a 10-h fasting period. The study was conducted in compliance with the Declaration of Helsinki, and the selected subjects agreed to the procedure by reviewing and signing the relevant, informed consensus.

Blood samples were collected into 10 mL test tubes containing EDTA from a subcutaneous vein using a permanent catheter inserted into the forearm at baseline (T_0) and 45, 90, 123, 150, 184, 247, 386, and 440 min. Samples were centrifuged at 1700× g for 10 min at 4 °C and the obtained plasma was aliquoted into test tubes containing citric acid (2 M, 10% v/v).

Urine samples were collected at baseline (T_0) and, after the intervention, at the following mean times: 3.45, 4.18, 5.14, 6.16, 8.19, 12, and 24 h in sterile, dark polystyrene tubes (100 mL) with screw caps with 10% L-ascorbic acid as a chemical preservative. Both plasma and urine samples were immediately shipped in dry ice to the Department of Chemical, Biological, Pharmaceutical and Environmental Sciences, University of Messina (Italy) for chemical analyses, stored at −80 °C and processed within 48 h.

2.3. Sample Preparation

Plasma and urine samples were processed, before and after hydrolysis, according to Alemán-Jiménez et al. [20], with some modifications. Briefly, plasma and urine samples were thawed at room temperature and centrifuged (10,000× g for 5 min). Sample supernatants (100 and 400 µL, respectively) were hydrolyzed by incubation with 300 UI (plasma) and 1500 UI (urine) of β-glucuronidase from *Helix pomatia* for 2 h at 37 °C, clarified with 200 µL of MeOH/HCl (0.2 M) and centrifuged at 10,000× g for 5 min. An SPE clean-up step, by using Strata X-AW cartridges (Phenomenex, Torrance, CA, USA) mounted on VacElut Cartridge Manifolds (Agilent Technologies, Inc., Santa Clara, CA, USA), was carried out. Cartridges were conditioned and equilibrated with 2 mL of MeOH/HCOOH (98:2, v/v) and 2 mL of water/HCOOH (98:2, v/v), respectively. After sample loading, SPE cartridges were washed with water/HCOOH (98:2, v/v). Analytes were eluted with 1 mL of MeOH/HCOOH (98:2, v/v) and dried by a gentle stream of nitrogen at room temperature. Extracts were recovered with 200 µL of the mobile phase used for the LC-DAD-ESI-MS/MS analyses (see Section 2.4). Quality control samples were prepared by spiking DOPET and metabolites (DOPAC, HVA, and MOPET) in baseline control plasma and urine samples at two different concentrations (1.2 ng/mL and 5.3 ng/mL) correspondent to the limit of quantification (LOQ) in plasma and urine samples, respectively. Both precision (CV < 10%) and accuracy (≥90%) recorded in three replicates were acceptable according to ICH and FDA guidelines.

2.4. Quali-Quantitative Determination of DOPET and Metabolites by LC-DAD-ESI-MS/MS

Plasma and urinary DOPET and metabolites were analyzed by LC-DAD-ESI-MS/MS (Agilent Technologies, Inc., Santa Clara, CA, USA). Chromatographic analysis was carried out by a Luna Omega PS C18 column (150 mm × 2.1 mm, 5 μm; Phenomenex, Torrance, CA, USA) at 25 °C by using a mobile phase consisting of 0.1% HCOOH (Solvent A) and methanol (Solvent B) according to the following elution program: 0–18 min, 5% B; 18–21 min, 95% B; 21–30 min, 5% B; 30–35 min, 5%. The injection volume was 10 μL, and the flow rate was 0.4 mL/min. The UV–Vis spectra were recorded, ranging from 190 to 400 nm, and chromatograms were acquired at 280 nm. The experimental parameters of the mass spectrometer (ion trap, model 6320, Agilent Technologies, Santa Clara, CA, USA) equipped with an electrospray ionization interface operating in the negative (ESI−) and positive (ESI+) ionization mode were set as follows: 3.5 kV capillary voltage, 40 psi nebulizer (N2) pressure, 350 °C drying gas temperature, 9 L/min drying gas flow, and 40 V skimmer voltage. The acquisition was carried out in full-scan mode (90–1000 m/z). Mass spectra were acquired using a fragmentation energy of 1.2 V (MS/MS). Data were acquired by Agilent ChemStation software version B.01.03 and Agilent trap control software version 6.2. Quantification was carried out by building external calibration curves of commercially available reference standards (see Section 2.1).

3. Results

In this study, a new pharmaceutical formulation containing 7.5 mg of DOPET conveyed in EVOO was administered orally to 20 healthy volunteers. The enrolled subjects' features are shown in Table 1.

Table 1. Features of enrolled healthy subjects.

Parameters	Values
Participants	20
Weight (kg)	65.1 ± 2.4
Height (cm)	169.2 ± 4.0
BMI (kg/m^2)	22.8 ± 1.0
Age (years)	49.6 ± 5.9
Sex (M/F)	9/11

Values were expressed as mean ± standard deviation (n = 20) for continuous variables. Abbreviations: Body Mass Index (BMI).

The quali-quantitative determinations of free DOPET and metabolites were carried out by LC-DAD-ESI-MS/MS analysis (Table 2) on plasma and urine samples after oral administration of 2 cps/day, corresponding to 15 mg or 97.3 μmole of DOPET. The LC-DAD-ESI-MS/MS parameters are shown in Table 2.

Table 2. LC-DAD-ESI-MS/MS parameters for the quali-quantitative determination of hydroxytyrosol (3,4-dihydroxy-phenylethanol, DOPET), 3,4-dihydroxyphenylacetic acid (DOPAC), 4-Hydroxy-3-methoxyphenethanol (MOPET) and homovanillic acid (HVA) in plasma and urine samples.

Analyte	RT (min)	ESI Mode	[M-H]$^-$/[M-H]$^+$ (m/z)	MS/MS (m/z)	λ_{max} (nm)
DOPAC	3.263	Positive	169/	123	280
DOPET	4.042	Negative	153/	123	280
HVA	5.054	Positive	/183	137	280
MOPET	5.431	Positive	/169	151	280

Three phase I metabolites were identified in plasma samples ($T_{0–440\ min}$): DOPAC, HVA, and MOPET. Moreover, sulfo-conjugated and glucurono-conjugated phase II derivatives have also been identified. As is possible to observe from Figure 1A,B, the chromatographic separation did not show any overlap between DOPET and metabolites, and no interference was found, at the retention times of analytes, from plasma and urine constituents.

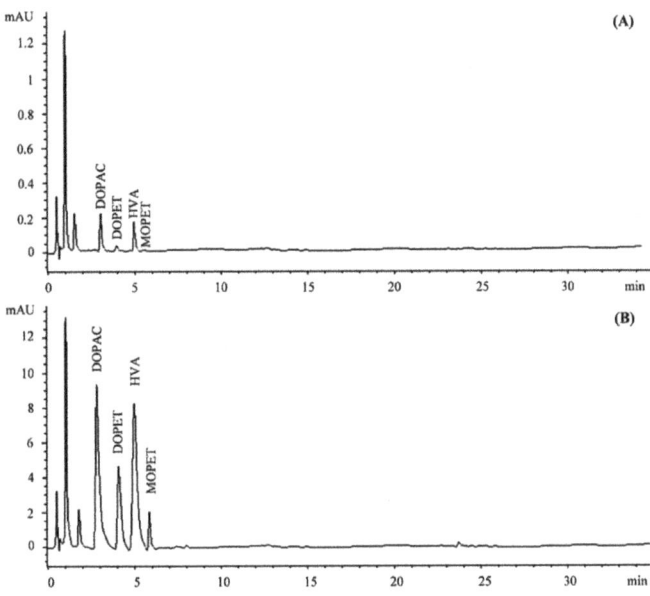

Figure 1. Representative chromatograms of plasma (**A**) and urine (**B**) samples acquired at 280 nm. DOPAC, 3,4-dihydroxyphenylacetic acid; DOPET, 3,4-dihydroxy-phenylethanol; homovanillic acid (HVA); 4-hydroxy-3-methoxy-phenylethanol (MOPET).

The plasma concentration versus time profiles of free DOPET, following ingestion of 2 cps containing 15 mg DOPET conveyed in EVOO, was analyzed by a non-compartmental approach using Phoenix-WinNonLin software (Certara, St. Louis, MO, USA). The results are shown in Figure 2.

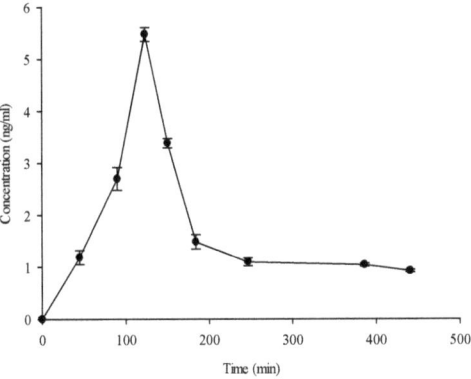

Figure 2. Mean plasma concentration-time profile after oral dose (15 mg) of hydroxytyrosol (3,4-dihydroxy-phenylethanol, DOPET). Results represent the concentration (ng/mL) expressed as mean ± standard deviation ($n = 20$).

The mean plasma concentration-time profile shows C_{max} and T_{max} values of 5.48 ng/mL and 123 min, respectively. The T_{max} value found is compatible with a gastro-resistant formulation, considering that gastric emptying occurs in about two hours. Using the time-course values, other pharmacokinetics parameters such as half-life time ($T_{1/2}$), the area under the curve ($AUC_{0-440\,min}$), AUC from T_0 to T_∞ ($AUC_{0-\infty}$), AUC extrapolated_predicted (AUC_{extrap_pred}), the concentration at T_{last} (440 min) (C_{last}), and first-order rate constant associated with the terminal (log-linear) portion of the curve (K_{el}) were calculated (Table 3). The $AUC_{0-440\,min}$ represents the time-averaged concentration of free DOPET circulating in the plasma compartment in the time-lapse, taking into account for pharmacokinetic study.

On the contrary, $AUC_{0-\infty}$ is the AUC from time 0 extrapolated to infinite time. This parameter is calculated using the following equation:

$$AUC_{0-\infty} = AUC_{0-440} + AUC_{440-\infty}$$

Assuming that DOPET is eliminated mono-exponentially after the last measurable concentration, and that no other process than elimination is involved, the terminal elimination rate of DOPET can be accurately estimated from the elimination constant calculated with the experimental data. This elimination rate is not affected by time or plasma concentrations of DOPET. Furthermore, assuming that other processes such as absorption and distribution in the terminal phase of the pharmacokinetic process are not involved, we can treat the extrapolated portion of the AUC like an IV bolus dose. Considering this, the AUC_{0-440} min can be calculated as the following:

$$AUC_{440-\infty} = \frac{C_{last}}{K_{el}}$$

This extrapolated AUC is then added to the observed AUC to give the total AUC value.

The small difference recorded between the $AUC_{0-440\,min}$ and $AUC_{0-\infty}$ shows that the adopted time course is enough to investigate the DOPET pharmacokinetic behavior in humans, because it highlights that, at $T_{440\,min}$, most of the free DOPET has been withdrawn from systemic circulation. For this purpose, another key parameter to calculate is the AUC_{extrap_pred} (%), the fraction of the total AUC that is due to the extrapolated AUC. Because the AUC_{extrap_pred} (%) value recorded in the present study was below 20% (mean value 18.23%), it indicates that sufficient sampling has been made for an accurate estimation of the elimination rate constant and the observed AUC.

Finally, it is possible to observe from Table 3 that, for each pharmacokinetic parameter considered, interindividual variability was recorded, although it was ≤10%.

According to what has been previously made for plasma samples, also the LC-DAD-ESI-MS/MS analyses of DOPET and metabolites in urine samples were performed both before and after hydrolysis. Figure 3 shows the mean concentration (μM)-time profile of DOPET and metabolites in urine samples after a DOPET oral dose of 15 mg (97.3 μmole).

In addition to free metabolites, sulfo-conjugated and glucurono-conjugated derivatives were also identified (Figure 3). Already from this figure, it is possible to observe as the sulfo-conjugated derivatives are the most abundant excreted metabolites followed by HVA, glucurono-conjugated derivatives, DOPAC, DOPET, and MOPET. Furthermore, it is possible to observe that the peak concentration of the parent compound and all identified metabolites, was reached approximately 6 h after DOPET administration, with 19.46, 18.39, 11.48, 9.93, 4.67, and 0.44 μmole as mean peak, respectively. Finally, expressing the cumulative results of metabolites distribution in urine (24 h) in terms of mean relative area percentage with respect to all identified and unidentified compounds (Figure 4), results do not change and, according to what mentioned above, sulfo-conjugated derivatives were found the most representative metabolites (31.32%), followed by HVA (28.58%), glucurono-conjugated derivatives (17.60%), DOPAC (13.48%), DOPET and MOPET (8.49% and 0.94%, respectively).

Table 3. Pharmacokinetic parameters (mean ± standard deviation) in humans following oral administration of 15 mg of hydroxytyrosol (3,4-dihydroxy-phenylethanol, DOPET) (n = 20).

Formulation	Subject	$T_{1/2}$ (min)	T_{max} (min)	C_{max} (ng/mL)	AUC_{0-t} (min*ng/mL)	$AUC_{0-\infty}$ (min*ng/mL)	$AUC_{t-\infty}$ (min*ng/mL)	AUC_{extrap_pred} (%)	C_{last} (ng/mL)	K_{el} (1/min)
Cps	1	149.933	123.000	5.294	712.679	892.913	157.173	19.306	0.761	0.005
	2	150.601	123.000	5.339	723.268	890.490	140.285	18.416	0.758	0.005
	3	148.323	123.000	5.478	695.670	880.506	149.079	17.557	0.732	0.005
	4	147.841	123.000	5.455	747.088	884.379	153.415	17.838	0.741	0.004
	5	149.380	123.000	5.398	706.174	902.077	154.248	17.937	0.744	0.005
	6	148.145	123.000	5.488	723.391	881.723	186.829	17.663	0.766	0.005
	7	151.791	123.000	5.610	776.967	902.792	158.029	17.517	0.730	0.005
	8	149.106	123.000	5.636	721.224	883.552	169.367	17.964	0.750	0.004
	9	151.339	123.000	5.547	744.207	877.017	157.389	17.496	0.761	0.005
	10	151.423	123.000	5.437	693.288	928.467	155.505	18.052	0.713	0.005
	11	150.435	123.000	5.492	693.742	889.982	173.295	18.456	0.734	0.005
	12	147.188	123.000	5.319	687.641	900.942	149.048	17.905	0.780	0.005
	13	145.501	123.000	5.540	730.696	869.484	124.409	18.387	0.731	0.005
	14	151.564	123.000	5.388	785.410	906.364	147.764	18.551	0.693	0.005
	15	147.207	123.000	5.650	723.804	892.232	181.822	18.185	0.751	0.005
	16	150.346	123.000	5.640	714.127	930.630	159.252	19.351	0.769	0.005
	17	147.919	123.000	5.502	716.517	907.057	180.365	18.262	0.735	0.005
	18	150.308	123.000	5.560	702.227	908.825	163.785	18.656	0.712	0.005
	19	152.516	123.000	5.548	728.582	881.112	155.566	18.511	0.748	0.005
	20	143.372	123.000	5.531	732.654	918.608	184.160	18.595	0.742	0.005
	N	20	20	20	20	20	20	20	20	20
	Mean	149.212	123.000	5.493	722.968	896.457	160.039	18.230	0.743	0.005
	SD	2.299	0.000	0.106	25.857	16.814	15.649	0.528	0.021	0.000
	CV%	1.541	0.000	1.928	3.576	1.876	9.778	2.895	2.859	6.282

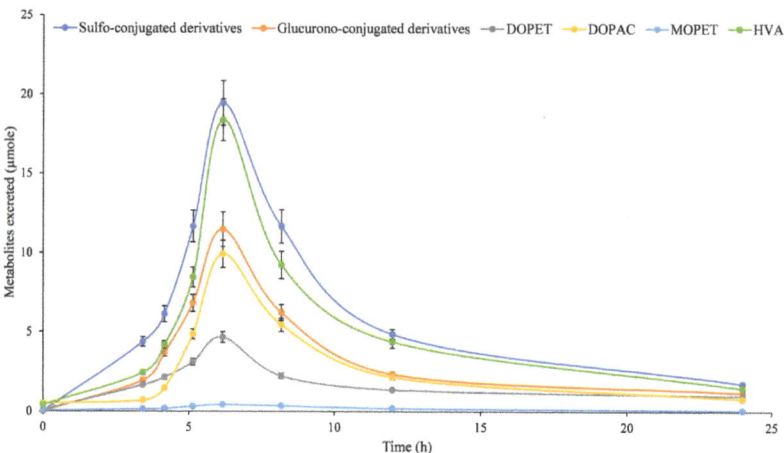

Figure 3. Mean concentration-time profile of metabolites present in urine after an oral dose (15 mg, 97.3 μmole) of hydroxytyrosol (3,4-dihydroxy-phenylethanol, DOPET). Results were expressed as mean amount (μmole) ± standard deviation (n = 20). DOPAC, 3,4-dihydroxyphenylacetic acid; DOPET, 3,4-dihydroxy-phenylethanol; homovanillic acid (HVA); 4-hydroxy-3-methoxy-phenylethanol (MOPET).

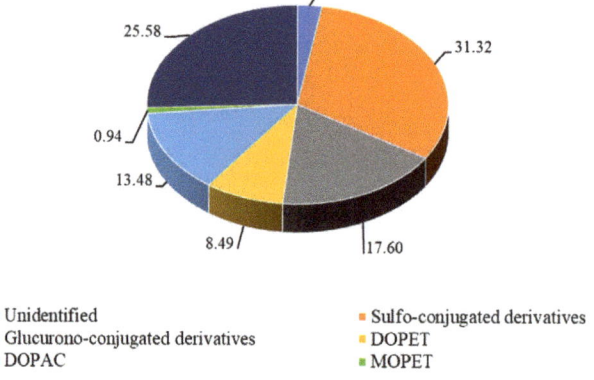

Figure 4. Cumulative percentage (24 h) of metabolites present in urine after oral dose (15 mg, 97.3 μmole) of hydroxytyrosol (3,4-dihydroxy-phenylethanol, DOPET). Results were expressed as mean relative area percentage (%) with respect to all identified and unidentified compounds. DOPAC, 3,4-dihydroxyphenylacetic acid; DOPET, 3,4-dihydroxy-phenylethanol; homovanillic acid (HVA); 4-hydroxy-3-methoxy-phenylethanol (MOPET).

Considering the results obtained in the present study, we can therefore predict, for the investigated formulation containing DOPET conveyed in EVOO, the following metabolic pathway shown in Figure 5.

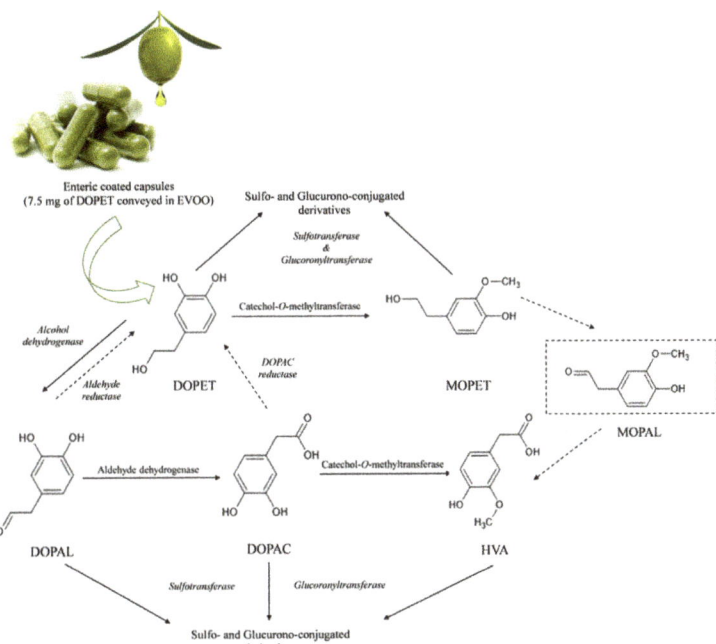

Figure 5. Human metabolic pathways of hydroxytyrosol (3,4-dihydroxy-phenylethanol, DOPET) conveyed in extra virgin olive oil (EVOO) and administered orally as enteric-coated capsules. 4-Hydroxy-3-methoxy-phenylethanol (MOPET); 3-methoxy-4-hydroxyphenylacetaldehyde (MOPAL); homovanillic acid (HVA); 3,4-dihydroxyphenylacetic acid (DOPAC); 3,4-Dihydroxyphenylacetaldehyde (DOPAL).

4. Discussion

Before discussing the pharmacokinetics of hydroxytyrosol, a premise must be made about the physical and chemical features of olive polyphenols (OP). They are structurally heterogeneous compounds with different polarities that influence their intestinal absorption. Specifically, DOPET is absorbed in the intestine by passive diffusion because of its amphiphilic properties. On the contrary, oleuropein, another abundant olive polyphenol, in its free form, is less absorbed by the enterocyte because of its hydrophobic structure and greater molecular weight. This implies that it can be degraded to DOPET [25] because of biotransformation during digestion and absorption processes, thereby raising the bioavailable content of DOPET and, in part, reaching the large intestine, where it is degraded by colonic microflora [26].

Recently, clinical trials to evaluate the pharmacokinetics of OP have increased. Accordingly, to give a clear picture in this sense, only the literature concerning human studies was discussed in the present study to identify the advantages or disadvantages deriving from a specific pharmaceutical formulation.

Gonzalez-Santiago et al. [27] analyzed the plasma concentrations of free DOPET in 10 subjects (8 males and 2 females, middle age 28 years) after an oral administration of a single dose (2.5 mg/kg b.w.) of DOPET isolated by an olive mill wastewater extract. DOPET reached the maximum plasma concentration at 13 min with a C_{max} of 1.11 μM. T_{max} and C_{max} values are compatible with those observed in the present study, considering the gastro-resistant formulation that, as such, requires about two hours from administration to make the DOPET available for absorption, and the different dose administered, about twelve times greater than that used in the present study.

Kountouri et al. [28] investigated DOPET bioavailability in 7 healthy men (middle-aged 35 years) who consumed 100 g of olives containing 76.73 mg of DOPET. Quantification of OP in plasma at different times pointed out that almost all polyphenols reached C_{max} at 1 h after olive consumption, with a plasma concentration of 3.15 µg/mL. This is the only study that reports a C_{max} so high compared to the administered dose. However, it should be emphasized that since we are dealing with 100 g of olives consumed as a single dose, and since this food is very rich in secoiridoids as well as simple phenols such as DOPET and tyrosol, this concentration could be more the result of metabolic transformations involving the more complex polyphenols which occur during gastrointestinal transit. This event, indeed, significantly increases the amount of DOPET available for absorption upstream, not to mention the effect of the food matrix, which could further facilitate the delivery of the bioactive compound. Regarding the absorption of DOPET from the food matrix, Miró-Casas et al. [29] investigated the absorption of DOPET from EVOO in 6 healthy volunteers (3 males and 3 females, middle age 36 years) showing a C_{max} and T_{max} of 25.83 ng/mL and 58 min, respectively after consumption of 25 mL of EVOO.

In another intervention study carried out on middle-aged healthy subjects (five males and four females), de Bock et al. [30] quantified the bioavailability of oleuropein and DOPET after oral administration of a pharmaceutical formulation containing an olive leaf extract as a liquid or encapsulated matrix. They showed that unlike oleuropein, the bioavailability of DOPET is not influenced by the matrix by which the polyphenols are administered, obtaining an almost overlap C_{max} (56 ng/mL vs. 59 ng/mL for the capsule and liquid matrix, respectively) and only a decrease of T_{max} of about 30 min, passing from encapsulated to the liquid formulation. Furthermore, the authors observed that HT-conjugated metabolites were the primary metabolites recovered in plasma and urine after supplementation and that gender difference in the OP bioavailability was observed.

However, recently, the influence of the food matrix on the rate of absorption and bioavailability of dietary DOPET was investigated by Alemán-Jiménez et al. [20] in a double-blind study carried out on 20 volunteers, who administered a single dose of 5 mg of DOPET through diverse food matrices: refined olive oil, flax oil, grapeseed oil, margarine, and pineapple juice. Interestingly, unlike what was stated earlier, the results revealed a strong impact of the matrices on the DOPET plasma concentration. Indeed, according to our results, while the C_{max} (3.79 ng/mL) was reached after 30 min of DOPET intake conveyed in EVOO, the intake of other matrices tested did not lead to a significant increase in the DOPET plasma concentration over time.

OP metabolic processing pathways have been extensively and deeply characterized by several animal and human studies [31]. Generally, these polyphenols undergo structural changes, mainly hydrolyzation processes by either digestive fluids in the stomach or intestines or phase I metabolic reactions [32,33] followed by phase II reactions, by which they are predominantly sulfated [32,33] or glucuronidated [29,34].

Concerning human trials, de Bock et al. [30] observed that oleuropein is extensively hydrolyzed, liberating DOPET and its aglycone and leading to an increase in the DOPET bio-accessibility. Metabolic phase II reactions cause the conjugation of DOPET, leading to a resulting high presence of sulfo- and glucuro-conjugated derivatives in plasma and urine. However, this behavior seems to be strictly dependent on the different compositions of phenolic compounds in the olive leaf extracts used in each study. Indeed, Kendall et al. [35], which carried out a study on 55 healthy young adults, who were given olive leaf supplements for 28 days, showed that neither oleuropein nor DOPET was detected in urine samples after chronic or acute consumption, suggesting that oleuropein escapes acid hydrolysis. Consequently, only oleuropein glucuronidated metabolites were identified in urine.

In confirmation of the fact that the polyphenolic composition can influence the activation of different metabolic pathways, another study carried out by Rubió et al. [33] on 12 healthy volunteers, in which EVOOs with different concentrations of phenolic content were given, showed that, after absorption, oleuropein has been extensively hydrolyzed by phase I metabolic reactions, triggering phase II metabolic reactions which have led predominantly, according to our results, to HT sulfo-conjugated. This is in accordance with García-Villalba et al. [34] and Suárez et al. [32], who revealed that oleuropein and ligstroside aglycones are hydrolyzed in the gastrointestinal tract as phase I metabolism, resulting in the polar phenols tyrosol and hydroxytyrosol. These are later conjugated by II phase metabolism and then excreted. It seems that the factor which plays a pivotal role in the activation of the metabolic reactions leading to sulfate and glucuronic acid conjugation may be the OP dosage administered [36]. Regarding OP such as oleuropein, which they are not absorbed in the small intestine, this effect is remarkable, because they reach the large intestine and, once there, is quickly transformed to DOPET by intestinal microbiota, leading to greater absorption by colon enterocytes [26]. It is well known, thanks to several animal and human studies carried out over time, that OP excretion is mainly performed via the kidneys through urine, except for compounds that escape intestinal absorption, which is directly excreted through feces per se, or after chemical transformations in the gastrointestinal tract [37]. Concerning human trials, Visioli et al. [38] investigated the presence of metabolites derived from OP in urine. For this purpose, olive oils enriched with four different phenolic extracts (20–84 µg/mL of DOPET and 36–140 µg/mL of tyrosol, respectively) was administered to 6 healthy male volunteers. Results expressed as a percentage of urine excretion with respect to the dose administered showed 29–40% for DOPET and 21–24% for tyrosol in 24 h [38]. Furthermore, Khymenets et al. [39], investigating the excretion rates of phenols and their conjugates in 24 h urine after a single dose of 50 mL of EVOO, observed the same trend with the maximum recovery of olive polyphenols' metabolites, according to our results, in 6 h urine samples. Alemán-Jiménez et al. [20] also quantified the free DOPET and relative metabolites in urine samples at 24 h after treatment with a single dose of 5 mg of DOPET through diverse food matrices in 20 subjects. Once again, the DOPET intake by its natural source (EVOO), showed, according to our results, significantly higher urinary levels of DOPET compared to basal urine, whereas DOPET metabolites did not show any significant changes depending on the matrix administered. Finally, confirming once again our results, no gender differences were found. These results were also confirmed by Khymenets et al. [40], who showed that urine levels of DOPET and its metabolites, after supplementation with 5 or 25 mg of DOPET/day for one week, accounted for 21 and 28% of the DOPET administered, respectively. Furthermore, according to our results, the predominant forms of DOPET excreted in urine were sulfo-conjugated (16.88–23.36%), followed by glucurono-conjugated (4.70–5.01%) and free DOPET form (0–0.02%). Finally, regarding the use of a pharmaceutical formulation, also de Bock et al. [30] confirmed what was previously observed evaluating the excretion of DOPET metabolites after the administration of an olive leaf extract. Indeed, the analysis of the DOPET's urinary metabolites revealed the predominance of sulfo- and glucurono-conjugates, whose concentration increases in the first 8 h after ingestion.

5. Conclusions

In conclusion, what emerges from the present and previous human studies is that, in addition to the dose of treatment and nutraceutical matrix (synthetic hydroxytyrosol, leaf extract, or olive fruit extract), another critical aspect that should be considered when designing a new pharmaceutical formulation is the vehicle within the DOPET is conveyed.

According to our results, the EVOO is the best vehicle, which leads to the major absorption of DOPET, ensuring greater bioavailability, about 2.5 times greater with respect to previous results at the same dose administered. Furthermore, in this regard, our study carried out on a greater number of subjects (20 vs. 7–10 subjects) confirms a negligible individual and gender variability in the DOPET bioavailability.

Author Contributions: Conceptualization, L.D.R. and D.T.; methodology, D.T. and A.S.; software, D.T.; validation, L.D.R., A.S. and D.T.; formal analysis, L.D.R., A.S., M.I. and P.G.; investigation, L.D.R., A.S. and D.T.; resources, D.T.; data curation, A.S. and D.T.; writing—original draft preparation, A.S., M.I. and D.T.; writing—review and editing, A.S. and D.T.; visualization, D.T.; supervision, A.S. and D.T.; project administration, D.T. funding acquisition, L.D.R. and D.T. All authors have read and agreed to the published version of the manuscript.

Funding: This research received no external funding.

Institutional Review Board Statement: The study was conducted in accordance with the Declaration of Helsinki and approved by the Ethics Committee of the Calabria Region Center Area Section (Register Protocol No. 146 17/05/2018). This trial is registered with ClinicalTrials.gov NCT01890070.

Informed Consent Statement: Informed consent was obtained from all subjects involved in the study.

Data Availability Statement: The data presented in this study are available on request from the corresponding author.

Acknowledgments: The authors would like to thank all participants.

Conflicts of Interest: The authors declare no conflict of interest.

References

1. Urquiaga, I.; Echeverría, G.; Dussaillant, C.; Rigotti, A. Origin, components and mechanisms of action of the Mediterranean diet. *Rev. Med. Chil.* **2017**, *145*, 85–95. [CrossRef] [PubMed]
2. Karković Marković, A.; Torić, J.; Barbarić, M.; Jakobušić Brala, C. Hydroxytyrosol, Tyrosol and Derivatives and Their Potential Effects on Human Health. *Molecules* **2019**, *24*, 2001. [CrossRef] [PubMed]
3. Robles-Almazan, M.; Pulido-Moran, M.; Moreno-Fernandez, J.; Ramirez-Tortosa, C.; Rodriguez-Garcia, C.; Quiles, J.L.; Ramirez-Tortosa, M. Hydroxytyrosol: Bioavailability, toxicity, and clinical applications. *Food Res. Int.* **2018**, *105*, 654–667. [CrossRef] [PubMed]
4. Mazzocchi, A.; Leone, L.; Agostoni, C.; Pali-Schöll, I. The Secrets of the Mediterranean Diet. Does [Only] Olive Oil Matter? *Nutrients* **2019**, *11*, 2941. [CrossRef] [PubMed]
5. Vilaplana-Pérez, C.; Auñón, D.; García-Flores, L.A.; Gil-Izquierdo, A. Hydroxytyrosol and potential uses in cardiovascular diseases, cancer, and AIDS. *Front. Nutr.* **2014**, *1*, 18.
6. Martínez-Zamora, L.; Peñalver, R.; Ros, G.; Nieto, G. Olive Tree Derivatives and Hydroxytyrosol: Their Potential Effects on Human Health and Its Use as Functional Ingredient in Meat. *Foods* **2021**, *10*, 2611. [CrossRef]
7. Hu, T.; He, X.W.; Jiang, J.G.; Xu, X.L. Hydroxytyrosol and its potential therapeutic effects. *J. Agric. Food Chem.* **2014**, *62*, 1449–1455. [CrossRef]
8. Martínez, L.; Ros, G.; Nieto, G. Hydroxytyrosol: Health Benefits and Use as Functional Ingredient in Meat. *Medicines* **2018**, *5*, 13. [CrossRef]
9. Romani, A.; Ieri, F.; Urciuoli, S.; Noce, A.; Marrone, G.; Nediani, C.; Bernini, R. Health Effects of Phenolic Compounds Found in Extra-Virgin Olive Oil, By-Products, and Leaf of *Olea europaea* L. *Nutrients* **2019**, *11*, 1776. [CrossRef]
10. D'Angelo, C.; Franceschelli, S.; Quiles, J.L.; Speranza, L. Wide Biological Role of Hydroxytyrosol: Possible Therapeutic and Preventive Properties in Cardiovascular Diseases. *Cells* **2020**, *9*, 1932. [CrossRef]
11. Peyrol, J.; Riva, C.; Amiot, M.J. Hydroxytyrosol in the Prevention of the Metabolic Syndrome and Related Disorders. *Nutrients* **2017**, *9*, 306. [CrossRef] [PubMed]
12. Echeverría, F.; Ortiz, M.; Valenzuela, R.; Videla, L.A. Hydroxytyrosol and Cytoprotection: A Projection for Clinical Interventions. *Int. J. Mol. Sci.* **2017**, *18*, 930. [CrossRef] [PubMed]
13. Rodríguez-Morató, J.; Boronat, A.; Kotronoulas, A.; Pujadas, M.; Pastor, A.; Olesti, E.; Pérez-Mañá, C.; Khymenets, O.; Fitó, M.; Farré, M.; et al. Metabolic disposition and biological significance of simple phenols of dietary origin: Hydroxytyrosol and tyrosol. *Drug Metab. Rev.* **2016**, *48*, 218–236. [CrossRef] [PubMed]
14. De la Torre, R.; Covas, M.I.; Pujadas, M.A.; Fitó, M.; Farré, M. Is dopamine behind the health benefits of red wine? *Eur. J. Nutr.* **2006**, *45*, 307–310. [CrossRef] [PubMed]
15. Colica, C.; Di Renzo, L.; Trombetta, D.; Smeriglio, A.; Bernardini, S.; Cioccoloni, G.; Costa de Miranda, R.; Gualtieri, P.; Sinibaldi Salimei, P.; De Lorenzo, A. Antioxidant Effects of a Hydroxytyrosol-Based Pharmaceutical Formulation on Body Composition, Metabolic State, and Gene Expression: A Randomized Double-Blinded, Placebo-Controlled Crossover Trial. *Oxid. Med. Cell. Longev.* **2017**, *2017*, 2473495. [CrossRef] [PubMed]
16. Nobili, V.; Alisi, A.; Mosca, A.; Crudele, A.; Zaffina, S.; Denaro, M.; Smeriglio, A.; Trombetta, D. The Antioxidant Effects of Hydroxytyrosol and Vitamin E on Pediatric Nonalcoholic Fatty Liver Disease, in a Clinical Trial: A New Treatment? *Antioxid. Redox Signal.* **2019**, *31*, 127–133. [CrossRef]

17. Mosca, A.; Crudele, A.; Smeriglio, A.; Braghini, M.R.; Panera, N.; Comparcola, D.; Alterio, A.; Sartorelli, M.R.; Tozzi, G.; Raponi, M.; et al. Antioxidant activity of Hydroxytyrosol and Vitamin E reduces systemic inflammation in children with paediatric NAFLD. *Dig. Liver Dis.* **2021**, *53*, 1154–1158. [CrossRef]
18. Panera, N.; Braghini, M.R.; Crudele, A.; Smeriglio, A.; Bianchi, M.; Condorelli, A.G.; Nobili, R.; Conti, L.A.; De Stefanis, C.; Lioci, G.; et al. Combination Treatment with Hydroxytyrosol and Vitamin E Improves NAFLD-Related Fibrosis. *Nutrients* **2022**, *14*, 3791. [CrossRef]
19. Smeriglio, A.; Denaro, M.; Mastracci, L.; Grillo, F.; Cornara, L.; Shirooie, S.; Nabavi, S.M.; Trombetta, D. Safety and efficacy of hydroxytyrosol-based formulation on skin inflammation: In vitro evaluation on reconstructed human epidermis model. *Daru* **2019**, *27*, 283–293. [CrossRef]
20. Alemán-Jiménez, C.; Domínguez-Perles, R.; Medina, S.; Prgomet, I.; López-González, I.; Simonelli-Muñoz, A.; Campillo-Cano, M.; Auñón, D.; Ferreres, F.; Gil-Izquierdo, Á. Pharmacokinetics and bioavailability of hydroxytyrosol are dependent on the food matrix in humans. *Eur. J. Nutr.* **2021**, *60*, 905–915. [CrossRef]
21. Bertelli, M.; Kiani, A.K.; Paolacci, S.; Manara, E.; Kurti, D.; Dhuli, K.; Bushati, V.; Miertus, J.; Pangallo, D.; Baglivo, M.; et al. Hydroxytyrosol: A natural compound with promising pharmacological activities. *J. Biotechnol.* **2020**, *309*, 29–33. [CrossRef] [PubMed]
22. Crudele, A.; Smeriglio, A.; Ingegneri, M.; Panera, N.; Bianchi, M.; Braghini, M.R.; Pastore, A.; Tocco, V.; Carsetti, R.; Zaffina, S.; et al. Hydroxytyrosol Recovers SARS-CoV-2-PLpro-Dependent Impairment of Interferon Related Genes in Polarized Human Airway, Intestinal and Liver Epithelial Cells. *Antioxidants* **2022**, *11*, 1466. [CrossRef] [PubMed]
23. López de las Hazas, M.C.; Piñol, C.; Macià, A.; Romero, M.P.; Pedret, A.; Solà, R.; Rubió, L.; Motilva, M.J. Differential absorption and metabolism of hydroxytyrosol and its precursors oleuropein and secoiridoids. *J. Funct. Foods* **2016**, *22*, 52–63. [CrossRef]
24. Nimmagadda, D.; Cherala, G.; Ghatta, S. Cytosolic sulfotransferases. *Indian J. Exp. Biol.* **2006**, *44*, 171–182. [PubMed]
25. Tuck, K.L.; Hayball, P.J. Major phenolic compounds in olive oil: Metabolism and health effects. *J. Nutr. Biochem.* **2002**, *13*, 636–644. [CrossRef] [PubMed]
26. Corona, G.; Tzounis, X.; Dessì, M.A.; Deiana, M.; Debnam, E.S.; Visioli, F.; Spencer, J.P.E. The fate of olive oil polyphenols in the gastrointestinal tract: Implications of gastric and colonic microflora-dependent biotransformation. *Free Radical Res.* **2006**, *40*, 647–658. [CrossRef]
27. González-Santiago, M.; Fonollá, J.; Lopez-Huertas, E. Human Absorption of a Supplement Containing Purified Hydroxytyrosol, a Natural Antioxidant from Olive Oil, and Evidence for Its Transient Association with Low-Density Lipoproteins. *Pharmacol. Res.* **2010**, *61*, 364–370. [CrossRef]
28. Kountouri, A.M.; Mylona, A.; Kaliora, A.C.; Andrikopoulos, N.K. Bioavailability of the phenolic compounds of the fruits (drupes) of Olea europaea (olives): Impact on plasma antioxidant status in humans. *Phytomedicine* **2007**, *14*, 659–667. [CrossRef]
29. Miro-Casas, E.; Covas, M.I.; Farre, M.; Fito, M.; Ortuño, J.; Weinbrenner, T.; Roset, P.; de la Torre, R. Hydroxytyrosol disposition in humans. *Clin. Chem.* **2003**, *49*, 945–952. [CrossRef]
30. De Bock, M.; Thorstensen, E.B.; Derraik, J.G.B.; Henderson, H.V.; Hofman, P.L.; Cutfield, W.S. Human Absorption and Metabolism of Oleuropein and Hydroxytyrosol Ingested as Olive (*Olea europaea* L.) Leaf Extract. *Mol. Nutr. Food Res.* **2013**, *57*, 2079–2085. [CrossRef]
31. Visioli, F.; Bernardini, E. Extra virgin olive oil's polyphenols: Biological activities. *Curr. Pharm. Des.* **2011**, *17*, 786–804. [CrossRef] [PubMed]
32. Suárez, M.; Valls, R.M.; Romero, M.P.; Macià, A.; Fernández, S.; Giralt, M.; Solà, R.; Motilva, M.J. Bioavailability of phenols from a phenol-enriched olive oil. *Br. J. Nutr.* **2011**, *106*, 1691–1701. [CrossRef] [PubMed]
33. Rubió, L.; Valls, R.M.; MacIà, A.; Pedret, A.; Giralt, M.; Romero, M.P.; De La Torre, R.; Covas, M.I.; Solà, R.; Motilva, M.J. Impact of olive oil phenolic concentration on human plasmatic phenolic metabolites. *Food Chem.* **2012**, *135*, 2922–2929. [CrossRef] [PubMed]
34. García-Villalba, R.; Carrasco-Pancorbo, A.; Nevedomskaya, E.; Mayboroda, O.A.; Deelder, A.M.; Segura-Carretero, A.; Fernández-Gutiérrez, A. Exploratory Analysis of Human Urine by LC-ESI-TOF MS after High Intake of Olive Oil: Understanding the Metabolism of Polyphenols. *Anal. Bioanal. Chem.* **2010**, *398*, 463–475. [CrossRef]
35. Kendall, M.; Batterham, M.; Callahan, D.L.; Jardine, D.; Prenzler, P.D.; Robards, K.; Ryan, D. Randomized Controlled Study of the Urinary Excretion of Biophenols Following Acute and Chronic Intake of Olive Leaf Supplements. *Food Chem.* **2012**, *130*, 651–659. [CrossRef]
36. Kotronoulas, A.; Pizarro, N.; Serra, A.; Robledo, P.; Joglar, J.; Rubió, L.; Hernaéz, Á.; Tormos, C.; Motilva, M.J.; Fitó, M.; et al. Dose-dependent metabolic disposition of hydroxytyrosol and formation of mercapturates in rats. *Pharmacol. Res.* **2013**, *77*, 47–56. [CrossRef]
37. Motilva, M.J.; Serra, A.; Rubió, L. Nutrikinetic studies of food bioactive compounds: From in vitro to in vivo approaches. *Int. J. Food Sci. Nutr.* **2015**, *66*, S41–S52. [CrossRef]
38. Visioli, F.; Galli, C.; Bornet, F.; Mattei, A.; Patelli, R.; Galli, G.; Caruso, D. Olive oil phenolics are dose-dependently absorbed in humans. *FEBS Lett.* **2000**, *468*, 159–160. [CrossRef] [PubMed]

39. Khymenets, O.; Farré, M.; Pujadas, M.; Ortiz, E.; Joglar, J.; Covas, M.I.; De La Torre, R. Direct Analysis of Glucuronidated Metabolites of Main Olive Oil Phenols in Human Urine after Dietary Consumption of Virgin Olive Oil. *Food Chem.* **2011**, *126*, 306–314. [CrossRef]
40. Khymenets, O.; Crespo, M.C.; Dangles, O.; Rakotomanomana, N.; Andres-Lacueva, C.; Visioli, F. Human Hydroxytyrosol's Absorption and Excretion from a Nutraceutical. *J. Funct. Foods* **2016**, *23*, 278–282. [CrossRef]

Disclaimer/Publisher's Note: The statements, opinions and data contained in all publications are solely those of the individual author(s) and contributor(s) and not of MDPI and/or the editor(s). MDPI and/or the editor(s) disclaim responsibility for any injury to people or property resulting from any ideas, methods, instructions or products referred to in the content.

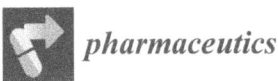

Article

Thermoresponsive Azithromycin-Loaded Niosome Gel Based on Poloxamer 407 and Hyaluronic Interactions for Periodontitis Treatment

Kunchorn Kerdmanee [1,2], Thawatchai Phaechamud [3] and Sucharat Limsitthichaikoon [1,*]

[1] Department of Pharmaceutical Technology, College of Pharmacy, Rangsit University, Pathum Thani 12000, Thailand
[2] Department of Periodontics, College of Dental Medicine, Rangsit University, Pathum Thani 12000, Thailand
[3] Department of Pharmaceutical Technology, Faculty of Pharmacy, Silpakorn University, Nakhon Pathom 73000, Thailand
* Correspondence: sucharat.l@rsu.ac.th; Tel.: +66-821415637

Citation: Kerdmanee, K.;
Phaechamud, T.; Limsitthichaikoon, S. Thermoresponsive Azithromycin-Loaded Niosome Gel Based on Poloxamer 407 and Hyaluronic Interactions for Periodontitis Treatment. *Pharmaceutics* 2022, 14, 2032. https://doi.org/10.3390/pharmaceutics14102032

Academic Editors: Gábor Vasvári and Ádám Haimhoffer

Received: 28 August 2022
Accepted: 21 September 2022
Published: 24 September 2022

Publisher's Note: MDPI stays neutral with regard to jurisdictional claims in published maps and institutional affiliations.

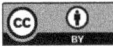

Copyright: © 2022 by the authors. Licensee MDPI, Basel, Switzerland. This article is an open access article distributed under the terms and conditions of the Creative Commons Attribution (CC BY) license (https://creativecommons.org/licenses/by/4.0/).

Abstract: Azithromycin (AZM) is a potential antimicrobial drug for periodontitis treatment. However, a potential sustained-release system is needed for intra-periodontal pocket delivery. This study focused on the development and evaluation of a thermoresponsive azithromycin-loaded niosome gel (AZG) to search for a desirable formulation for periodontitis treatment. AZG was further developed from an AZM-loaded niosomal formulation by exploiting the advantages of poloxamer 407 (P407) and hyaluronic acid (HA) interactions. The results showed that the addition of HA decreased the gelation temperature and gelation time of AZG. HA was found to increase the viscosity as well as mucoadhesive and tooth-root surface adhesive properties. The AZG solution state was injectable and exhibited pseudoplastic shear-thinning behavior. P407–HA interactions in AZG could contribute to gel strength. AZG showed 72 h of continuous drug release following the Korsmeyer–Peppas model and potentially enhanced drug permeation. The formulations apparently presented more efficient antibacterial activity against major periodontal pathogens than the standard AZM solution. AZM intra-periodontal pocket formulation and the remarkable properties of niosomes exhibited potential characteristics, including ease of administration, bioadhesion to the anatomical structure of the periodontal pocket, and sustained drug release with competent antimicrobial activity, which could be beneficial for periodontitis treatment.

Keywords: periodontal pocket drug delivery; poloxamer 407; hyaluronic acid; periodontitis; thermoresponsive niosome gel

1. Introduction

Periodontitis is a destructive disease affecting the tooth-supporting structure or the periodontium. The reported prevalence of periodontal disease is 20–50% of the global population [1]. As described in the contemporary pathogenesis of periodontitis, the disease is initiated by the invasion of periodontal pathogens. When triggered by microbes, defensive host immunity retaliates via the destructive weapon known as the inflammatory process, which aims to remove microbes. Dysbiosis (the conflict between host and microbes) emerges and is aggravated by host environmental and genetic factors. Collateral damage is inevitable on every battlefield, and, in this context, periodontium results in the destruction of the tooth-supporting bone and periodontal pocket formation [2]. Severe periodontitis can cause multiple tooth losses, which deteriorates the patient's quality of life. The gold standard of periodontitis treatment in the initial phase is mechanical debridement in conjunction with oral hygiene instruction [3]. However, this treatment modality yields limited outcomes, highlighting the need for potential adjunctive therapy [4]. The formation of the periodontal pocket is a clinical sign of periodontitis, which is the deepening of the gap between the tooth and gum. The depths of the periodontal pocket are difficult to adequately clean with self-care measures. Hence, the build-up of dental plaque biofilm containing pathogenic bacteria leads to the severe progression of periodontal disease. Although periodontal pockets are undesirable in maintaining health, this unique pathologic feature may be useful as a route for local drug delivery [5]. The active drugs could be directly delivered to the target site of the disease without passing through systemic metabolism. The local antibiotic application should avoid unwanted systemic side effects, such as nausea, vomiting, diarrhea, and bacterial resistance [6]. In the past decade, intra-periodontal pocket administration was utilized for various topical dosage forms.

Azithromycin (AZM) is a macrolide antibiotic with fascinating therapeutic properties. Apart from its susceptibility to major periodontal pathogens, its anti-inflammatory effects are well documented [7]. AZM's dual effects could be beneficial for the pathogenesis of periodontal disease in respect to bacterial elimination and the modulation of the host inflammatory response. However, the poor solubility of AZM, which is in BCS class II, could affect its bioavailability in biological tissues [8]. Drug dissolution must be improved to enable the local delivery of AZM for intra-periodontal pocket administration. In our previous study, AZM was successfully prepared in a niosomal formulation to enhance its solubility, stability, and releasing properties [9]. With the advantages of niosomal vesicles, AZM could also be delivered through the lipid bilayer of periodontal tissues to eliminate the residing pathogens. For example, in periodontitis conditions, pathogenic microbes, such as *Aggregatibacter actinomycetemcomitans* (*Aa*.) and *Porphyromonas gingivalis* (*Pg*.), were not only colonized in the periodontal pocket but also infiltrated the subjacent connective tissue level of the gingiva [10,11]. Because a potential carrier for delivering AZM-loaded niosomes into the periodontal pocket is needed, a thermoresponsive azithromycin-loaded niosome gel (AZG) was formulated based on the interactions of poloxamer 407 (P407) and hyaluronic acid (HA). Injectable gel formulations are widely used in dentistry as various kinds of dental material. Dentists are familiar with this dosage form. Thus, the gel formulation could be effortlessly administered to patients. However, for the treatment of chronic diseases involving bacterial infections, such as periodontitis, formulation development should focus on the long retention time and sustained release of drugs at the active site. The formulation, which can transform into a semi-solid state, could be advantageous for this purpose because it tolerates the dynamic changes in the oral environment. Accordingly, P407, which exhibited phase transformation properties, was chosen. P407 is a thermoresponsive co-polymer with the ability to transform into a gel state upon increasing temperature. P407 is categorized as an inactive ingredient by the FDA and, because of its biocompatibility and biodegradability, is applied in various kinds of pharmaceutical formulations, including periodontal formulations [12,13]. Poloxamer-based hydrogels have well-documented low cytotoxicity and biodegradability [14]. Another crucial property that could contribute to the retention time is the adhesion of the formulation to biological tissues [15]. However, the drawbacks of P407 are low mucoadhesiveness, a weak hydrogel structure, and its rapid dissolution in water [16]. The imperfections of P407 can be corrected by the addition of other polymers.

HA is a naturally occurring biopolymer produced by hyaluronan synthase from the plasma membrane and is commonly found in the extracellular matrix of human epithelial and connective tissues. Therefore, as a member of the glycosaminoglycan family, HA has excellent biocompatibility and non-immunogenicity. Additionally, HA is readily biodegradable by hyaluronidases and oxidative species available in the human body [17]. HA possesses favorable mucoadhesive [18] and other beneficial properties for periodontal treatment, such as anti-inflammatory and accelerated wound-healing effects [19]. Consequently, HA was included in this formulation's development. Recent studies showed that the coupling of P407–HA improved the textural integrity, rheological, and sustained drug release properties of the hydrogel matrix [15,20]. The selection of P407 and HA for AZM-loaded niosomes would favor the invention of a potential formulation with sustained antimicrobial activity for periodontitis treatment.

Therefore, the objective of this study was to develop a thermoresponsive azithromycin-loaded niosome gel for intra-periodontal pocket administration to improve the bioavailability of AZM in periodontal tissues. The physicochemical and mechanical properties of the formulations regarding the influence of P407–HA interactions were investigated to acquire a better understanding of the thermoresponsive gel based on P407 and HA. Drug release, mucosal permeation, and antibacterial studies were conducted to develop a desirable formulation for periodontitis treatment.

2. Materials and Methods

2.1. Materials

Azithromycin (AZM) was provided as a gift from Siam Chemi-Pharm (1997) Co., Ltd., Bangkok, Thailand. Poloxamer 407 (P407), cholesterol (CHL), Span® 60 (S60), Nile red (9-diethylamino-5H-benzo[alpha]phenoxazine-5-one), type II mucin from the porcine stomach (Sigma-Aldrich, St. Louis, MO, USA), and sodium hyaluronate (HA) 2.05×10^6 Da MW (SpecKare™, Nanjing, China) were purchased from local suppliers and used as received.

2.2. Preparation of Thermoresponsive Niosome Gel

AZG formulations were further developed from our previous study of AZM-loaded niosomes [9]. The niosomal suspension of AZM was fabricated by entrapping it into the niosomes of S60 and CHL utilizing the modified reverse-phase evaporation method. The amounts of S60 and CHL at the molar ratio of 3:3 (0.42 and 0.38 g, respectively, in the preparation of 30 mL niosomal suspension) and 1% of AZM were dissolved with absolute ethanol and submerged in an ultrasonic bath (POWERSONIC CP230T, Crest Ultrasonics, Ewing Township, NJ, USA) for 30 min. Then, deionized water as a secondary solvent was added and the mixture was continuously ultrasonicated for 30 min. After a homogeneous mixture was obtained, ethanol was eradicated by a rotary evaporator (N-1001, Eyela, Tokyo, Japan). The niosomal suspension was kept at 4 °C for 24 h to allow vesicle maturation. The niosomes were dyed with Nile red and we observed the vesicle staining under a confocal laser scanning microscope (DMi8, Leica, Wetzlar, Germany). Afterward, the thermoresponsive niosome gel formulations were prepared by adding HA and homogeneously mixing them with a propeller stirrer at 200 rpm (RW 20 digital, IKA, Staufen, Germany). Then, P407 was incorporated into the formulations by the cold method. Accurately weighed amounts of P407 were gradually added to the pre-mix of AZM-loaded niosomes and HA, which had been equilibrated at 4 °C. The amounts of HA and P407 varied, as presented in Table 1.

Table 1. Composition of thermoresponsive azithromycin-loaded niosome gels (AZG).

Formulation	Niosomes of Azithromycin		Thermoresponsive Gel Compositions	
	AZM (% w/v)	S60:CHL (Molar Ratio)	P407 (% w/v)	HA (% w/v)
AZG1	1	3:3	17	0.2
AZG2	1	3:3	17	1.1
AZG3	1	3:3	17	2.0
AZG4	1	3:3	18	0.2
AZG5	1	3:3	18	1.1
AZG6	1	3:3	18	2.0
AZG7	1	3:3	19	0.2
AZG8	1	3:3	19	1.1
AZG9	1	3:3	19	2.0

The mixtures of AZG formulations were stored overnight at 4 °C. The formulations were intermittently stirred until uniform mixtures were acquired. The pH of each formulation was examined using a digital pH meter (Eutech pH 700, Eutech Instruments Pte Ltd., Singapore). The prepared formulations were maintained at 4 °C in sealed containers.

2.3. Drug Content

To determine the total AZM content in the prepared formulations, one mL of each formulation was pipetted into a 10 mL volumetric flask. The volume was composed of methanol as the extraction solvent. The solution was left for 24 h. Then, the gel formulation was completely dissolved, which produced a clear solution. The extracted samples of each formulation were quantitatively investigated for drug content by a modified HPLC method (n = 3) [21]. The analysis was carried out on an HPLC system (LC-10, Shimadzu, Kyoto, Japan) equipped with a C18 column (Zorbax Eclipse XDB-C18, Agilent Technologies, Santa Clara, CA, USA). The mobile phase was composed of 80% of MeOH and 20% of 0.3 M KH_2PO_4 pH 7.56, under the conditions of a 1 mL/min flow rate, 50 °C, and 210 nm of the diode array detector. The injection volume was 20 µL.

2.4. Gelation Temperature

The phase transition temperature of the prepared thermoresponsive formulations was determined using a Brookfield viscometer (DV-II+ viscometer, Brookfield Engineering Laboratories, Middleborough, MA, USA). A sample container connected with a temperature-controlled jacket was filled with the formulations. The viscometer probe was set at 10 rpm, a fixed rotational speed, to measure the alteration in viscosity. The temperature of the system was controlled to increase from 3 °C to 40 °C, while the viscosity of the formulation was monitored. A significant elevation in viscosity at a specific temperature was observed and recorded as the gelation temperature of each formulation (n = 3).

2.5. Gelation Time

The time duration that the formulation needed for phase transformation from solution to gel state was examined by the test tube inversion method. Thin-walled scintillation glass vials were filled with the formulations and submerged in a temperature-controlled water bath, which was set to 37 °C. The phase transformation was visually observed. The total time needed for the meniscus of the formulation to stop moving upon tilting was recorded as the gelation time of each formulation (n = 3).

2.6. Gel Viscosity

The viscosity of the prepared formulations was evaluated using a Brookfield viscometer (DV-II+ viscometer, Brookfield Engineering Laboratories, USA). The sample container was connected to a temperature-controlled jacket. The viscometer was set at 10 rpm, a fixed rotational speed. The measurements of the solution and gel states of the formulation were conducted at 4 °C and 37 °C, respectively (n = 3).

2.7. Injectability of the Formulations

The prepared formulations were loaded into 1 mL syringes with a 22-gauge stainless-steel needle (0.7 mm diameter) intended for use in clinical situations. The syringe was fixed with a vertical holder aligned at the base platform of the texture analyzer (TA.XT PlusC, Stable Micro Systems, Surrey, UK). A cylindrical probe (Model P/0.5, 12.7 mm diameter) was directed downward to push the plunger rod of the syringe at a speed of 10 mm/s. The maximum force applied to inject the formulation from the syringe barrel through the needle tip was measured. The measurements were conducted immediately after each formulation was brought from the refrigerator, while the formulation was in the solution state (4 ± 5 °C).

2.8. Rheological Study

The rheological behavior of the solution state AZG was determined using the Kinexus pro rheometer (Malvern Instruments Ltd., Worcestershire, UK) with a PL20 stainless-steel parallel plate (20 mm diameter). The temperature during measurement was controlled at 4 °C. Shear stress was measured as a function of shear rate (n = 3), which varied from 0.1 to 100 s^{-1}, and the obtained data were analyzed by rSpace Rheometry software for

Kinexus version 1.75.2326. Flow profiles were fitted with various rheological equations, such as the Newtonian (Equation (1)), power law (Equation (2)), Bingham (Equation (3)), Hershel–Bulkley (Equation (4)), and Casson models (Equation (5)).

$$\tau = \eta \gamma \quad (1)$$

$$\tau = K \cdot \gamma^n \quad (2)$$

$$\tau = \tau_0 + \eta_p \cdot \gamma \quad (3)$$

$$\tau = \tau_0 + K \cdot \gamma^n \quad (4)$$

$$\tau^{0.5} = \tau_0^{0.5} + K \cdot \gamma^{0.5} \quad (5)$$

where τ is shear stress, η is viscosity, γ is the shear rate, η_p is plastic viscosity, K is the consistency index, τ_0 is the yield value, and n is the flow index.

2.9. Mucoadhesive Property

The mucoadhesion of each formulation was evaluated using the mucin disc model, with slight modifications [22,23]. The mucoadhesive force was measured with a texture analyzer (TA.XT PlusC, Stable Micro Systems, Surrey, UK). The mucin discs were prepared with 250 mg of crude mucin powder by utilizing a 13-mm-diameter die with the vacuum ring compression set at 10 tons for 30 s. One mucin disc was attached at the center of a 60 mm Petri dish, which was held to the base platform of the texture analyzer. Another mucin disc was attached to the cylindrical probe tip of the texture analyzer while the formulation was applied between the two mucin discs at 0.1 mL. The probe was moved downward until a 1 mm space between the discs was reached. The formulation was induced to form a gel state. Subsequently, the probe was directed to compress and held for 30 s, before moving upward at a rate of 10 mm/s. The maximum force used to separate the mucin discs from each other was measured as the mucoadhesion force of each formulation (n = 3).

2.10. Tooth-Root Surface Adhesion

Tooth-root surface specimens were prepared from extracted human teeth, with slight modifications from the previous study [23]. The flat-surface roots were equally sectioned into 6.6 × 6.6 mm pieces with a thickness of 1.5 mm, with a micro motor (Strong 90, Saeshin, Daegu, Korea) equipped with a diamond cutting disc. Three of the root specimens were attached to a 25 × 25 mm acrylic plate with cyanoacrylate glue (UHU Super Glue, UHU GmbH & Co. KG, Bühl, Germany). The acrylic plate was fixed at the center of a 60 mm Petri dish, which was held at the base platform of the texture analyzer. Three more root specimens were prepared in the same way and attached to an identical acrylic plate. The second acrylic plate was attached to the cylindrical probe of the texture analyzer in the same alignment. The formulation was applied between the tooth-root surface specimens. The tooth-root surface adhesive force of each formulation was evaluated by the texture analyzer in the same manner as in the mucoadhesive study (n = 3).

2.11. Texture Profile Analysis

The gel state of the prepared formulations was investigated for texture profile properties by the texture analyzer (TA.XT PlusC, Stable Micro Systems, Surrey, UK). Each formulation was loaded in a 55 mm culture dish and induced to form a gel state. The double compression method was utilized [23]. The probe of the texture analyzer was moved downward at a speed of 2 mm/s until it contacted the surface of the gel formulation. Then, the probe was directed to penetrate the gel matrix for half of its height, and the probe was withdrawn upward to the first surface-contact position. The probe was held at this position for 15 s before running the second compression in the same manner as the first. The hardness, springiness, and resilience values of each formulation were calculated from the force–time graphs provided by the texture analyzer software (n = 3).

2.12. In Vitro Drug Release Study

The drug release characteristics of the prepared formulations were investigated with the Franz diffusion cell apparatus. The dialysis membrane with a 12 kDa MW cutoff (Sigma-Aldrich, St. Louis, MO, USA) was utilized. The surface area of the diffusive interface was 176.625 mm². One mL of each formulation was accurately pipetted and applied to the donor compartment. The receptor compartment (11 mL volume) was filled with the dissolution medium, which was a phosphate buffer of pH 6.8, and magnetically stirred at 300 rpm. The system temperature was controlled at 37 °C. Samples of the medium containing the released drug were withdrawn for 1 mL at predetermined time points and refilled with the equivalent volume of fresh medium. The sink condition was maintained throughout the experiment. The quantities of released AZM in each sample were analyzed using the HPLC method, as previously described. The drug release profiles were plotted and mathematically fitted with kinetic models—for example, the zero-order (Equation (6)), first-order (Equation (7)), Higuchi (Equation (8)), and Korsmeyer–Peppas models (Equation (9)).

$$Q_t = K_0 \cdot t \tag{6}$$

$$\ln Q_t = \ln Q_0 - K_1 \cdot t \tag{7}$$

$$Q_t = K_H \cdot t^{1/2} \tag{8}$$

$$D_t / D_\infty = K_{KP} \cdot t^n \tag{9}$$

where Q_t is the amount of drug released at time t; Q_0 is the initial amount of the drug in the formulation; and K_0, K_1, and K_H are the release rate constants of the zero-order, first-order, and Higuchi models, respectively. In Equation (9), D_t/D_∞ is the proportion of drug released at time t, K_{KP} is the kinetic constant, and n is the release exponent.

2.13. Ex Vivo Permeation Study

Mucosal permeation behavior was observed using the Franz diffusion cell apparatus method. Porcine esophagus mucosa was used as a permeation membrane [24]. Fresh porcine esophagi of comparable size and appearance were purchased from the local slaughterhouse. The esophagus was resected to remove the muscle and excised to obtain mucosal specimens with sizes of 30 × 30 mm and with 2 mm thickness. The epithelium side of the mucosal membrane was positioned facing the donor compartment, whereas the connective tissue side was positioned facing the receptor compartment. The diffusive surface area was 176.625 mm². The receptor compartment was fully filled with 11 mL of phosphate buffer of pH 6.8 as a dissolution medium. The donor compartment was loaded with 1 mL of AZG formulation. The system was continuously stirred at 300 rpm at 37 °C. One mL of medium sample was collected at predetermined time points and refilled with an equal amount of fresh medium. The sink condition was maintained. Permeated drugs in the sample were quantified with HPLC, as previously mentioned (n = 3).

2.14. Antibacterial Studies

AZG formulations were evaluated for an antibacterial assay against *Aggregatibacter actinomycetemcomitans* (*Aa.*, ATCC 43718) and *Porphyromonas gingivalis* (*Pg.*, ATCC 33277) using the agar well diffusion method. The lyophilized bacterial strains were grown in tryptic soy broth (TSB, Himedia Laboratories, Mumbai, India) for 36 h at 37 °C in an anaerobic jar with GasPak (Becton, Dickinson, and Company, Sparks, MD, USA). The organism turbidity of the broth suspensions was checked using the 0.5 McFarland standard. The standardized inocula of *Aa.* and *Pg.* were prepared at the concentration of 1.5×10^8 cells/mL and swabbed on the surface of sheep blood agar (Medex Solutions Ltd., Saraburi, Thailand). A sterile cork borer was used to create an 8-mm-diameter well on the inoculated agar before introducing 0.1 mL of formulation to the well. The equivalent concentration of AZM in a phosphate buffer pH 6.8 solution-soaked disc was used for comparison. The tested samples were incubated in an anaerobic incubator for 24 h. Then, the inhibition zone of each formulation was measured (n = 3).

2.15. Statistical Analysis

All measurements were performed in a triplicate manner. All categorical variable data were evaluated as percentages (n = 3). Continuous variable data are described as mean and standard deviation (SD). A *p*-value of <0.05 was taken as statistical significance and analyzed using SPSS 13 software (SPSS Inc., Chicago, IL, USA).

3. Results and Discussion
3.1. Formulation Preparation

AZM is a potential drug for periodontitis treatment [7]. However, because of its poor water solubility, it is classified as a BCS class II drug. This may affect the bioavailability of AZM in periodontal tissue for a localized dosage form. Therefore, an appropriate delivery system is needed. In this investigation, a niosome template was applied to formulate an efficient carrier for AZM. Practically, the niosomal vesicle system increases the solubility of hydrophobic drugs, enhances drug permeation, and improves the stability of the formulation [25,26]. AZM niosomes were prepared based on the modified reverse-phase evaporation method. AZM was successfully loaded into niosomes with nano-sized particles, charge stability, and biocompatibility [9]. Figure 1a presents confocal images of Nile-red-stained unilamellar niosomal vesicles obtained by confocal laser scanning microscopy. The hypothesized niosome vesicle structure is displayed in Figure 1b.

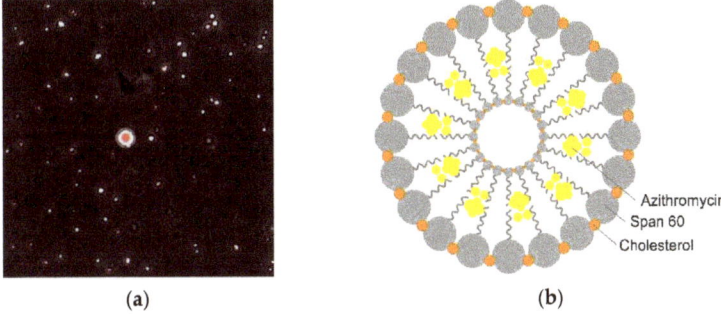

Figure 1. (**a**) Visualization of prepared AZM-loaded niosomes stained with Nile red dye that indicated lipid droplet as a red-stained vesicle under confocal laser scanning microscope; (**b**) schematic illustration of AZM-loaded niosomes prepared from cholesterol and Span® 60 (adapted from Moghassemi and Hadjizadeh 2014 [25]).

The vesicle consists of a double layer of S60, which is stabilized by CHL [25]. AZM was entrapped within the hydrophobic tails of S60. In this work, AZM-loaded niosomes were further developed into the form of a thermoresponsive gel for intra-periodontal pocket administration in clinical applications. To study the physical interaction of P407 and HA with the niosomal formulation, AZG was successfully prepared into nine different formulations by varying the concentrations of P407 (17–19% w/v) and HA (0.2–2% w/v) (Table 1). The prepared formulations appeared as a homogenous white, opaque solution owing to the appearance of the niosomal suspension prepared from CHL and S60. All formulations remained in uniformed mixtures that were not reliant on the concentrations of P407 and HA.

The measured pH of all prepared formulations was in the range of 6.89 ± 0.01 to 6.92 ± 0.04 (Table 2). The pH of the AZG formulation was slightly reduced from that of the prepared AZM-loaded niosomes, which were 7.04 ± 0.06. In periodontitis conditions, the pH of the periodontal pocket could decrease from the mean value of 6.92 ± 0.03 [27]. Therefore, the prepared formulations should be compatible with the periodontal pocket environment, without causing irritation to the biological tissues of the patient. Drug content data revealed the percentage of loaded AZM as ranging from 93.09 ± 0.94 to

94.49 ± 0.81 (Table 2). The drug content of AZG regarded the entrapment efficiency of AZM-loaded niosomes.

Table 2. Physicochemical properties of AZG formulations (mean ± SD, n = 3).

Physical Properties	Gelation Temperature (°C)	Gelation Time (seconds)	pH	Drug Content (%)	Viscosity (cps) 4 °C	Viscosity (cps) 37 °C
Formulation						
AZG1	40.33 ± 0.06	227.00 ± 3.61	6.91 ± 0.02	93.86 ± 0.81	2.24 ± 0.25	162.77 ± 5.75
AZG2	36.60 ± 0.10	171.67 ± 3.51	6.90 ± 0.03	94.02 ± 1.28	29.86 ± 0.44	194.20 ± 10.14
AZG3	36.23 ± 0.15	87.33 ± 3.06	6.92 ± 0.04	93.90 ± 1.18	124.67 ± 13.51	216.07 ± 11.47
AZG4	34.20 ± 0.10	200.67 ± 3.05	6.89 ± 0.01	94.38 ± 0.56	2.60 ± 0.52	189.03 ± 4.28
AZG5	32.43 ± 0.38	125.33 ± 2.52	6.89 ± 0.01	93.87 ± 1.23	36.98 ± 4.43	195.10 ± 6.30
AZG6	33.10 ± 0.10	85.00 ± 4.58	6.90 ± 0.01	94.49 ± 0.81	125.30 ± 6.85	241.53 ± 9.56
AZG7	32.67 ± 0.15	173.33 ± 3.06	6.90 ± 0.02	93.09 ± 0.94	2.55 ± 0.30	218.97 ± 12.62
AZG8	29.60 ± 0.20	107.00 ± 3.00	6.90 ± 0.02	93.37 ± 0.92	34.73 ± 3.23	247.23 ± 13.21
AZG9	27.83 ± 0.55	68.00 ± 2.00	6.92 ± 0.01	93.64 ± 1.37	143.53 ± 15.55	283.77 ± 3.75

3.2. Thermoresponsive Properties

AZG was designed to convert from solution to gel state after being injected into the periodontal pocket, which accounted for the addition of P407 to the composition. The phase transformation of the formulations was evaluated in terms of gelation temperature and gelation time (Table 2). The average gelation temperature varied from 27.83 ± 0.5 to 40.33 ± 0.06 °C. In the formulation groups with an equal amount of HA, the influences of P407 were observed. The incremental increase in P407 concentration significantly reduced the gelation temperature ($p < 0.01$). P407 is a triblock co-polymer composed of double hydrophilic polyethylene oxide (PEO) sandwiching with single hydrophobic polypropylene oxide (PPO) in between. Upon temperature increase, PPO groups interact with each other with van der Waals forces and form hydrophobic cores, while PEO groups build up the hydrophilic shells of micelles with hydrogen bonds to the water molecule [12]. Upon further temperature increases, micelles aggregate at a certain temperature and arrange into 3D cubic forms to achieve gel-state transformation. The increase in P407 concentration resulted in the abundance of co-polymers to facilitate micelle formation [28].

Gelation time, which represents the setting time of the formulation, was in the range of 68.00 ± 2.00 to 227.00 ± 3.61 s. Similar to the gelation temperature, the increase in P407 concentration from 17 to 19% significantly reduced the gelation time ($p < 0.01$). However, AZG1 was unable to form a gel state because the gelation temperature was higher than 37 °C. In the formulation groups with an equal amount of P407, the increase in HA concentration from 0.2 to 1.1% significantly reduced the gelation temperature ($p < 0.01$). The increase in HA from 1.1 to 2% showed no significant changes in the gelation temperature, except in the group with 19% of P407, which exhibited a significant reduction in the gelation temperature ($p < 0.01$). Moreover, the increase in HA concentration was found to significantly decrease the gelation time ($p < 0.01$). However, in the group with 2% of HA, the increase in P407 concentration from 17 to 18% only showed a trend of reduction.

The addition of HA in the formulation exhibited the tendency to reduce the AZG gelation temperature and gelation time. This phenomenon could be explained by the incorporation of high-molecular-weight HA caused by the high-density packing of HA and P407 molecules, which could facilitate the micellization process of P407 [29]. Moreover, the additives in the P407 formulation, which could form non-covalent bonds with P407, reduced the gelation temperature by decreasing the interaction of P407 with water [12,28]. In this situation, the availability of the hydroxyl and carboxyl groups of HA could form hydrogen bonds with P407 [20]. This resulted in dehydration, which could facilitate the micellization process because there were fewer water molecules to interfere with the joining of PPO in the hydrophobic cores of the micelles [30]. Another possible explanation could be that the strong hydrophilicity of HA, a powerful humectant, attracted the water fraction from the molecular chain of the poloxamer, contributing to the reduction in gelation time [31]. There are many phase transformation mechanisms that could be utilized in formulation development, such as pH, temperature, and solvent exchange. Among others, temperature is a common physiological state of the human body, and it may be regarded as the simplest triggering mechanism. The prepared formulation would readily perform phase transformation at the active site. In clinical practice, the dosage-form setting time should not take too long; otherwise, the formulation might prematurely dislodge from the periodontal pocket.

3.3. Viscosity and Injectability

The viscosity of all formulations is displayed in Table 2. At 4 °C, the formulations were in the solution state. The measured viscosity was in the range of 2.24 ± 0.25 to 143.53 ± 15.55 cps. The viscosity was found to increase significantly upon the increase in HA concentration from 17 to 18% ($p < 0.05$) and 18 to 19% ($p < 0.01$). On the other hand, the increase in P407 showed no significant changes in the viscosity as no micellization occurred.

At 37 °C, all formulations transformed into the gel state. The viscosity was elevated to the range of 162.77 ± 5.75 to 283.77 ± 3.75 cps. The increases in HA concentration were found to significantly enhance the viscosity of the gel-state AZG ($p < 0.05$). Except in the group of 17% P407, the changes in HA from 1.1 to 2% only presented an increasing trend. The influence of P407 indicated that the increase in P407 concentration from 17 to 18% showed an increasing trend but was not statistically significant, whereas the increase from 18 to 19% exhibited significantly elevated gel-state viscosity ($p < 0.05$). The higher viscosity in each formulation was influenced by the increased concentration of both P407 and HA in the formulation. Phase transformation of P407 via micellization directly affected the gel-state viscosity. The influence of HA on the increase in viscosity was clearly present in the formulation solution state as a result of the high molecular weight of HA included in AZG (2.05×10^6 Da).

Then, the solution state of all formulations was evaluated for injectability (Table 3). The force used to inject the formulation showed a similar trend to the viscosity of each formulation. However, the maximum force used to expel the formulations through the needle tip of the syringe was less than 2 N in all formulations. Therefore, all formulations were considered injectable. This should facilitate intra-periodontal pocket administration. Thus, clinicians could conveniently inject the formulation into the narrow space of the periodontal pocket with minimal pressure.

Table 3. Injectability and textural properties of AZG (mean ± SD, n = 3).

Mechanical Properties	Injectability (N)	Texture Profile Analysis		
		Hardness (mN)	Springiness (Ratio)	Resilience (Ratio)
Formulation				
AZG1	0.78 ± 0.01	249.80 ± 6.90	0.25 ± 0.01	0.002 ± 0.00
AZG2	0.94 ± 0.01	418.89 ± 18.60	0.24 ± 0.00	0.002 ± 0.00
AZG3	1.26 ± 0.06	554.96 ± 1.04	0.24 ± 0.00	0.003 ± 0.00
AZG4	1.24 ± 0.03	378.39 ± 4.14	0.25 ± 0.00	0.002 ± 0.01
AZG5	1.32 ± 0.03	472.05 ± 14.37	0.24 ± 0.00	0.002 ± 0.00
AZG6	1.50 ± 0.04	562.11 ± 0.03	0.24 ± 0.01	0.002 ± 0.01
AZG7	1.13 ± 0.03	400.60 ± 5.85	0.25 ± 0.00	0.002 ± 0.00
AZG8	1.55 ± 0.41	508.22 ± 12.91	0.24 ± 0.00	0.002 ± 0.00
AZG9	1.94 ± 0.04	617.29 ± 14.31	0.24 ± 0.00	0.003 ± 0.01

3.4. Rheological Behavior

The AZG solution state was investigated for flow behavior. The shear stress and shear rate curves of the prepared formulations are displayed in Figure 2. All AZG formulations exhibited a non-Newtonian fluid flow according to the nonlinear relationship between shear stress and shear rate. The slope of the curves indicated that the viscosity of the AZG formulations decreased upon the shear force applied, which demonstrated pseudoplastic behavior [32]. The viscosity and shear stress increases are attributed to the increased concentrations of P407 and HA in the formulation.

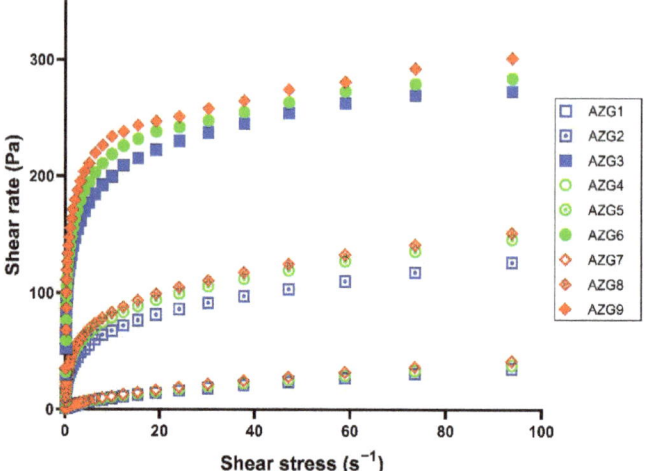

Figure 2. Shear stress and shear rate plots indicating rheological behavior of the solution state of AZG formulations (mean value).

When the plots were analyzed with rheological equations, it was discovered that rheological data were best fitted with the Herschel–Bulkley model, which is typical for non-Newtonian fluids. The flow index (n value) from the Herschel–Bulkley equation of all formulations was in the range of 0.189 ± 0.003 to 0.585 ± 0.023, which indicated shear-thinning flow behavior (n value < 1). Regarding the injectable dosage form, pseudoplastic behavior was considered desirable. Force is needed for pseudoplastic fluids to flow. When the shear force was applied to the formulation, the entangled molecular structure changed and was oriented toward the direction of the force [33]. Then, the formulation could flow through the syringe barrel and the needle tip to the target site. After injection, the formulation could spread into the complicated anatomical structure of the periodontal pocket by the injection force, which reduced the viscosity of the pseudoplastic formulation. After thoroughly spreading into the target site, the formulation should reinstitute its viscosity and remain in the periodontal pocket without dripping due to the pseudoplastic shear-thinning effect [34].

3.5. Bioadhesive Properties

Aside from the phase transformation feature, the adhesion of the formulation to the biological tissues extends the retention time of the formulation. Based on histopathology, one side of the periodontal pocket is bordered by the pocket epithelium and the other side is the tooth-root surface, and the junctional epithelium is located at the base of the pocket [35]. In this study, the bioadhesive properties of AZG were examined for both sides of the periodontal pocket territory, which involved mucoadhesion to the pocket epithelium and the adhesion of AZG to the tooth-root surface.

3.5.1. Mucoadhesion

The evaluation of the mucoadhesive properties of all AZG formulations is displayed in Figure 3. The mucoadhesive force was in the range of 0.45 ± 0.02 to 1.27 ± 0.02 N. A higher concentration of HA in the formulation resulted in a significantly greater mucoadhesive force ($p < 0.01$). In the formulation with the same amount of HA, the higher amount of P407 also significantly increased the mucoadhesive force of each formulation ($p < 0.01$). This illustrates the synergistic effect between P407 and HA on mucoadhesive enhancement. Despite being a versatile excipient, the bioadhesion of P407 alone was weak, which could affect the potential of topical formulations [16]. In poloxamer-based formulations, additives are needed in order to improve the mucoadhesive properties. In this regard, HA can be employed as a mucoadhesive biopolymer, which can help to improve the mucoadhesive properties in various dosage forms [36–38]. HA mucosal bonding can be explained with mucoadhesive theories. First, the HA molecular structure results in hydrogen bonding with biological surfaces [39]. Second, the HA coil structures entangle the mucous membranes [40]. High-molecular-weight HA possesses multiple coil structures, which accommodate the entanglement process. Therefore, high-molecular-weight HA exhibited higher mucoadhesive force than low-molecular-weight HA [18].

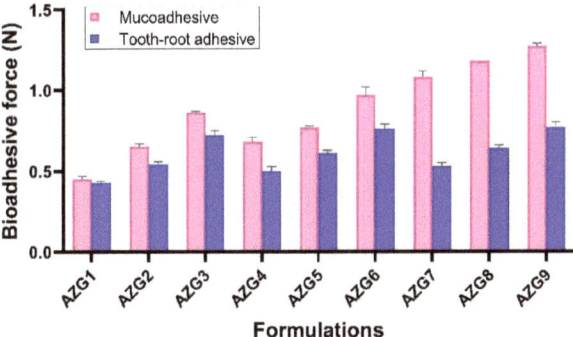

Figure 3. Bioadhesive force of AZG formulations representing adhesion to mucosa and tooth-root surface (mean ± SD, n = 3).

In this study, the synergistic effects of P407 and HA in mucoadhesion were observed. The surfactant role and the hydrophilicity of P407 during the solution state could facilitate the penetration and entanglement of HA into the mucoadhesive interface and set up stronger adhesion [41]. The oral environment is a challenging condition for dosage-form development due to the various dynamic changes, such as saliva flow and the movement of the tongue and mastication muscles. In addition, the formulation for intra-periodontal pocket administration must further withstand the gingival crevicular fluid (GCF) flow, which is secreted from the junctional epithelium at the bottom of the periodontal pocket. The reported flow of GCF is 0.33–0.5 µL/min, which tends to flush out the periodontal pocket [42]. Therefore, a formulation with high bioadhesive properties could overcome these unfavorable oral environment conditions.

3.5.2. Tooth-Root Surface Adhesion

The adhesive force of AZG on the tooth-root surface specimens was in the range of 0.43 ± 0.01 to 0.77 ± 0.03 N (Figure 3). The increase in HA concentration resulted in significantly higher adhesion ($p < 0.01$). An increase in P407 was only found to significantly enhance tooth-root adhesion in the group with 0.2 and 1% of HA; the increment in P407 from 17 to 18% significantly increased the adhesion ($p < 0.05$), while the other groups showed no significant statistical differences upon varying the P407 concentrations. In contrast to the mucoadhesive study, the results revealed that the adhesion to the tooth-root surface was mainly dependent on the concentration of HA. The mechanism of adhesion to the tooth-root surface can be explained by mechanical theory. The mucoadhesive substance filled and adhered to the rough or irregular surfaces with an increased contact area of the adhesive interface [43].

The root surface of the human tooth is covered by cementum, which is porous in structure. The formulation adhesiveness was possibly improved by penetrating and entangling the coil structures of HA into the microporosity of the root surface. In clinical situations, mucin from saliva infiltrates the root microporosity, which would further aid in the formulation's adhesion. Formulation adhesion to the tooth structure is currently being researched. According to the histopathologic features of the periodontal pocket, the pocket lining epithelium was ulcerated due to the inflammatory stage of periodontitis. The repairing epithelium was turned over at a high rate, and the shedding of the fragile epithelium layer could remove the adhered formulation from the periodontal pocket [23]. Therefore, the adhesion to the tooth-root surface prevents formulation dislodgement. Increased HA concentrations apparently increase the AZG formulation's tooth-root surface adhesion.

3.6. Texture Profile Analysis

Texture profile analysis is widely used in food sciences for characterizing textural properties, such as hardness, springiness, and resilience. These properties are also useful in the pharmaceutical technology field. Thus, many recently published studies adopted this technique to analyze invented dosage forms [22,23,30]. Gel-state AZG was investigated for its textural properties to understand the gel behavior during residence in the periodontal pocket (Table 3). Hardness is the maximum force of the first compression to penetrate the gel formulation [44]. It was discovered that the increase in HA significantly increased the gel-state hardness ($p < 0.01$). When determining the influence of P407, it was found that the increase in the concentration of P407 significantly increased the gel hardness ($p < 0.05$). However, in the 0.2 and 2% HA group, the increase in P407 from 17 to 18% only showed an increasing trend of hardness but was not statistically significant. The results indicated that the hardness of the gel state was directly dependent on the formulation's concentration of P407 and HA. Hardness represents the strength of the gel matrix, which was in the range of 249.80 ± 6.90 to 617.29 ± 14.31 mN. The gel strength of all prepared formulations was comparable to other periodontal formulation studies [23,30]. Although P407 could perform phase transformation, the obtained gel matrix is limited in its pharmaceutical application due to structural weaknesses and its rapid dissolution in water. The P407 matrix gel strength could be improved by the addition of a second polymer, or by the modification of its chemical structure [16].

In this study, the AZG matrix was reinforced by the addition of HA. The coupling of P407 and HA resulted in P407–HA interactions, which occurred by secondary bonds, such as hydrogen bonds, and the formation of large micelles embedded into the coil structures of HA, which improved the rheological properties of the hydrogel matrix [20]. The stronger matrix could be effectively maintained in the periodontal pocket. However, the gel should not be too hard, which would allow deformity inside the periodontal pocket. Otherwise, the gel state may hinder the periodontium repair process. Additionally, springiness is how well a product physically "springs back after it has been deformed". Resilience is how well a product "fights to regain its original height" [44]. It was found that springiness was in the range of 0.24 to 0.25, while resilience was low and in the range of 0.002 to 0.003. The data indicated that the gel state of all prepared formulations exhibited no bounce-back behavior. Increased P407 and HA concentrations showed no influence on the springiness and resilience. These results were in accordance with previous textural studies [23]. The AZG gel state should be able to deform within the periodontal pocket. Therefore, AZG should not interfere with periodontal tissue growth during the healing process.

All AZG formulations prepared in this study were able to perform phase transformation at physiological temperatures using different gelation times. These formulations could be used for intra-periodontal pocket administration. However, when considering its clinical application as a dental material, the long setting time would be impractical. In terms of viscosity and rheology, the formulations that had low viscosity and pseudoplastic properties could be difficult to manipulate during injection because of the free-flowing fluids. The formulations with moderate viscosity could facilitate administration by injection, enabling clinicians to control the volume of the formulation administered. In terms of the rheological aspect, the moderate-viscosity formulation needs a higher injection force, which should help to push the formulation to efficiently penetrate through the narrow gap of the soft tissue inside the periodontal pocket. Furthermore, the formulations that exhibited high mucoadhesive and tooth-root adhesion forces could potentially achieve a long retention time and sustained drug release within the periodontal pocket. Therefore, considering all the above-mentioned factors, AZG3, 6, 8, and 9 were high-potential formulations and were chosen for further examinations.

3.7. In Vitro Drug Release and Kinetic Profiles

The cumulative release plots of AZM for 72 h from AZG3, 6, 8, and 9 are displayed in Figure 4. The release profiles of the four formulations were similar in behavior and there was no lag time presented in all formulations. It was found that AZG8 exhibited the highest drug release rate, followed by AZG3, 6, and 9. In the fourth hour, AZG8's release considerably increased, becoming higher than others, and continued for 72 h. The cumulative release plots differentiate the release profile into three phases: (1) fast release at the first 12 h; (2) sustained release from 12 to 48 h; and (3) steady state of release at 48–72 h [45]. The development of AZG formulations for periodontitis treatment was expected to feature fast drug release after administration, and then maintained release, which would achieve antimicrobial activity inside the periodontal pocket for 72 h according to the AZM oral administration dosage [7]. Data from the cumulative plots revealed that all tested formulations exhibited similar release profiles with prompted and sustained AZM release for up to 72 h. However, AZG8 presented the highest release rate compared with other formulations.

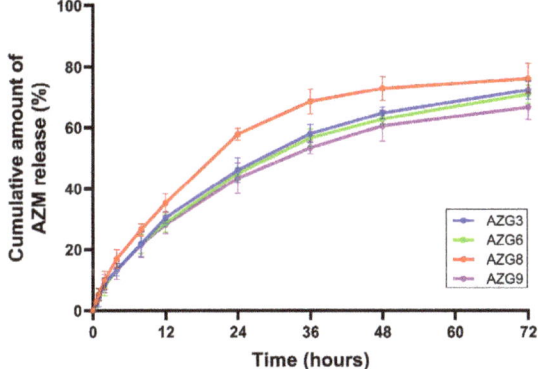

Figure 4. Percent cumulative drug release of AZG formulations. Data are mean ± SD, n = 3.

The cumulative drug release data were analyzed with various kinetic models, such as the zero-order, first-order, Higuchi, and Korsmeyer–Peppas models. The results of linear regression with the equation parameters of each formulation are displayed in Table 4. The AZG formulation release rates were best fitted to the Korsmeyer–Peppas model, which indicated that the AZG formulation drug release was provided by polymeric matrix drug delivery [46]. When considering the release exponent (n) of the Korsmeyer–Peppas equation, the n-values were in the range of $0.45 < n < 0.89$ [47]. Therefore, the drug is released in a non-Fickian diffusion manner. AZM formulation release was from both polymeric matrix diffusion and erosion [48]. The physical properties of AZG played an important role in the release behavior. AZG8, which yielded the highest release rate, consisted of 18% P407 and 1.1% HA. Decreased concentrations of P407 and HA resulted in lower hardness in the tested group. Consequently, the AZG8 gel matrix easily eroded, allowing faster drug release. A similar explanation could be applied to the releases of AZG3, 6, and 9. These formulations were equally composed of 2% HA, and the hardness of the gel matrices was solely dependent on the concentrations of P407. AZG3, with 17%

P407, had the lowest gel hardness compared with AZG6 (18% of P407) and 9 (19% of P407). Therefore, AZG3 exhibited the highest drug release rate, followed by AZG6 and 9.

Table 4. Kinetic model fitting of AZG formulations.

Kinetic Models	Zero-Order		First-Order		Higuchi		Korsmeyer–Peppas		
Formulation	K_0	r^2	K_1	r^2	K_H	r^2	K_{KP}	n	r^2
AZG3	2.699	0.964	0.032	0.982	7.756	0.944	4.797	0.741	0.998
AZG6	2.600	0.953	0.030	0.975	7.505	0.952	4.905	0.715	0.998
AZG8	3.186	0.954	0.039	0.980	9.191	0.950	5.972	0.718	0.998
AZG9	2.567	0.938	0.030	0.963	7.452	0.963	5.211	0.681	0.999

K_0, K_1, K_H, K_{KP} are equation parameters of zero-order, first-order, Higuchi, Korsmeyer–Peppas, respectively. The n values are release exponents of Korsmeyer–Peppas equation.

As mentioned in the texture profile analysis, the interactions between P407 and HA created a stronger hydrogel matrix [20]. The P407–HA hydrogel matrix could be used as a controlled-release device to sustain and slow the release of drugs because of its improved structural integrity and stability [15]. Regarding the AZM oral regimen, 500 mg is provided orally once a day for 3 days, which is considered a short course of administration [7]. Therefore, the efficient sustained-release system would be able to deliver AZM with a single application. This should encourage patient compliance and would potentially reduce dental visits for periodontal treatment, especially during the COVID-19 pandemic.

3.8. Ex Vivo Permeation Study

The amount of AZM permeated through the mucosal specimen is displayed in Figure 5. The permeated AZM was highest in AZG8, owing to its lowest HA loading compared with other tested formulations, followed by 9, 6, and 3. Therefore, the obtained molecular structure was loosely packed and combined with low textural hardness, and was also prone to erosion. Moreover, AGZ8's high mucoadhesion also contributed to the high permeation rate due to its formation of a strong mucoadhesive interface, which adhered closer to the mucous [49]. When making comparisons between AZG3, 6, and 9, which had equivalent amounts of HA (2%), AZG9 with 19% of P407 showed the highest permeation rate, followed by 6 (18% of P407) and 3 (17% of P407). The P407 concentration could be responsible for the high permeation rate. It was found that P407 increased transmucosal drug delivery [50]. Apart from this, AZG9 also possessed the highest mucoadhesive properties.

In this study, the porcine esophagus was utilized as a mucosal permeation model because of its structural properties that resemble the human oral mucosa. The preparations to obtain the standardized esophageal specimens were uncomplicated compared with the porcine buccal mucosa, which might be destroyed by mastication, are varying in texture, and have limited availability [24]. The log P value of AZM, which is 3.98, indicated that AZM is limitedly soluble in water and tends to disperse in lipids [51]. This suggests that the low number of permeated drugs was due to AZM being mostly distributed in the lipid bilayer of the mucosal specimen. This situation would be beneficial for periodontitis treatment. As a role of topical formulation, it was expected that the formulation would provide slow drug release within the periodontal pocket, deliver the drugs permeating through the periodontal pocket epithelium, and then maintain the drugs within the epithelium and connective tissue of the gingiva to eliminate the infiltrated periodontal pathogens.

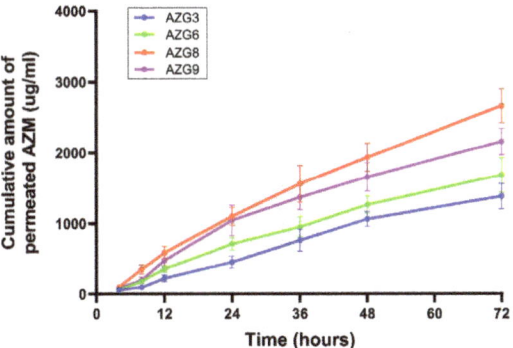

Figure 5. Cumulative permeated drug from ex vivo mucosal permeation model. Data are mean ± SD, n = 3.

3.9. Antibacterial Activity

AZG formulations were evaluated for antibacterial properties against major periodontal pathogens, namely *Aa.* and *Pg.* (Figure 6).

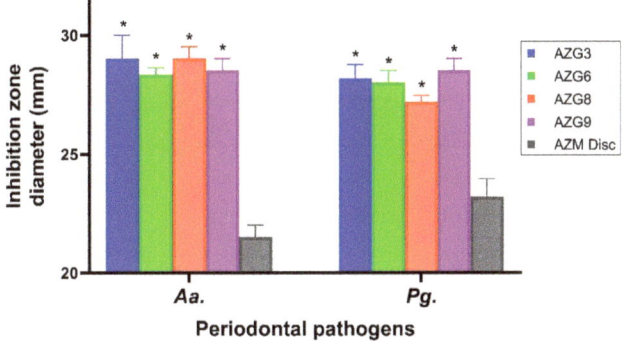

Figure 6. Antibacterial activity of AZG against major periodontal pathogens, namely *Aggregatibacter actinomycetemcomitans* (*Aa.*) and *Porphyromonas gingivalis* (*Pg.*). Data are mean ± SD, n = 3. Asterisks indicate statistically significant differences compared with AZM disc ($p < 0.01$).

The results of the inhibition zone indicated that all AZG formulations exhibited significantly higher antibacterial activity ($p < 0.05$) than the AZM solution at the equivalent concentration. This might be due to the hydrogel matrix of AZG, which facilitated the diffusion of the drugs. The results were consistent with both pathogens. However, when comparisons were made between each AZG formulation, no considerable difference in antibacterial activity was found. The inhibition zone was absent in the blank niosomal gel samples comparable to the negative control, which was phosphate buffer. *Aa.* and *Pg.* are both recognized as major periodontal pathogens associated with severe forms of periodontitis [52]. Their infiltration into the sub-epithelium and connective tissue causes a persistent infection that is problematic for conventional treatment. Even scaling and root planing, the gold standards of periodontitis treatment, cannot remove all residing pathogens. The local delivery of antibiotics could eliminate the remaining bacteria. However, the formulation should exhibit a long retention time in the periodontal pocket and enhance transmucosal drug delivery.

Considering the results obtained, it is possible to conclude that after administration to the intricate gap of the periodontal pocket, AZG transformed into a gel state. The hydrogel matrix of P407–HA gradually eroded. AZM-loaded niosomes were released from the matrix by means of diffusion and erosion for more than 72 h. AZM should be delivered to the periodontal pocket and permeated to the surrounding periodontal tissues through the advantages provided by niosomes, to eliminate residing periodontal pathogens. Based on overall performance, AZG9 would be the most desirable formulation for periodontitis treatment. The selection of AZM as a model drug, along with HA as an additive, was considered on account of the anti-inflammatory properties of AZM and the wound healing properties of HA. These effects are advantageous for periodontitis treatment and will be further investigated in our upcoming study.

4. Conclusions

The primary outcome of this study was to invent a desirable formulation suitable for injection into the periodontal pocket for adjunctive periodontitis treatment. The developed AZG based on P407–HA interactions and AZM-loaded niosomes provided acceptable properties, such as ease of administration and sustained drug release with enhanced drug permeation, and improved the bioavailability of AZM in periodontal tissue. The invented formulations were effective in eliminating pathogenic bacteria. Therefore, within the limits of this study, AZG exhibited potential efficiency for periodontitis treatment, which should be further investigated in future research.

Author Contributions: Conceptualization, K.K. and S.L.; methodology, K.K. and S.L.; validation, K.K. and S.L.; formal analysis, K.K. and S.L.; investigation, K.K. and S.L.; resources, S.L. and T.P.; data curation, K.K. and S.L.; writing—original draft preparation, K.K. and S.L.; writing—review and editing, K.K., T.P. and S.L.; supervision, S.L. All authors have read and agreed to the published version of the manuscript.

Funding: This research received no external funding.

Institutional Review Board Statement: Not applicable.

Informed Consent Statement: Not applicable.

Data Availability Statement: Not applicable.

Acknowledgments: The authors would like to thank Paul Mines for the English language review.

Conflicts of Interest: The authors declare no conflict of interest.

References

1. Sanz, M. European workshop in periodontal health and cardiovascular disease. *Eur. Heart J. Suppl.* **2010**, *12*, B2. [CrossRef]
2. Meyle, J.; Chapple, I. Molecular aspects of the pathogenesis of periodontitis. *Periodontol. 2000* **2015**, *69*, 7–17. [CrossRef]
3. Cobb, C.M. Clinical significance of non-surgical periodontal therapy: An evidence-based perspective of scaling and root planing. *J. Clin. Periodontol.* **2002**, *29* (Suppl. 2), 6–16. [CrossRef] [PubMed]
4. Tomasi, C.; Leyland, A.H.; Wennström, J.L. Factors influencing the outcome of non-surgical periodontal treatment: A multilevel approach. *J. Clin. Periodontol.* **2007**, *34*, 682–690. [CrossRef]
5. Nair, S.C.; Anoop, K.R. Intraperiodontal pocket: An ideal route for local antimicrobial drug delivery. *J. Adv. Pharm. Technol. Res.* **2012**, *3*, 9. [CrossRef] [PubMed]
6. Jepsen, K.; Jepsen, S. Antibiotics/antimicrobials: Systemic and local administration in the therapy of mild to moderately advanced periodontitis. *Periodontol. 2000* **2016**, *71*, 82–112. [CrossRef] [PubMed]
7. Hirsch, R.; Deng, H.; Laohachai, M.N. Azithromycin in periodontal treatment: More than an antibiotic. *J. Periodontal Res.* **2012**, *47*, 137–148. [CrossRef] [PubMed]
8. Idkaidek, N.M.; Najib, N.; Salem, I.; Jilani, J. Physiologically-based IVIVC of azithromycin. *Am. J. Pharmacol. Sci.* **2014**, *2*, 100–102. [CrossRef]
9. Kerdmanee, K.; Limsitthichaikoon, S. Fabrication and characterization of azithromycin-loaded niosomes for periodontitis treatment. *Key Eng. Mater.* **2021**, *901*, 55–60. [CrossRef]
10. Pin-Chuang, L.; Walters, J.D. Relative effectiveness of azithromycin in killing intracellular *Porphyromonas gingivalis*. *Clin. Exp. Dent. Res.* **2016**, *2*, 35–43. [CrossRef]
11. Pin-Chuang, L.; Walters, J.D. Azithromycin kills invasive *Aggregatibacter actinomycetemcomitans* in gingival epithelial cells. *Antimicrob. Agents Chemother.* **2013**, *57*, 1347–1351. [CrossRef]
12. Dumortier, G.; Grossiord, J.L.; Agnely, F.; Chaumeil, J.C. A review of poloxamer 407 pharmaceutical and pharmacological characteristics. *Pharm. Res.* **2006**, *23*, 2709–2728. [CrossRef] [PubMed]

13. Carvalho, F.C.; Bruschi, M.L.; Evangelista, R.C.; Gremião, M.P.D. Mucoadhesive drug delivery systems. *Braz. J. Pharm. Sci.* **2010**, *46*, 1–17. [CrossRef]
14. Carvalho, G.C.; Araujo, V.H.S.; Fonseca-Santos, B.; de Araújo, J.T.C.; de Souza, M.P.C.; Duarte, J.L.; Chorilli, M. Highlights in poloxamer-based drug delivery systems as strategy at local application for vaginal infections. *Int. J. Pharm.* **2021**, *602*, 120635. [CrossRef] [PubMed]
15. Jung, Y.; Park, W.; Park, H.; Lee, D.-K.; Na, K. Thermo-Sensitive injectable hydrogel based on the physical mixing of hyaluronic acid and pluronic F-127 for sustained NSAID delivery. *Carbohydr. Polym.* **2017**, *156*, 403–408. [CrossRef] [PubMed]
16. Abou-Shamat, M.A.; Calvo-Castro, J.; Stair, J.L.; Cook, M.T. Modifying the properties of thermogelling poloxamer 407 solutions through covalent modification and the use of polymer additives. *Macromol. Chem. Phys.* **2019**, *220*, 1900173. [CrossRef]
17. Liao, Y.-H.; Jones, S.A.; Forbes, B.; Martin, G.P.; Brown, M.B. Hyaluronan: Pharmaceutical characterization and drug delivery. *Drug Deliv.* **2005**, *12*, 327–342. [CrossRef] [PubMed]
18. Snetkov, P.; Zakharova, K.; Morozkina, S.; Olekhnovich, R.; Uspenskaya, M. Hyaluronic acid: The influence of molecular weight on structural, physical, physico-chemical, and degradable properties of biopolymer. *Polymers* **2020**, *12*, 1800. [CrossRef]
19. Dahiya, P.; Kamal, R. Hyaluronic acid: A boon in periodontal therapy. *N. Am. J. Med. Sci.* **2013**, *5*, 309–315. [CrossRef]
20. Mayol, L.; Biondi, M.; Quaglia, F.; Fusco, S.; Borzacchiello, A.; Ambrosio, L.; La Rotonda, M.I. Injectable thermally responsive mucoadhesive gel for sustained protein delivery. *Biomacromolecules* **2011**, *12*, 28–33. [CrossRef]
21. Al-Rimawi, F.; Kharoaf, M. Analysis of azithromycin and its related compounds by RP-HPLC with UV detection. *J. Chromatogr. Sci.* **2010**, *48*, 86–90. [CrossRef] [PubMed]
22. da Silva, J.B.; de Souza Ferreira, S.B.; Reis, A.V.; Cook, M.T.; Bruschi, M.L. Assessing mucoadhesion in polymer gels: The effect of method type and instrument variables. *Polymers* **2018**, *10*, 254. [CrossRef] [PubMed]
23. Agossa, K.; Lizambard, M.; Rongthong, T.; Delcourt-Debruyne, E.; Siepmann, J.; Siepmann, F. Physical key properties of antibiotic-free, PLGA/HPMC-based in-situ forming implants for local periodontitis treatment. *Int. J. Pharm.* **2017**, *521*, 282–293. [CrossRef] [PubMed]
24. Diaz del Consuelo, I.; Pizzolato, G.-P.; Falson, F.; Guy, R.H.; Jacques, Y. Evaluation of pig esophageal mucosa as a permeability barrier model for buccal tissue. *J. Pharm. Sci.* **2005**, *94*, 2777–2788. [CrossRef] [PubMed]
25. Moghassemi, S.; Hadjizadeh, A. Nano-niosomes as nanoscale drug delivery systems: An illustrated review. *J. Control. Release Soc.* **2014**, *185*, 22–36. [CrossRef]
26. Damrongrungruang, T.; Paphangkorakit, J.; Limsitthichaikoon, S.; Khampaenjiraroch, B.; Davies, M.J.; Sungthong, B.; Priprem, A. Anthocyanin complex niosome gel accelerates oral wound healing: In vitro and clinical studies. *Nanomedicine* **2021**, *37*, 102423. [CrossRef]
27. Eggert, F.M.; Drewell, L.; Bigelow, J.A.; Speck, J.E.; Goldner, M. The pH of gingival crevices and periodontal pockets in children, teenagers and adults. *Arch. Oral Biol.* **1991**, *36*, 233–238. [CrossRef]
28. Giuliano, E.; Paolino, D.; Fresta, M.; Cosco, D. Mucosal applications of poloxamer 407-based hydrogels: An overview. *Pharmaceutics* **2018**, *10*, 159. [CrossRef]
29. Pereira, G.G.; Dimer, F.A.; Guterres, S.S.; Kechinski, C.P.; Granada, J.E.; Cardozo, N.S.M. Formulation and characterization of poloxamer 407®: Thermoreversible gel containing polymeric microparticles and hyaluronic acid. *Quim. Nova* **2013**, *36*, 1121–1125. [CrossRef]
30. da Silva, J.B.; Cook, M.T.; Bruschi, M.L. Thermoresponsive systems composed of poloxamer 407 and HPMC or NaCMC: Mechanical, rheological and sol-gel transition analysis. *Carbohydr. Polym.* **2020**, *240*, 116268. [CrossRef]
31. Choi, H.; Lee, E.; Kim, M.; Kim, C. Effect of additives on the physicochemical properties of liquid suppository bases. *Int. J. Pharm.* **1999**, *190*, 13–19. [CrossRef]
32. Srivastava, M.; Kohli, K.; Ali, M. Formulation development of novel in situ nanoemulgel (NEG) of ketoprofen for the treatment of periodontitis. *Drug Deliv.* **2016**, *23*, 154–166. [CrossRef]
33. Swain, G.P.; Patel, S.; Gandhi, J.; Shah, P. Development of moxifloxacin hydrochloride loaded in-situ gel for the treatment of periodontitis: In-vitro drug release study and antibacterial activity. *J. Oral Biol. Craniofacial Res.* **2019**, *9*, 190–200. [CrossRef] [PubMed]
34. Ghica, M.V.; Hîrjău, M.; Lupuleasa, D.; Dinu-Pîrvu, C.-E. Flow and thixotropic parameters for rheological characterization of hydrogels. *Molecules* **2016**, *21*, 786. [CrossRef] [PubMed]
35. Bartold, P.M.; Walsh, L.J.; Narayanan, A.S. Molecular and cell biology of the gingiva. *Periodontol. 2000* **2000**, *24*, 28–55. [CrossRef] [PubMed]
36. Mayol, L.; Quaglia, F.; Borzacchiello, A.; Ambrosio, L.; La Rotonda, M.I. A novel poloxamers/hyaluronic acid in situ forming hydrogel for drug delivery: Rheological, mucoadhesive and in vitro release properties. *Eur. J. Pharm. Biopharm.* **2008**, *70*, 199–206. [CrossRef]
37. Hsieh, H.Y.; Lin, W.Y.; Lee, A.L.; Li, Y.C.; Chen, Y.J.; Chen, K.C.; Young, T.H. Hyaluronic acid on the urokinase sustained release with a hydrogel system composed of poloxamer 407: HA/P407 hydrogel system for drug delivery. *PLoS ONE* **2020**, *15*, e0227784. [CrossRef]
38. Trombino, S.; Servidio, C.; Curcio, F.; Cassano, R. Strategies for hyaluronic acid-based hydrogel design in drug delivery. *Pharmaceutics* **2019**, *11*, 407. [CrossRef]

39. Pritchard, K.; Lansley, A.B.; Martin, G.P.; Helliwell, M.; Marriott, C.; Benedetti, L.M. Evaluation of the bioadhesive properties of hyaluronan derivatives: Detachment weight and mucociliary transport rate studies. *Int. J. Pharm.* **1996**, *129*, 137–145. [CrossRef]
40. Russo, E.; Selmin, F.; Baldassari, S.; Gennari, C.G.M.; Caviglioli, G.; Cilurzo, F.; Minghetti, P.; Parodi, B. A Focus on mucoadhesive polymers and their application in buccal dosage forms. *J. Drug Deliv. Sci. Technol.* **2016**, *32*, 113–125. [CrossRef]
41. Ensign, L.M.; Lai, S.K.; Wang, Y.-Y.; Yang, M.; Mert, O.; Hanes, J.; Cone, R. Pretreatment of human cervicovaginal mucus with pluronic F127 enhances nanoparticle penetration without compromising mucus barrier properties to herpes simplex virus. *Biomacromolecules* **2014**, *15*, 4403–4409. [CrossRef] [PubMed]
42. Medlicott, N.J.; Rathbone, M.J.; Tucker, I.G.; Holborow, D.W. Delivery systems for the administration of drugs to the periodontal pocket. *Adv. Drug Deliv. Rev.* **1994**, *13*, 181–203. [CrossRef]
43. Leung, S.-H.S.; Robinson, J.R. Polymer structure features contributing to mucoadhesion. II. *J. Control. Release* **1990**, *12*, 187–194. [CrossRef]
44. Texture Profile Analysis. Texture Technologies. Available online: https://texturetechnologies.com/resources/texture-profile-analysis (accessed on 24 May 2022).
45. Jain, R.A.; Rhodes, C.T.; Railkar, A.M.; Malick, A.W.; Shah, N.H. Controlled release of drugs from injectable in situ formed biodegradable PLGA microspheres: Effect of various formulation variables. *Eur. J. Pharm. Biopharm.* **2000**, *50*, 257–262. [CrossRef]
46. Mhlanga, N.; Ray, S.S. Kinetic models for the release of the anticancer drug doxorubicin from biodegradable polylactide/metal oxide-based hybrids. *Int. J. Biol. Macromol.* **2015**, *72*, 1301–1307. [CrossRef] [PubMed]
47. Korsmeyer, R.W.; Gurny, R.; Doelker, E.; Buri, P.; Peppas, N.A. Mechanisms of solute release from porous hydrophilic polymers. *Int. J. Pharm.* **1983**, *15*, 25–35. [CrossRef]
48. Ritger, P.L.; Peppas, N.A. A simple equation for description of solute release II. Fickian and anomalous release from swellable devices. *J. Control. Release* **1987**, *5*, 37–42. [CrossRef]
49. Pedreiro, L.N.; Cury, B.S.F.; Chaud, M.V.; Gremião, M.P.D. A novel approach in mucoadhesive drug delivery system to improve zidovudine intestinal permeability. *Braz. J. Pharm. Sci.* **2016**, *52*, 715–725. [CrossRef]
50. Bodratti, A.M.; Alexandridis, P. Formulation of poloxamers for drug delivery. *J. Funct. Biomater.* **2018**, *9*, 11. [CrossRef]
51. Vanić, Ž.; Rukavina, Z.; Manner, S.; Fallarero, A.; Uzelac, L.; Kralj, M.; Amidžić Klarić, D.; Bogdanov, A.; Raffai, T.; Virok, D.P.; et al. Azithromycin-liposomes as a novel approach for localized therapy of cervicovaginal bacterial infections. *Int. J. Nanomed.* **2019**, *14*, 5957–5976. [CrossRef]
52. Torrungruang, K.; Jitpakdeebordin, S.; Charatkulangkun, O.; Gleebbua, Y. *Porphyromonas gingivalis, Aggregatibacter actinomycetemcomitans,* and *Treponema denticola/Prevotella intermedia* co-infection are associated with severe periodontitis in a Thai population. *PLoS ONE* **2015**, *10*, e0136646. [CrossRef] [PubMed]

MDPI AG
Grosspeteranlage 5
4052 Basel
Switzerland
Tel.: +41 61 683 77 34

Pharmaceutics Editorial Office
E-mail: pharmaceutics@mdpi.com
www.mdpi.com/journal/pharmaceutics

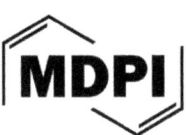

Disclaimer/Publisher's Note: The statements, opinions and data contained in all publications are solely those of the individual author(s) and contributor(s) and not of MDPI and/or the editor(s). MDPI and/or the editor(s) disclaim responsibility for any injury to people or property resulting from any ideas, methods, instructions or products referred to in the content.

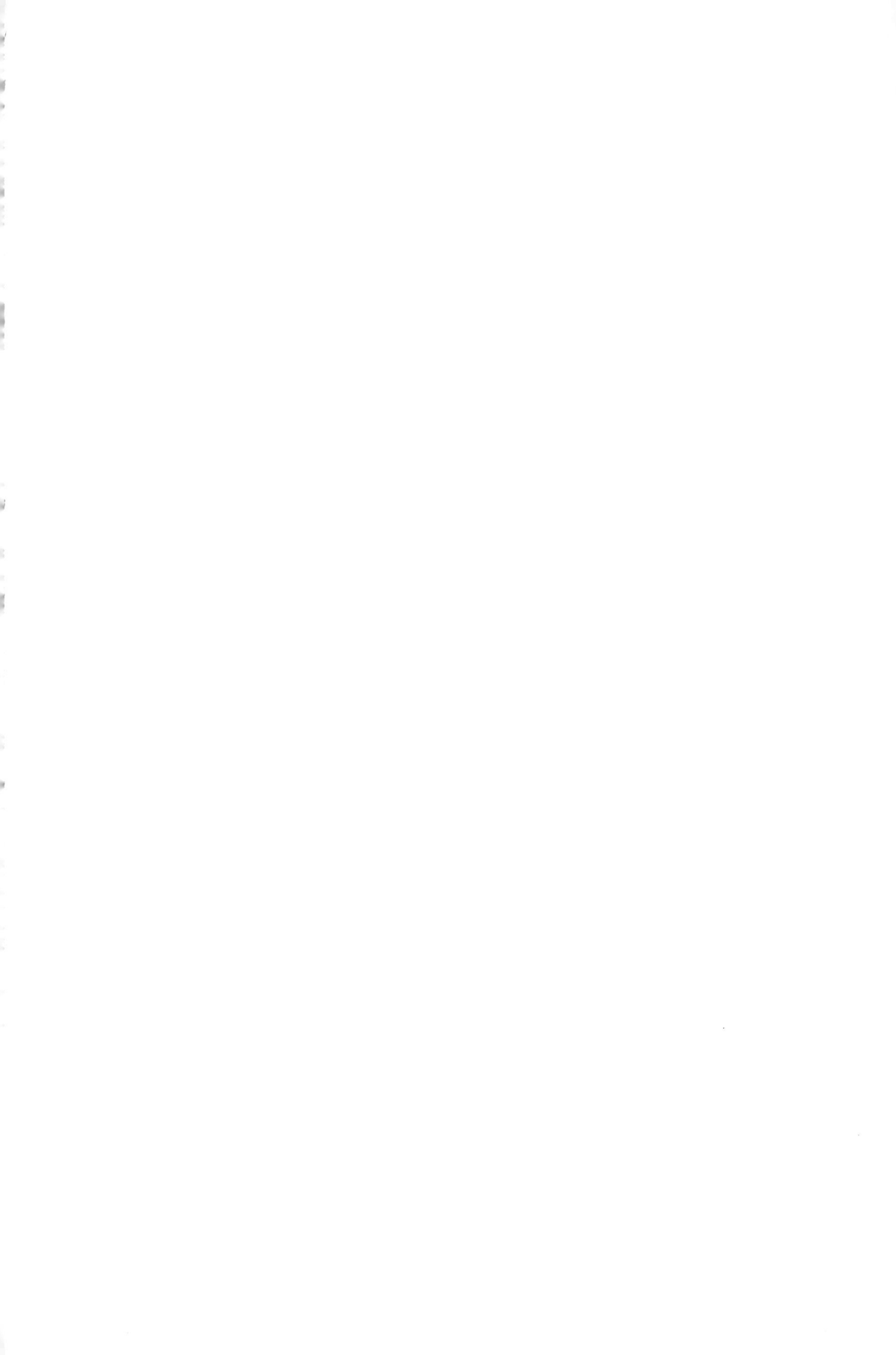